Cognitive Behavior Therapy and Eating Disorders

Cognitive Behavior Therapy and Eating Disorders

Christopher G. Fairburn

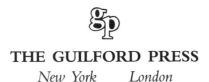

THE GUILFORD PRESS
New York   London

© 2008 The Guilford Press
A Division of Guilford Publications, Inc.
72 Spring Street, New York, NY 10012
www.guilford.com

Printed in the United States of America

This book is printed on acid-free paper.

Last digit is print number: 9   8   7   6   5   4

Library of Congress Cataloging-in-Publication Data

Fairburn, Christopher G.
  Cognitive behavior therapy and eating disorders / by Christopher G. Fairburn.
    p. ;   cm.
  Includes bibliographical references and index.
  ISBN: 978-1-59385-709-7 (hardcover : alk. paper)
  1. Eating disorders—Treatment.   2. Cognitive therapy.   I. Title.
  [DNLM: 1. Eating Disorders—therapy.   2. Cognitive Therapy.   WM 175 F164c 2008]
  RC552.E18F36 2009
  616.85'2606—dc22

                                                                2008002971

To Guy and Sarah

Contributors

Christopher G. Fairburn, DM, FMedSci, FRCPsych, is Wellcome Principal Research Fellow and Professor of Psychiatry at the University of Oxford. He is a well-known international authority on eating disorders and has a particular interest in the development and evaluation of psychological treatments. He has twice been a Fellow at Stanford's Center for Advanced Study in the Behavioral Sciences and is a Fellow of the U.K. Academy of Medical Sciences. He is a Governor of the Wellcome Trust, the largest international biomedical research foundation.

Sarah Beglin, DPhil, DClinPsych, Adult Eating Disorder Service, Cambridge and Peterborough Mental Health Partnership NHS Trust, Addenbrooke's Hospital, Cambridge, United Kingdom

Kristin Bohn, DPhil, Dipl-Psych, Clinical Psychology Department, Royal Holloway University of London, London, United Kingdom

Zafra Cooper, DPhil, DipPsych, Oxford University Department of Psychiatry, Oxford, United Kingdom

Riccardo Dalle Grave, MD, Villa Garda Hospital Department of Eating and Weight Disorder, Garda (Verona), Italy

Deborah M. Hawker, PhD, DClinPsych, Psychological Health Services, Inter-Health, London, United Kingdom

Rebecca Murphy, DClinPsych, Oxford University Department of Psychiatry, Oxford, United Kingdom

Marianne E. O'Connor, BA, Oxford University Department of Psychiatry, Oxford, United Kingdom

Roz Shafran, PhD, School of Psychology and Clinical Language Sciences, University of Reading, Reading, United Kingdom

Anne Stewart, MB, BS, BSc, MRCPsych, Child and Adolescent Mental Health Service, Oxfordshire and Buckinghamshire Mental Health Partnership NHS Trust, and Oxford University Department of Psychiatry, Oxford, United Kingdom

Suzanne Straebler, APRN-Psychiatry, MSN, Oxford University Department of Psychiatry, Oxford, United Kingdom

Deborah Waller, MB, BChir, MRCGP, 19 Beaumont Street Medical Practice, Oxford, United Kingdom

Acknowledgments

Particular thanks to all those who have contributed to the development of the treatment described in this book, most especially,

Zafra Cooper and Roz Shafran
Kristin Bohn and Debbie Hawker
Rebecca Murphy and Suzanne Straebler

And thanks to my two longstanding colleagues,

Mara Catling and Marianne O'Connor

And to my two mentors,

Michael Gelder and Robert Kendell

Thanks also to the Wellcome Trust for their personal support and for funding the research that led to the development of this treatment.

Contents

ADAPTATIONS OF CBT-E

POSTSCRIPT

APPENDICES

INTRODUCTION

CHAPTER 1

This Book and How to Use It

Christopher G. Fairburn

As a clinician one is lucky to work with patients with eating disorders. Although these patients have a reputation for being difficult to treat, the great majority can be helped and many, if not most, can make a full and lasting recovery. One can transform these people's lives: one can really make a difference.

> One is lucky to work with patients with eating disorders.

This book is about how to help patients: how to make a difference. It describes how to practice "enhanced" cognitive behavior therapy (CBT-E), the latest version of the leading empirically supported treatment for eating disorders. It has been written by clinicians of various professional backgrounds and varying levels of clinical experience. All, however, are experts at delivering CBT-E and all work in real-world clinical settings. The book is based on our combined clinical experience. It describes the treatment in fine detail from the very beginning when one first meets the patient through to post-treatment review appointments, and it explains how the treatment may be adapted to suit particular patient subgroups and settings.

The title of the book is no accident. It is about CBT-E *and* eating disorders. It opens with a detailed and novel "transdiagnostic" account of eating disorder psychopathology and the processes that are responsible for it being self-perpetuating. It then goes on to explain how to identify the processes that are operating in the individual patient and on this basis create a bespoke tailor-made treatment that fits the patient's psychopathology.

The book is designed to be a practical guide, and it has been written with the practicing clinician in mind. (I prefer the word "guide" to the more widely used term "manual." This is because the former conveys the notion that the book is providing guidance [which it is] whereas the latter implies that it is prescribing a set series of procedures [which it is not].) The book is intended to be easy to use. For the sake of clarity it has been kept almost totally free from research findings and in-text references. At the end of each chapter, however, there is a section on "Recommended Reading" that lists key articles and books that are likely to be of interest. (The Recommended Reading pertaining to Chapters 5–12 is placed at the end of Chapter 12 to avoid duplication.)

Background to the Development of CBT-E

In some ways this book has taken 30 years to write, as CBT-E has its origins in the late 1970s when it was developed as a theory-driven, outpatient-based treatment for adults with bulimia nervosa (CBT-BN; Fairburn, 1981). At that stage bulimia nervosa was just being recognized and had been described as "intractable" (Russell, 1979). Through the 1980s and 1990s CBT-BN was progressively refined and was the subject of a succession of randomized controlled trials, the findings of which consistently supported both the treatment and the theory upon which it was based.

By the late 1990s it was clear that CBT-BN was the leading treatment for bulimia nervosa, but it was equally clear that it needed to be enhanced because less than half the patients made a full and lasting recovery. This led me and my colleagues Zafra Cooper and Roz Shafran to examine in detail, patient by patient, why some patients did well and others did not. Eventually we identified some consistent obstacles to change. The challenge was to see if they could be overcome by modifying the treatment. There followed a period of trial and error during which we experimented with new versions of the treatment. At the same time we extended the cognitive behavioral theory of bulimia nervosa to all eating disorders and on this basis made the treatment "transdiagnostic" in its scope (Fairburn, Cooper, & Shafran, 2003; see Chapter 2). This preparatory work culminated in a 5-year transdiagnostic treatment trial based at two treatment centers in the United Kingdom (Oxford and Leicester). The trial has now been completed and its findings suggest that CBT-E is indeed more potent than CBT-BN, and that it can be used across the full range of eating disorders (Fairburn et al., 2009). Now other clinical teams in the United Kingdom and abroad have started to use CBT-E and are reporting equally positive results. Hence the need for this book.

This Book

This book is designed to provide a comprehensive, yet fine-grain, account of how to implement CBT-E. It needs to be read as a whole as it is assumed in each chapter that the reader is familiar with the preceding ones (although there is extensive cross-referencing to help readers move around within the book). Its structure is as follows:

Chapter 2: This chapter describes the psychopathology of eating disorders. It adopts a transdiagnostic perspective, thereby providing the rationale for transdiagnostic treatment. It also describes the cognitive behavioral theory that underpins the strategies and procedures that characterize CBT-E.

Chapter 3: This chapter provides a general overview of CBT-E. It outlines its strategy and structure, and how it differs from other forms of CBT. It also highlights certain points about the implementation of the treatment.

Chapter 4: This is concerned with the assessment of patients and how to prepare them for treatment. It also discusses the medical management of patients from the perspective of non-medical therapists.

Chapters 5–12: These chapters provide the details of how to implement the main "focused" form of CBT-E.

Chapters 13–16: These closing chapters describe the various adaptations of CBT-E, including its "broad" version; its use with adolescents; its use in inpatient and day patient settings; and two outpatient forms of CBT-E (intensive outpatient CBT-E and group CBT-E); and finally the use of CBT-E with "complex cases."

Appendices A–C: These appendices provide the latest versions of three assessment measures: the Eating Disorder Examination (EDE 16.0), the Eating Disorder Examination Questionnaire (EDE–Q 6.0) and the Clinical Impairment Assessment Questionnaire (CIA 3.0).

It is important to note what the book does not aim to accomplish. It does not provide a comprehensive account of what is known about eating disorders, nor does it attempt to discuss every aspect of their management. What it does provide is a complete account of how to manage and treat patients using CBT-E. Some readers may be surprised to find few references to eating disorder diagnoses (e.g., anorexia nervosa, bulimia nervosa; see Chapter 2). This is because we find that they are of little relevance to our clinical practice.

Nor is this book a generic guide to CBT. This knowledge is assumed. Excellent CBT guides exist, some of which are listed in the Recommended Reading section at the end of this chapter.

> Some readers may be surprised to find few references to eating disorder diagnoses. This is because we find that they are of little relevance to our clinical practice.

Learning to Practice CBT-E

No specific professional qualifications are required to practice CBT-E, but certain background knowledge and experience are important. With regard to the former, the therapist should be well informed about psychopathology in general and eating disorder psychopathology in particular (see Chapter 2). The therapist should also be aware of the medical complications of eating disorders and be able to manage them appropriately (see Chapter 4). As regards prior experience, the therapist should have had some training in cognitive behavior therapy (CBT) and, ideally, experience working with patients with eating disorders. With this background many therapists will be able to implement CBT-E by simply following the guidelines in this book.

There has been remarkably little research on how to train people to implement psychological treatments. Current practice in this regard is more or less evidence-free. Workshops given by expert clinicians — preferably ones who actually practice the treatment — are useful adjuncts to written treatment guides, but far better is ongoing case supervision, although it is difficult to obtain. Regular peer supervision is a valuable substitute and should be sought if at all possible.

Recommended Reading

Background to the Development of CBT-E

Fairburn, C. G. (1981). A cognitive behavioural approach to the treatment of bulimia. *Psychological Medicine, 11,* 707–711.

Fairburn, C. G. (1985). Cognitive-behavioral treatment for bulimia. In D. M. Garner & P. E.

Garfinkel (Eds.), *Handbook of treatment for eating disorders* (pp. 160–192). New York: Guilford Press.

Fairburn, C. G., Cooper, Z., & Shafran, R. (2003). Cognitive behaviour therapy for eating disorders: A "transdiagnostic" theory and treatment. *Behaviour Research and Therapy, 41*, 509–528.

Fairburn, C. G., Marcus, M. D., & Wilson, G. T. (1993). Cognitive-behavioral therapy for binge eating and bulimia nervosa: A comprehensive treatment manual. In C. G. Fairburn & G. T. Wilson (Eds.), *Binge eating: Nature, assessment, and treatment* (pp. 361–404). New York: Guilford Press.

Garner, D. M., & Bemis, K. M. (1982). A cognitive-behavioral approach to anorexia nervosa. *Cognitive Therapy and Research, 6*, 123–150.

Garner, D. M., Vitousek, K. M., & Pike, K. M. (1997). Cognitive-behavioral therapy for anorexia nervosa. In D. M. Garner & P. E. Garfinkel (Eds.), *Handbook of treatment for eating disorders* (2nd ed., pp. 94–144). New York: Guilford Press.

Effectiveness of CBT-E

Byrne, S. M., Fursland, A., Allen, K. L., & Watson, H. (2011). The effectiveness of enhanced cognitive behavioural therapy for eating disorders: An open trial. *Behaviour Research and Therapy, 49*, 219–226.

Fairburn, C. G., Cooper, Z., Doll, H. A., O'Connor, M. E., Bohn, K., Hawker, D. M., Wales, J. A., & Palmer, R. L. (2009). Transdiagnostic cognitive behavioral therapy for patients with eating disorders: A two-site trial with 60-week follow-up. *American Journal of Psychiatry, 166*, 311–319.

Guides to the Practice of CBT

Beck, J. S. (1995). *Cognitive therapy: Basics and beyond.* New York: Guilford Press.

Beck, J. S. (2005). *Cognitive therapy for challenging problems: What to do when the basics don't work.* New York: Guilford Press.

Bennett-Levy, J., Butler, G., Fennell, M., Hackman, A., Mueller, M., & Westbrook, D. (2004). *Oxford guide to behavioural experiments in cognitive therapy.* Oxford: Oxford University Press.

Leahy, R. L. (2001). *Overcoming resistance in cognitive therapy.* New York: Guilford Press.

Leahy, R. L. (2003). *Cognitive therapy techniques: A practitioner's guide.* New York: Guilford Press.

Leahy, R. L., & Holland, S. J. (2000). *Treatment plans and interventions for depression and anxiety disorders.* New York: Guilford Press.

Ledley, D. R., Marx, B. P., & Heimberg, R. G. (2005). *Making cognitive-behavioral therapy work.* New York: Guilford Press.

Padesky, C. A., & Greenberger, D. (1995). *Clinician's guide to mind over mood.* New York: Guilford Press.

Persons, J. B. (1989). *Cognitive therapy in practice: A case formulation approach.* New York: Norton.

Other Articles of Relevance to Chapter 1

National Institute for Clinical Excellence. (2004). *Eating disorders: Core interventions in the treatment and management of anorexia nervosa, bulimia nervosa and related eating disorders.* London: National Institute for Clinical Excellence.

Russell, G. F. M. (1979). Bulimia nervosa: An ominous variant of anorexia nervosa. *Psychological Medicine, 9*, 429–448.

Wilson, G. T., Grilo, C. M., & Vitousek, K. M. (2007). Psychological treatment of eating disorders. *American Psychologist, 62*, 199–216.

CHAPTER 2

Eating Disorders: The Transdiagnostic View and the Cognitive Behavioral Theory

Christopher G. Fairburn

The way eating disorders are classified encourages the view that there are a number of distinct conditions, each requiring its own form of treatment. There are strong reasons to question this stance. In the first part of this chapter the transdiagnostic perspective on eating disorders is presented, both with regard to their psychopathology and treatment, thereby providing the rationale for transdiagnostic treatment. In the second part of the chapter the cognitive behavioral theory of the maintenance of eating disorders is outlined — the theory that provides the foundation for CBT-E.

The Way Eating Disorders Are Classified

The leading scheme for classifying and diagnosing eating disorders, the American Psychiatric Association's *Diagnostic and Statistical Manual of Mental Disorders — Fourth Edition* (DSM-IV), recognizes two eating disorders, anorexia nervosa and bulimia nervosa, together with a residual diagnostic category termed "eating disorder not otherwise specified" (eating disorder NOS). Diagnostic criteria are provided for anorexia nervosa and bulimia nervosa (outlined in Table 2.1) but none for eating disorder NOS: Instead, it is a residual diagnosis reserved for eating disorders of clinical severity that do not meet the diagnostic criteria for anorexia nervosa or bulimia nervosa.

Figure 2.1 shows in diagrammatic form the relationship between these three diagnoses. The two overlapping inner circles represent anorexia nervosa (the smaller circle) and bulimia nervosa (the larger circle) respectively, the area of potential overlap being that occupied by those people who would meet the diagnostic criteria for both disorders but for the "trumping" convention that gives the diagnosis anorexia nervosa prece-

TABLE 2.1. Diagnostic Criteria for the Eating Disorders

Anorexia Nervosa

In essence, three features need to be present to make a diagnosis of anorexia nervosa:
1. Over-evaluation of shape and weight and their control; that is, judging self-worth largely, or even exclusively, in terms of shape and weight and the ability to control them.
2. Active maintenance of an unduly low body weight (typically defined as maintaining a body weight less than 85% of that expected or a body mass index of 17.5 or below[a]).
3. Amenorrhea (in post-pubertal females). The value of this criterion is questionable and it is likely to be dropped in DSM-V. This is because the majority of female patients who meet the other two diagnostic criteria are also amenorrheic, and those who are not closely resemble those who are.

Bulimia Nervosa

Three features also need to be present to make a diagnosis of bulimia nervosa:
1. Over-evaluation of shape and weight and their control, as in anorexia nervosa.
2. Recurrent binge eating. A "binge" is an episode of eating during which an objectively large amount of food is eaten, given the circumstances, and there is a sense of loss of control at the time.
3. Extreme weight-control behavior (e.g., sustained dietary restriction, recurrent self-induced vomiting or laxative misuse).

In addition, there is an exclusionary criterion; namely that the diagnostic criteria for anorexia nervosa should not be met. This criterion ensures that it is not possible for patients to receive both diagnoses at one time.

Eating Disorder NOS

There are no diagnostic criteria for eating disorder NOS. Rather, it is a residual category for eating disorders of clinical severity that do not meet the diagnostic criteria for anorexia nervosa or bulimia nervosa.

Binge Eating Disorder

Recurrent binge eating in the absence of the extreme weight-control behavior seen in bulimia nervosa. In DSM-IV it is a form of eating disorder NOS, although its status may change in DSM-V.

---

[a]Body mass index (BMI) is a widely used way of representing weight adjusted for height. It is weight (in kg) divided by height squared (in m) (i.e., Wt/Ht^2). See Table 2.3 for further information about the BMI and its use with patients with eating disorders.

dence over that of bulimia nervosa (see Table 2.1). Surrounding these two circles is an outer circle that defines the boundary of eating disorder "caseness"; that is, the boundary between having an eating disorder — a state of clinical significance — and having a lesser, non-clinical problem with eating. It is this boundary that demarcates what is, and is not, an eating disorder. Within the outer circle, but outside the two inner circles, lies eating disorder NOS.

The relative prevalence of the three diagnoses is not what would be expected from the literature on eating disorders. Most common is the relatively neglected diagnosis of eating disorder NOS: it comprises between 50 and 60% of adult outpatients. Next is bulimia nervosa, which comprises about 30% of cases, and least common is anorexia nervosa, which comprises the remaining 10–15%. Less is known about the distribution of the three diagnoses among adolescents, but it seems that eating disorder NOS is the

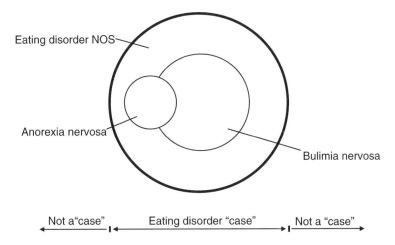

FIGURE 2.1. A schematic representation of the relationship between anorexia nervosa, bulimia nervosa and eating disorder NOS. From Fairburn and Bohn (2005). Copyright 2005 by Elsevier. Reprinted with permission.

most common diagnosis among them too, followed by anorexia nervosa and then bulimia nervosa.

Figure 2.2 illustrates the relative prevalence of the three diagnoses among adult outpatients. Included in the figure is binge eating disorder, a relatively new diagnostic concept that has provisional status within DSM-IV (and is technically a form of eating disorder NOS). It denotes an eating problem characterized by recurrent binge eating in the absence of the extreme weight-control behavior seen in bulimia nervosa (i.e., extreme dietary restriction, self-induced vomiting or laxative misuse). It commonly co-occurs with obesity.

Conceptually, it is helpful to distinguish three subgroups within eating disorder NOS, although there is no sharp boundary between them. The first subgroup comprises cases that closely resemble anorexia nervosa or bulimia nervosa but just fail to

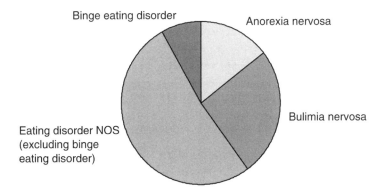

FIGURE 2.2. The relative prevalence of the three main eating disorder diagnoses (plus binge eating disorder) in adult outpatients.

meet their diagnostic criteria; for example, body weight may be marginally above the threshold for anorexia nervosa or the frequency of binge eating may be just too low for a diagnosis of bulimia nervosa. These cases are best viewed as "subthreshold" forms of anorexia nervosa or bulimia nervosa respectively, and might be better included within these diagnoses. Indeed, it is not unlikely that the boundaries of anorexia nervosa and bulimia nervosa will be expanded in DSM-V to embrace such cases. The second and largest subgroup consists of cases in which the clinical features of anorexia nervosa and bulimia nervosa are combined in a different way to that seen in the two prototypic disorders. Such states are best described as "mixed." Patients with "binge eating disorder" form the third and smallest subgroup (comprising less than 10% of eating disorder cases).

It has recently been suggested that a new eating disorder diagnosis be recognized, termed "purging disorder." This is intended for patients who have recurrent episodes of purging but do not binge eat. There are many problems with this concept. For example, the relationship between purging disorder and bulimia nervosa is far from clear because many people with purging disorder have "subjective binges" (defined below) and are therefore similar to people with bulimia nervosa. More important, however, is the fact that there is no evidence that the diagnosis has any prognostic or therapeutic implications. There are no data to suggest that patients with purging disorder differ from other patients with eating disorder NOS, or patients with bulimia nervosa, in either their course or response to treatment.

One other eating disorder diagnosis should be mentioned for completeness. This is "night eating syndrome." It refers to a state in which there is recurrent nocturnal awakening accompanied by eating. In contrast with the eating that sometimes co-occurs with sleep disorders, the eating in night eating syndrome takes place while the person is fully awake. Typically people with night eating syndrome eat relatively little in the day. Night eating syndrome is not a formally recognized diagnosis and its definition is a matter of debate. It is quite distinct from the three main eating disorder diagnoses of anorexia nervosa, bulimia nervosa and eating disorder NOS.

Clinical Reality: Shared and Evolving Psychopathology

What is most striking about anorexia nervosa, bulimia nervosa and eating disorder NOS is not what distinguishes them but how similar they are. More or less the same psychopathology is seen across the eating disorder diagnoses, and its severity is much the same too. There is an arbitrariness to the way this psychopathology is carved up to create the three diagnostic concepts.

> What is most striking about anorexia nervosa, bulimia nervosa and eating disorder NOS is not what distinguishes them but how similar they are.

The psychopathology of eating disorders may be meaningfully categorized into "specific" and "general" components, the former comprising features only seen in the eating disorders and the latter consisting of features seen in other psychiatric conditions. As many of the terms used to describe the specific psychopathology overlap with words in common usage, an eating disorder glossary is provided in Table 2.2.

TABLE 2.2. A Glossary of Key Terms Used to Describe the Psychopathology of Eating Disorders

Anorexia — Loss of appetite

Binge eating — A "binge" is an episode of eating during which an objectively large amount of food is eaten, given the circumstances, and there is a sense of loss of control at the time.

- *Subjective binge eating* — A "binge" in which the amount eaten is not unusually large, given the circumstances
- *Objective binge eating* — A true "binge" as defined above

Body image disparagement — The view that one's body is loathsome or repulsive. Commonly accompanied by body shape avoidance.

Body shape dissatisfaction — Dislike of one's appearance or body. This is common, unlike over-evaluation of shape and weight.

Calorie-counting — The continuous monitoring of calorie intake and the calculation of a running total. Generally the person is trying to keep under a daily calorie limit but often the calorie-counting is inaccurate. Underweight patients tend to over-estimate their intake whereas the opposite is more typical of overweight patients.

Core psychopathology — A widely used term to denote the characteristic over-evaluation of shape and weight and their control seen in most patients with eating disorders

Debting — The creation of an energy deficit or "debt" (typically through exercising) to accommodate subsequent eating

Delayed eating — Postponing eating as a means of weight control or resisting binge eating

Dietary guidelines — General dietary objectives that are flexible in nature

Dietary restraint — Attempting to limit the amount eaten

Dietary restriction – True undereating in a physiological sense

Dietary rules — Highly specific dietary goals

Driven exercising — A particular form of excessive exercising in which there is a subjective sense of being driven or compelled to exercise, the giving of exercise precedence over other activities and exercising when it might do physical harm.

Excessive exercising — Exercising to an undue extent, either in terms of physical health or psychosocial adjustment, or both

Food avoidance — The purposeful avoidance of certain foods (generally because they are perceived as fattening or because they tend to trigger binges)

Grazing — A term sometimes used to describe the tendency to pick more or less continuously at food. It is pejorative and best avoided.

Over-evaluation of shape and weight and their control — The judging of self-worth largely, or even exclusively, in terms of shape and weight and the ability to control them

Purging — A collective noun used to denote self-induced vomiting or the misuse of laxatives or diuretics.

- *Compensatory purging* — Episodes of purging designed to compensate for specific episodes of perceived or actual overeating
- *Non-compensatory purging* — Episodes of purging that are not in response to specific episodes of perceived or actual overeating.

Specific Psychopathology

The "Core Psychopathology" of Eating Disorders

Eating disorders are essentially "cognitive disorders," as anorexia nervosa and bulimia nervosa and most cases of eating disorder NOS share a distinctive "core psychopathology" that is cognitive in nature. This psychopathology is the over-evaluation of shape and weight and their control. (For a full description of this psychopathology and its expressions, see Chapter 8.) Whereas the majority of people evaluate themselves on the basis of their perceived performance in a variety of domains of life (e.g., the quality of their relationships; their work performance; their sporting prowess), people with eating disorders judge their self-worth largely, or even exclusively, in terms of their shape and weight and their ability to control them. This psychopathology is peculiar to the eating disorders (and, in a modified form, to body dysmorphic disorder) and is the same in females and males, adults and adolescents. However, it is uncommon in the general population. The over-evaluation of shape and weight needs to be distinguished from body shape dissatisfaction, which refers to dislike of one's appearance. Body shape dissatisfaction is widespread in the general population; its presence is sometimes referred to as "normative discontent."

> **Eating disorders are essentially "cognitive disorders."**

The core psychopathology is expressed in a variety of ways: Indeed, most features of these disorders appear to be secondary to it and its effects. Thus most patients with this psychopathology are intensely concerned about their weight. Many weigh themselves frequently and as a result become preoccupied with trivial changes in their weight, whereas others switch to actively avoiding knowing their weight while nevertheless remaining highly concerned about it. Similar behavior is seen with respect to body shape, with many patients repeatedly checking and scrutinizing their bodies, focusing on parts that they dislike, whereas others actively avoid seeing themselves assuming that they look fat and disgusting (body image disparagement). Such checking and avoidance tends to maintain the overconcern about shape and weight. Many repeatedly compare their shape with that of others and in a way that makes them conclude that they are unattractive. Most are afraid of weight gain and fatness, and many repeatedly "feel fat," which they tend to equate with being fat whatever their actual shape. Not surprisingly, these concerns about appearance have a profound effect on social functioning and intimate relationships. Socializing may be difficult or avoided altogether; undressing in front of others may be impossible; and many patients dislike their body being touched.

In a subgroup of patients the core psychopathology takes a different form (and one that is not described in DSM-IV). Rather than there being over-evaluation of shape and weight and their control, there is over-evaluation of control over eating per se, although the two forms of psychopathology may co-exist. When this variant is present in isolation, patients show little body checking, body avoidance or feeling fat: instead, they diet intensely (i.e., control their eating) and engage in various forms of dietary checking (e.g., calorie-counting) and avoidance (e.g., food avoidance). Many strongly value the sense of self-control that they get from engaging in these forms of behavior. This presentation is most common in young patients in the early stages of an eating disorder, and in patients who are underweight. It is also seen in non-Western cases.

The dieting of patients with eating disorders may be driven by additional motives too, including asceticism, competitiveness, and a desire to attract attention from others, but these motives are quite different from the over-evaluation of shape and weight and their control that is peculiar to the eating disorders.

Eating Habits, Weight–Control Behavior and Body Weight

The core psychopathology has a major impact on eating habits. It results in sustained and extreme attempts to limit food intake ("dietary restraint"). This is one of the most prominent characteristics of people with eating disorders and is seen across the eating disorder diagnoses (other than in binge eating disorder). The form that the dieting takes is unlike everyday dieting. Rather than having general guidelines about how they should eat, people with eating disorders set themselves multiple demanding, and highly specific, dietary rules designed to limit the amount that they eat. These rules vary in nature but typically concern when they should eat (e.g., not before 6 P.M.), how much they should eat (e.g., less than 600 kcals per day) and, most especially, what they should eat, with most patients having a large number of foods that they are attempting not to eat at all ("food avoidance"). As a result of these rules, their eating becomes restricted in nature and inflexible. Such behavior is profoundly impairing, although because patients adjust their lives accordingly they lose sight of how impaired they are. Concentration is affected as a result of what is almost constant preoccupation with thoughts about food and eating. Eating at home becomes difficult, and eating out may be impossible. Some patients insist on eating on their own as this allows them to eat in the way that they want and to concentrate on what they are doing. Many have great difficulty deciding what to eat if faced with choices and some avoid this by eating the same things every day. Some have to know precisely what is in the food that they are eating. Typically these patients weigh their food and keep a running total of their daily calorie intake. Social eating may be especially difficult: birthdays, Thanksgiving, and other celebrations tend to be dreaded for months in advance because of the pressure to eat more than usual and to do so in front of others.

The attempts to limit the amount eaten may, or may not, be successful. It is far from invariable that the attempts result in true undereating in a physiological sense ("dietary restriction"). If they are successful — which tends to be the case in the initial stages of an eating disorder — weight is lost and the patient may become significantly under-weight, developing adverse physical and psychosocial effects as a result. (This outcome occurs in patients who meet diagnostic criteria for anorexia nervosa and in those patients with eating disorder NOS who are underweight; see Chapter 11). These secondary effects are important for three main reasons: First, some are life-threatening (e.g., the cardiovascular effects) or difficult to reverse (e.g., the effects on bones); second, some tend to cause the eating disorder to persist and so encourage the patient to continue undereating (e.g., the preoccupation with food and eating, social withdrawal, heightened fullness); and third, many are profoundly impairing (e.g., reduced concentration, poor sleep, heightened obsessionality, and indecisiveness). Generally there is no true "anorexia" (loss of appetite) as such.

Some patients also engage in excessive exercising — a practice that is seen across the eating disorders, although it is most common in underweight patients. It is a particular problem in inpatient settings where patients are unable to be physically active. The exercising takes various forms, including excessive daily activity (e.g., standing rather than sitting, walking everywhere); exercising in a normal manner but to an extreme extent (e.g., going to the gym three times every day); and exercising in an abnormal manner (e.g., doing very large numbers of push-ups or sit-ups). "Driven exercising" is a particular form of excessive exercising that has the following additional characteristics: a subjective sense of being driven or compelled to exercise, giving exercise precedence over other activities (e.g., socializing) and exercising even when it might do physical harm (e.g., after having been injured; when risking fractures if very underweight). The motives behind excessive exercising vary. In most instances it is a form of weight control or a means of altering shape, but in some it is also used to modulate mood (see Chapter 10).

Binge eating is another characteristic feature of patients with eating disorders, a "binge" being an episode of eating during which an objectively large amount of food is eaten, given the circumstances, accompanied by a sense of loss of control at the time. Binge eating is seen across the eating disorders, although it is least common in anorexia nervosa. In almost all patients other than those with binge eating disorder, the binge eating takes place against the background of severe dietary restraint with or without accompanying dietary restriction. The frequency of binge eating varies from once or twice a week (the latter being the DSM-IV diagnostic threshold) to several times a day, and the amount eaten per episode varies but is typically between 1,000 and 2,000 kilocalories (kcals). In most cases each binge is followed by self-induced vomiting or the misuse of laxatives or diuretics, although there are patients who do not "purge" afterward. (Purging is the collective noun for self-induced vomiting or the misuse of laxatives or diuretics). Most patients find binge eating aversive and distressing (and expensive), and it is often the reason that they seek help. Some patients find that binge eating helps them modulate their mood (see Chapter 10).

In addition to true binges, there are "subjective binges" in which the amount eaten is not truly large, given the circumstances. This type of binge eating tends to get overlooked in accounts of the psychopathology of eating disorders, yet such binges are not uncommon and can be just as distressing and impairing as true ("objective") binges. Most of the binges seen in anorexia nervosa tend to be of this type. Subjective binges may, or may not, be followed by purging.

Purging also occurs across the eating disorders, except for binge eating disorder (by definition). Purging may be "compensatory" or "non-compensatory." Compensatory purging is the use of purging to minimize the effects on weight of specific episodes of eating that the patient views as excessive. If the purging is compensatory it is linked to these episodes, follows them, and only occurs when they occur. In non-compensatory purging the behavior functions as a more "routine" form of weight control, akin to dieting, in which case the link with episodes of "excessive" eating is not so close. Like binge eating and intense exercising, purging may function as a means of mood modulation (see Chapter 10). A variant of purging is the repeated spitting out of food, which may be viewed as a form of non-compensatory purging.

Binge eating apart, overeating is not common among patients with eating disorders, the exception being those with binge eating disorder. These patients have recurrent episodes of binge eating, much as in bulimia nervosa, but their eating habits outside the binges are quite different in that they have a general tendency to overeat. Indeed, their eating habits resemble those of people with obesity, albeit with binges superimposed. By definition, extreme dieting, purging and excessive exercising are not present in binge eating disorder.

It is not widely recognized that most patients with an eating disorder have an unremarkable body weight. This is because the effects of any undereating and binge eating tend to cancel each other out. Thus most patients with bulimia nervosa and eating disorder NOS have a body mass index (BMI) in the healthy range (between 20.0 and 24.9). (See Table 2.3 for discussion of the BMI and its use with patients with eating disorders.) By definition, patients with anorexia nervosa are significantly underweight, and this is also true of a proportion of those with eating disorder NOS. At the other end of the weight spectrum, the great majority of patients with binge eating disorder are either overweight or have co-existing obesity (BMI 30 or more) reflecting their general tendency to overeat.

TABLE 2.3. The Body Mass Index (BMI) and Its Use with Patients with Eating Disorders

- The BMI is a convenient way of representing weight adjusted for height. It is weight (in kg) divided by height squared (in m) (i.e., Wt/Ht^2). It was proposed by Quetelet in 1835, a Belgian astronomer and mathematician.

- The chart on the inside of the front cover of the book provides a simple means of determining a person's BMI based on his or her height and weight. The figures given apply to adults of either sex between the ages of 18 and 60 years. BMI centile charts are available for younger patients (e.g., www.cdc.gov/growthcharts).

- In general the BMI works well as a way of classifying people's weight adjusted for their height. Below are the BMI thresholds used in this book. These thresholds differ somewhat from those derived from research on obesity and its associated medical complications. Instead, they are specifically designed to take account of the health implications of lower BMIs for people with eating disorders.

Significantly underweight[a]	17.5 or below
Underweight[b]	17.6–18.9
Low weight[c]	19.0–19.9
Healthy weight[d]	20.0–24.9
Overweight[e]	25.0–29.9
Obesity[f]	30.0 or more

[a]At a BMI of 17.5 or below people are subject to marked adverse physical and psychosocial effects of being underweight (see Chapter 11).

[b]At a BMI between 17.6 and 18.9 most people experience some adverse physical and psychosocial effects of being underweight. Few people in Western societies (other than some of Asian origin) can maintain a BMI below 19.0 without actively restricting what they eat.

[c]A BMI between 19.0 and 19.9 is low but generally not unhealthy.

[d]A BMI between 20.0 and 24.9 is widely viewed as optimal from a health point of view. Some sources view a BMI between 18.5 and 24.9 as being healthy, but (as noted above) this broader BMI range does not take account of the health implications of lower BMIs for people with eating disorders.

[e]A BMI between 25.0 and 29.9 is associated with increased health risks.

[f]A BMI of 30.0 or more is associated with markedly increased health risks.

General Psychopathology

Like the specific psychopathology, the general psychiatric features are similar across the eating disorders. Depressive and anxiety features are particularly common and, indeed, most patients meet criteria for one or more mood or anxiety disorders. Depressive features are especially common among patients who binge eat, whereas anxiety features tend to be more characteristic of patients who have high levels of dietary restraint. In patients who are underweight obsessional features tend to be especially prominent and are in part a consequence of being underweight (see Chapter 11). Some patients engage in repeated self-injury (especially cutting), and an overlapping group have problems with substance misuse (especially excessive alcohol intake). These features are seen across the eating disorders but are most common among those who binge eat.

It is difficult to assess the personality of patients with eating disorders because many features of interest are directly affected by the presence of the eating disorder. Making personality disorder diagnoses is particularly hazardous in these patients as most will have had no period of adulthood free from the presence of the eating disorder (i.e., there is no eating disorder-free period available on which

> **Making personality disorder diagnoses is particularly hazardous in patients with eating disorders.**

to judge their personality).[1] Nevertheless, personality disorder diagnoses are commonly made: For example, those patients who engage in self-injury or substance misuse often attract the diagnosis of borderline personality disorder. Two personality traits are thought to be particularly common — perfectionism and low self-esteem — and typically both will have been in evidence well before the eating disorder began.

Physical Problems

Almost all the physical problems encountered in patients with eating disorders can be attributed to their behavior. Those seen in anorexia nervosa are largely due to these patients' undereating and low weight, and equivalent abnormalities are seen in underweight patients with eating disorder NOS. Purging, if frequent, results in fluid and electrolyte disturbance, whatever the eating disorder diagnosis, and vomiting eventually results in dental damage, again whatever the eating disorder diagnosis. (The medical management of patients with eating disorders is discussed in Chapter 4.)

How Eating Disorder Psychopathology Evolves

> **If the distinctions between the eating disorders seem arbitrary when viewed cross-sectionally, they seem even more so if a longitudinal view is taken.**

If the distinctions between the eating disorders seem arbitrary when viewed cross-sectionally, they seem even more so if a longitudinal view is taken.

Anorexia nervosa typically starts in mid-teenage years with the onset of

---

[1]Note that "A Personality Disorder should be diagnosed only when the defining characteristics appeared before early adulthood, are typical of the individual's long-term functioning, and do not occur exclusively during an episode of an Axis I disorder" (American Psychiatric Association, 1994, p. 632).

dietary restriction. This restriction becomes progressively more extreme and inflexible and, as a result, weight is lost and the person becomes significantly underweight. However, a frequent occurrence is the development of binge eating, weight regain, and progression to bulimia nervosa (in about half the cases) or a mixed form of eating disorder NOS.

Bulimia nervosa has a slightly later age of onset, typically in late adolescence or early adulthood. It usually starts in much the same way as anorexia nervosa: Indeed, in about a quarter of cases the diagnostic criteria for anorexia nervosa are met for a time. It is highly self-perpetuating: Patients often present with an unremitting history of 8 or more years of disturbed eating, and even 5–10 years after presentation between a third and a half still have an eating disorder of clinical severity, although in many cases it has changed from bulimia nervosa into a mixed form of eating disorder NOS.

There has been little research on the development and course of eating disorder NOS. As in bulimia nervosa, most patients present in their adolescence or 20s, and with a comparable length of history. Between a quarter and a third have had anorexia nervosa or bulimia nervosa in the past.

Binge eating disorder has a rather different course compared to the other eating disorders. Most patients are middle-age and a third or more are male. This profile is quite unlike patients with anorexia nervosa, bulimia nervosa and eating disorder NOS, who are generally adolescent or young adult females. Binge eating disorder also tends to be intermittent rather than persistent, with most patients reporting sustained periods when they are prone to binge eat and other times when they are in control of their eating. Throughout, these patients have a general tendency to overeat and gain weight. Few report a history of anorexia nervosa or bulimia nervosa.

In summary, and putting binge eating disorder aside, one of the most striking characteristics of eating disorders is the diagnostic migration. While a small subgroup of patients retains a constant clinical picture, the great majority migrate between the eating disorders diagnoses. This migration is not random, however. It reflects the fact that eating disorders tend to start with dietary restraint and restriction, but patients' control over eating typically breaks down and binge eating develops. Thus those who meet diagnostic criteria for anorexia nervosa tend to do so early in the course of the disorder and then progress to bulimia nervosa or eating disorder NOS. Others either meet diagnostic criteria for bulimia nervosa or eating disorder NOS from the outset and move between the two.

These diagnostic movements beg the question "Do the changes in diagnosis truly reflect recovery from one psychiatric disorder and the development of another, as the DSM-IV scheme would suggest, or do they reflect the evolution of a single eating disorder?" If a patient with eating disorder NOS, who had a history of anorexia nervosa and bulimia nervosa, were told that she had suffered from three different psychiatric disorders, two of which she had recovered from, she would react with surprise and skepticism.

> **Do the changes in eating disorder diagnosis truly reflect recovery from one psychiatric disorder and the development of another, or do they reflect the evolution of a single eating disorder?**

From her perspective she has had a single evolving eating disorder — and, surely, this is indeed the case?

The Transdiagnostic View

As noted at the beginning of this chapter, the DSM-IV scheme for classifying eating disorders encourages the view that there are a number of distinct eating disorders. Consideration of their clinical features and course challenges this view, however. Patients with anorexia nervosa, bulimia nervosa and eating disorder NOS have a great many features in common, and studies of their course indicate that they migrate between these diagnoses. These two characteristics suggest that there is a case for viewing eating disorders as a single diagnostic category rather than as separate disorders.

The implication of the DSM-IV scheme is that each of the eating disorders requires its own form of treatment. This too may be questioned. The fact that eating disorders persist but evolve in form (but do not evolve into other psychiatric disorders) suggests that "transdiagnostic" mechanisms play a major role in maintaining eating disorder psychopathology. In other words, it seems that there are mechanisms that lock patients into having an eating disorder but not a particular eating disorder. If this is the case, treatments that are capable of addressing these mechanisms should be effective with all eating disorders rather than just one. Both our clinical experience with CBT-E and the research findings to date suggest that this is indeed the case.

The Cognitive Behavioral Theory

The theory that underpins CBT-E is concerned with the processes that maintain eating disorder psychopathology rather than those responsible for its initial development, although the two may overlap. This focus on currently operating maintaining mechanisms is common to almost all empirically supported cognitive behavioral treatments.

The theory that formed the basis for CBT-BN is the one that has been most extensively studied and hence it is described first.

The Cognitive Behavioral Theory of Bulimia Nervosa

According to the cognitive behavioral theory of bulimia nervosa, central to the maintenance of the disorder is these patients' core psychopathology: their dysfunctional scheme for self-evaluation. As explained above, most other features seen in the eating disorders can be understood as stemming directly from it, including the dietary restraint (see pathway a, Figure 2.3), the other forms of weight-control behavior, the various forms of body checking and avoidance, and the preoccupation with thoughts about shape, weight and eating.

The only feature of bulimia nervosa that is not obviously a direct expression of the core psychopathology is these patients' binge eating. The cognitive behavioral theory proposes that binge eating is largely a product of their form of dietary restraint. Rather than adopting general guidelines about how they should eat, these patients try to adhere to multiple demanding and highly specific dietary rules. Accompanying these rules is the tendency to react in an extreme and negative fashion to the (almost inevitable) breaking of them, such that even minor dietary slips are viewed as evidence of lack of self-control. Patients respond to such rule-breaking by temporarily abandoning their

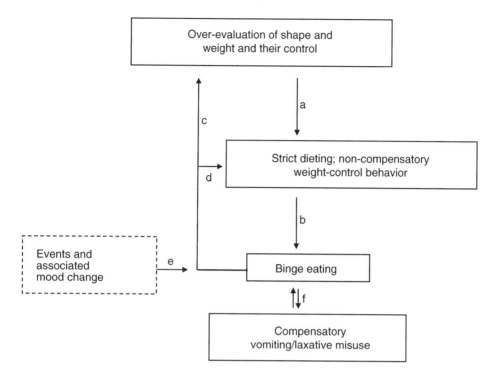

FIGURE 2.3. The cognitive behavioral theory of bulimia nervosa.

From *Cognitive Behavior Therapy and Eating Disorders* by Christopher G. Fairburn. Copyright 2008 by The Guilford Press. This figure is available online at www.psych.ox.ac.uk/credo/cbt_and_eating_disorders.

dietary restraint — and, as a result, succumb to the urge to eat that arises from the restraint (and any accompanying dietary restriction), the result being a short-lived period of uncontrolled eating (i.e., an episode of subjective or objective binge eating; pathway b). This produces the distinctive pattern of eating that characterizes bulimia nervosa in which attempts to restrict eating are interrupted by repeated episodes of binge eating. The binge eating in turn maintains the core psychopathology by intensifying patients' concerns about their shape and weight (pathway c). It also encourages yet greater dietary restraint, thereby increasing the risk of further binge eating (pathway d).

To this account should be added the undoubted fact that these patients' dietary slips and binges do not come "out of the blue"; rather, they are particularly likely to occur in response to adverse day-to-day events and negative moods. In part this is because it is difficult to maintain dietary restraint under such circumstances, and in part because binge eating temporarily ameliorates negative mood states and distracts patients from thinking about their difficulties (pathway e).

A further process maintains binge eating among those who practice compensatory purging. These patients' belief in the ability of purging to minimize weight gain results in a major deterrent against binge eating being undermined. They do not realize that vomiting only retrieves part of what has been eaten, and laxatives have little or no effect (see Chapter 6).

This well-supported cognitive behavioral theory of the maintenance of bulimia

nervosa has clear implications for treatment. It suggests that if treatment is to have a lasting impact on patients' binge eating and purging — the one aspect of their disorder that
most patients want to change — then it also needs to address their extreme dieting, their
over-evaluation of shape and weight, and any tendency for their eating to change in
response to adverse events and negative moods.

The Transdiagnostic Cognitive Behavioral Theory

The cognitive behavioral theory of bulimia nervosa may be extended to all eating disorders. This is warranted as anorexia nervosa and most forms of eating disorder NOS have
much in common with bulimia nervosa. As already noted, they share essentially the
same distinctive core psychopathology and this psychopathology is expressed in similar
attitudes and behavior. Thus patients with anorexia nervosa attempt to restrict their food
intake in the same rigid and extreme way as patients with bulimia nervosa, and they too
may vomit, misuse laxatives or diuretics, and over-exercise. Nor does binge eating distinguish the two diagnoses, for there is a subgroup of patients with anorexia nervosa who
binge eat (with or without compensatory purging). The major difference between
anorexia nervosa and bulimia nervosa lies in the relative balance of the undereating and
overeating, and its effect on body weight. In bulimia nervosa body weight is usually
unremarkable because the overeating and undereating cancel each other out. However,
in anorexia nervosa the attempts to restrict eating are more successful with the result
that undereating predominates and the patient remains significantly underweight and
has secondary physical and psychosocial features as a result. Certain of these secondary
features serve to maintain the undereating, thereby locking patients into a self-
perpetuating state (see Chapter 11). Figure 2.4 illustrates the cognitive behavioral theory
of the maintenance of the classic "restricting" form of anorexia nervosa.

The processes that maintain bulimia nervosa and anorexia nervosa also appear to
maintain the clinical presentations seen in eating disorder NOS. Figure 2.5 shows the
composite transdiagnostic cognitive behavioral theory, which is essentially a combination of the bulimia nervosa and restricting anorexia nervosa theories. In our experience,
this composite theory represents well the range of processes that serve to maintain any
eating disorder, whatever its exact form, the specific processes operating in any individual depending upon the exact psychopathology present. In some cases only a limited
number of these processes are active, as in many cases of binge eating disorder, whereas
in others the majority are operating, as in cases of anorexia nervosa in which there is
binge eating and purging. Like the cognitive behavioral theory of bulimia nervosa, the
transdiagnostic theory highlights the processes that need to be tackled in treatment and
it is these that are addressed in CBT-E.

Recommended Reading

Clinical Features of the Eating Disorders

Fairburn, C. G., & Harrison, P. J. (2003). Eating disorders. *Lancet, 361,* 407–416.
Garner, D. M. (1997). Psychoeducational principles in treatment. In D. M. Garner & P. E.

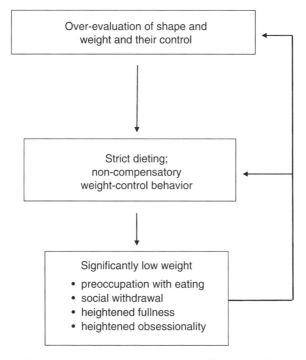

FIGURE 2.4. The cognitive behavioral theory of ("restricting") anorexia nervosa.

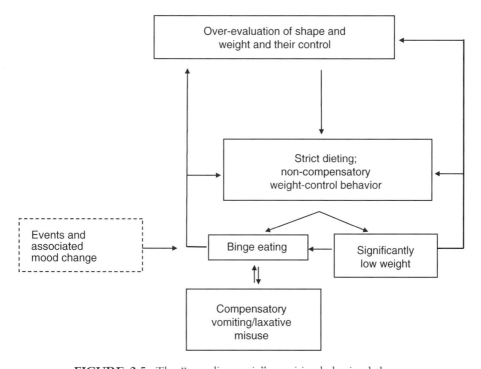

FIGURE 2.5. The "transdiagnostic" cognitive behavioral theory.

From *Cognitive Behavior Therapy and Eating Disorders* by Christopher G. Fairburn. Copyright 2008 by The Guilford Press. These figures are available online at www.psych.ox.ac.uk/credo/cbt_and_eating_disorders.

Garfinkel (Eds.), *Handbook of treatment for eating disorders* (2nd ed., pp. 145–177). New York: Guilford Press.

Grilo, C. M. (2006). *Eating and weight disorders.* New York: Psychology Press.

Palmer, R. (2000). *Helping people with eating disorders: A clinical guide to assessment and treatment.* Chichester: Wiley.

Diagnosis and Classification of Eating Disorders

American Psychiatric Association. (1994). *Diagnostic and statistical manual of mental disorders* (4th ed.). Washington, DC: Author.

Commission on Adolescent Eating Disorders. (2005). Eating disorders. In D. L. Evans et al. (Eds.), *Treating and preventing adolescent mental health disorders* (pp. 257–332). New York: Oxford University Press.

de Zwaan, M., Roerig, D. B., Crosby, R. D., & Mitchell, J. E. (2006). Nighttime eating: A descriptive study. *International Journal of Eating Disorders, 39,* 224–232.

Fairburn, C. G., & Bohn, K. (2005). Eating disorder NOS (EDNOS): An example of the troublesome "not otherwise specified" (NOS) category in DSM-IV. *Behaviour Research and Therapy, 43,* 691–701.

Fairburn, C. G., & Cooper, Z. (2007). Thinking afresh about the classification of eating disorders. *International Journal of Eating Disorders, 40,* 5107–5111.

Fairburn, C. G., Cooper, Z., & Shafran, R. (2003). Cognitive behaviour therapy for eating disorders: A "transdiagnostic" theory and treatment. *Behaviour Research and Therapy, 41,* 509–528.

Keel, P. K. (2007). Purging disorder: Subthreshold variant or full-threshold eating disorder. *International Journal of Eating Disorders, 40,* 589–594.

Striegel-Moore, R. H., Franko, D. L., May, A., Ach, E., Thompson, D., & Hook, J. M. (2006). Should night eating syndrome be included in the DSM-IV? *International Journal of Eating Disorders, 39,* 544–549.

Wonderlich, S. A., Joiner, T. E., Keel, P. K., Williamson, D. A., & Crosby, R. D. (2007). Eating disorder diagnoses: Empirical approaches to classification. *American Psychologist, 62,* 167–180.

CHAPTER 3

Enhanced Cognitive Behavior Therapy for Eating Disorders ("CBT-E"): An Overview

Christopher G. Fairburn, Zafra Cooper and Roz Shafran

Eating disorders and CBT are a perfect match.

Eating disorders and CBT are a perfect match because eating disorders are fundamentally "cognitive disorders" and CBT is of its very nature designed to produce cognitive change. This chapter provides an overview of "enhanced" cognitive behavior therapy for eating disorders (CBT-E). It opens with an outline of its strategy and structure, then provides an account of the adaptations that have been devised to suit particular patient subgroups and settings. This is followed by a brief description of the types of cognitive behavioral procedures used together with some thoughts about therapist characteristics. The chapter ends by highlighting certain points about the implementation of the treatment.

Treatment Strategy and Structure

CBT-E is a treatment for eating disorder psychopathology, rather than an eating disorder diagnosis. It was designed as a treatment for adults, although it can be adapted for use with younger patients (see Chapter 14). It is equally

CBT-E is a treatment for eating disorder psychopathology, rather than an eating disorder diagnosis.

suitable for males and females. Patients do not need to be particularly intelligent, well-educated or psychologically minded to benefit from CBT-E: Indeed some of the hardest patients to help are those highly intelligent patients who are prone to intellectualize.

The strategy underpinning CBT-E is to construct a "formulation" (or set of hypotheses) of the processes that are maintaining the patient's psychopathology and use it to identify the features that need to be targeted in treatment. Thus, a personalized formulation is constructed at the very outset, although this is revised as treatment proceeds. In this way a bespoke tailor-made treatment is created that fits the individual patient's evolving psychopathology and changes with it. This said, there are some standard aspects of CBT-E. First, it is generally of fixed length, with the great majority of patients receiving 20 treatment sessions over 20 weeks. Second, it uses certain well-specified strategies and procedures to address the targeted psychopathology. These are described in Chapters 5 to 12. And third, it has four relatively well-defined stages. Table 3.1 shows how the appointments are typically distributed across them.

> **In CBT-E a bespoke treatment is created that fits the individual patient's psychopathology.**

Stage One is an intensive initial stage and appointments are twice-weekly. Research on a range of disorders, including eating disorders, has shown that the magnitude of change in the first few weeks of treatment is a potent predictor of outcome. It is therefore crucial that treatment starts well. The aims of Stage One are to engage the patient in treatment and change, to jointly create a personalized formulation, to provide relevant education, and to introduce two potent CBT-E procedures that are of relevance to all patients with an eating disorder. These are "in-session weighing" and "regular eating." By the end of Stage One patients should be engaged in treatment; be well informed about weight, weighing and weight change; and be learning to eat regular meals and

TABLE 3.1. The Temporal Pattern of Appointments in the 20-Session Version of CBT-E

Stage in treatment	Week in treatment	Session number
Stage One	1	Initial session, 1
	2	2, 3
	3	4, 5
	4	6, 7
Stage Two	5	8
	6	9
Stage Three	7	10
	8	11
	9	12
	10	13
	11	14
	12	15
	13	16
	14	17
Stage Four	15	
	16	18
	17	
	18	19
	19	
	20	20
Review session	20 weeks post-treatment	

snacks without eating between them. These are the foundations upon which other changes are built. To the extent that these goals are achieved, the patient will be in an excellent state to start addressing the core processes that maintain the eating disorder.

Stage Two is a brief transitional stage in which the therapist and patient take stock, review progress, identify any emerging barriers to change, modify the formulation as needed, and plan Stage Three. With patients who are not underweight (as defined below) appointments are weekly from this point. The Stage Two review has several purposes, one of which is to detect patients who are not doing well. This is important because unless the cause of their poor response is identified and addressed, it is unlikely that these patients will have a good outcome. The review and reformulation is also designed to encourage therapists to adjust their treatment to suit the evolving nature of the eating disorder. It is at this point that CBT-E becomes highly individualized.

Stage Three is the main body of treatment and the aim is to address the main mechanisms that are maintaining the patient's eating disorder. Precisely how this is done varies considerably from patient to patient. There are eight weekly appointments.

Stage Four is the final stage of treatment and the focus shifts to the future. There are two aims; the first to ensure that the changes are maintained (over the subsequent 20 weeks until a review appointment is held), and the second to minimize the risk of relapse in the long-term. The appointments are scheduled at 2-week intervals.

The Various Forms of CBT-E

There are various forms of CBT-E, as summarized in Table 3.2. There is the main "focused" version that concentrates exclusively on the eating disorder psychopathology. This is suitable for the majority of patients and should be viewed as the default version. In addition, there is a "broad" version that is designed to address mechanisms "external" to the core eating disorder that contribute to its maintenance in some patients (see Chapter 13). This version has three additional treatment "modules" that address clinical perfectionism, low self-esteem and interpersonal difficulties, respectively. The fourth of the original modules — addressing mood intolerance — has been incorporated into the focused version of the treatment (see Chapter 10).

TABLE 3.2. The Various Forms of CBT-E

Two versions
- Focused version (the core treatment) — see Chapters 5–12.
- Broad version (with modules addressing clinical perfectionism, core low self-esteem and interpersonal difficulties) — see Chapter 13.

Two intensities
- 20-session version (for patients with a BMI over 17.5) — see Chapters 5–10 and 12.
- 40-session version (for patients with a BMI between 15.0 and 17.5) — see Chapter 11.

Version for younger patients (under 18 years) — see Chapter 14.

Intensive version (for inpatient and intensive outpatient use) — see Chapter 15.

Group version — see Chapter 15.

CBT-E has also been adapted to suit younger patients (see Chapter 14) and those who need inpatient treatment (see Chapter 15). In addition, there are two variants of the standard outpatient approach, an intensive version and a group version (see Chapter 15).

As generally used, and as evaluated in research trials, CBT-E is a time-limited treatment. For patients who are not significantly underweight (defined in this context as having a BMI over 17.5) 20 treatment sessions over 20 weeks are generally sufficient. For patients below this weight, treatment needs to be modified and extended. Given the relative prevalence of underweight and non-underweight patients, the 20-session version is appropriate for over 80% of adult outpatients. The adaptations for underweight patients are described in Chapter 11.

The fact that CBT-E is generally time-limited might be thought to be inconsistent with the claim that it is individualized. To an extent this is true but there are major advantages to working within a fixed time frame, and in our view these outweigh the potential disadvantage of standardization of treatment length. The main advantage is that a fixed time frame concentrates the mind of both the patient and the therapist. It encourages the establishment of the "therapeutic momentum" that is needed early on to make inroads into the eating disorder, and it helps ensure that the therapist and patient keep working hard at achieving change. It also makes it much more likely that treatment will have a formal ending, rather than merely fizzling out as sometimes happens when treatment is open-ended. Having a definite end ensures that important future-oriented topics are covered in the final sessions of treatment.

There are circumstances under which it is appropriate to adjust the length of treatment. It rarely needs to be shortened, although this does sometimes apply in cases of binge eating disorder if the binge eating rapidly ceases and there is little other psychopathology to address. More often there is a case for extending treatment. The indications for doing this are discussed toward the end of the chapter (see page 33).

The principal point to note is that in the vast majority of cases treatment can and should end on time. This was not the first author's original practice. He used to keep treating patients until they were virtually asymptomatic. This was unnecessary and

> **In the vast majority of cases treatment can and should end on time.**

possibly not in the patients' interests. So long as patients have got to the point where the main maintaining mechanisms have been disrupted, they continue to improve after treatment has ended. Under these circumstances treatment can and should finish. Otherwise, patients (and therapists) tend to ascribe any continuing improvement to the ongoing therapy rather than the progress that the patient has made. In practice this means that it is acceptable to end treatment with patients who are still dieting to an extent, perhaps binge eating and vomiting on occasions, and often having residual concerns about shape and weight.

CBT-E Treatment Procedures

CBT-E is a form of cognitive behavior therapy (CBT). As noted in Chapter 2, in common with most other empirically supported forms of CBT, it is primarily concerned with the processes that are maintaining the patient's psychopathology, with cognitive processes being viewed as of paramount importance. To this end CBT-E uses cognitive and behavioral strategies and procedures, integrated with relevant education.

The style of CBT-E resembles that of other forms of CBT and it is therefore a definite advantage if the therapist has had CBT training. As in other forms of CBT establishing a collaborative working relationship is of fundamental importance, the goal being that the therapist and patient work together as a team to help the patient overcome the eating problem. This is particularly important with patients who have eating disorders because "being in control" is of great importance to them. Therapists need to ensure that these patients, and especially the underweight ones, understand what is happening in treatment and are active participants in it. If they feel that they are being controlled, coerced or misled, patients will resist change. (Further details on the engagement of underweight patients are given in Chapter 11.) It should be made clear to patients that overcoming an eating problem is difficult, but worthwhile, and that treatment will need to be given priority. In common with other forms of CBT, ongoing self-monitoring and the successful accomplishment of strategically planned homework tasks are of fundamental importance, and to ensure that these tasks are undertaken, the therapeutic relationship should be such that the therapist can be firm at times. This is important because some of the tasks are difficult and anxiety-provoking.

Two principles underpin CBT-E. First, simpler procedures are preferred over more complex ones; and second, it is better to do a few things well rather than many things badly (the principle of parsimony). However, the bottom line with CBT-E is whether a strategy or procedure is effective or not.

> **The principle of parsimony: It is better to do a few things well than many things badly.**

Although CBT-E uses a variety of generic cognitive behavioral strategies and procedures (e.g., cognitive biases such as dichotomous thinking and selective attention are addressed in the usual way), CBT-E differs from certain forms of CBT. It does not use conventional thought records, although one column of the standard monitoring record is available for this purpose and at points patients are asked to record their thoughts and feelings about particular topics (e.g., when addressing body checking and feeling fat; see pages 103 and 113, respectively). CBT-E does not make much use of formal cognitive restructuring, and some readers may be taken aback to find no reference to certain widely used CBT concepts; specifically, automatic thoughts, assumptions, core beliefs and schemas. In this particular patient population we do not find that these methods or concepts are needed to produce the changes that are required. Rather, as is generally the case, the most powerful way of achieving cognitive change is by helping patients change the way that they behave and then analyzing the effects and implications of those changes. It may also surprise readers that there is also almost no reference in this book to the concept of "personality disorder." It is important to note that we do, of course, see the types of patient who tend to be given personality disorder diagnoses. We do not use this concept ourselves mainly for the reasons specified in Chapter 2 (see page 16). Guidance on the management of these patients is to

> **The most powerful way of achieving cognitive change is by helping patients make changes to the way that they behave and then analyzing the effects and implications of these changes.**

be found throughout the book but especially in Chapters 10 and 13 in the context of describing the "broad" version of the treatment.

While CBT-E employs the general therapeutic style of collaborative empiricism characteristic of CBT, and exploratory questioning is used to help patients clarify their thinking, we do not view so-called "Socratic questioning" as essential, although it can be helpful at times. (As an aside, it is interesting to note that the term is a misnomer given what is known about Socrates; see Table 3.3.) In our view, and again referring to these particular patients, the same end can very often be achieved using simpler and more efficient means. We also make limited use of *formal* behavioral experiments as (once again referring to this particular patient population) they tend to be hard to interpret.[1] In part this is because the outcomes of greatest relevance to the core psychopathology of eating disorders (i.e., changes in shape or weight) do not lend themselves to short-term experimentation. For this reason different strategies are needed. Lastly, we do not provide patients with recordings of their treatment sessions as in our experience doing so tends trigger persistent and unhelpful ruminative thinking.

What we do view as essential is that patients learn to de-center from their eating problem. We want them to become interested in it, to understand how it works and why it is self-maintaining. We encourage them to observe themselves enacting their formulation live, and to become intrigued by the effects, and implications, of trying different ways of behaving. Later in treatment, when the processes maintaining the eating disorder have been sufficiently disrupted for patients to have periods when they think quite differently, we help them spot shifts in their mindset (see Chapter 8). In this way they learn to manipulate their frame of mind and thereby deal more effectively with setbacks that might otherwise develop into full-scale relapses.

> We encourage patients to observe themselves enacting their formulation live, and to become intrigued by the effects, and implications, of trying different ways of behaving.

TABLE 3.3. Socrates and Socratic Questioning

It is unlikely that Socrates engaged in the type of questioning that CBT therapists ascribe to him. His mode of questioning was probing and persistent, and prone to confuse the person questioned. An excellent description of how it felt to be questioned by Socrates comes from Plato's *Meno* (402 B.C.):

"You know, people kept telling me, Socrates, even before I met you, that all you do is go around being baffled by things and baffling everyone else. And now that I have met you, sure enough, I feel as though you're bewitching me, and jinxing me, and casting some strange spell over me, to the point where I'm about as baffled as can be."

Note. Quote from Plato's *Meno.* Translated by A. Beresford. Penguin, London, 2005 (p. 99). We are grateful to Professor David Charles for identifying this source.

---

[1]A contrast may be drawn between formal behavioral experiments of the hypothesis-testing variety, of which we make limited use, and helping patients make strategic changes to the way that they behave that are designed to produce cognitive change and are justified and interpreted in the context of the patient's formulation.

Therapist Characteristics

As mentioned in Chapter 1, no specific professional qualifications are required to practice CBT-E. However, the ideal therapist should have had training in CBT and prior experience working with patients with eating disorders. The therapist should also be aware of the medical complications of eating disorders and be able to manage them appropriately (see Chapter 4).

In contrast with many other applications of CBT, the gender of the therapist is relevant to treatment. Most patients with eating disorders are female and as a result female therapists have certain advantages. They may be viewed by patients as being more likely to understand their difficulties and, in addition, they may serve as a role model in terms of acceptance of shape and weight.

> In contrast with many other applications of CBT, the gender of the therapist is relevant to treatment.

Nevertheless, therapists' competence at delivering CBT-E is the critical issue and of far greater importance than their gender.

A subject rarely discussed is the appearance of the therapist. This is of little relevance if the therapist is middle-age or of the opposite gender, as the patient is unlikely to be interested in his or her appearance, but it is relevant if the patient and therapist are of the same gender and similar in age. Patients with eating disorders are acutely aware of the shape of other relevant people, and this includes that of their therapist. Therapists who are very thin may find themselves at a disadvantage when trying to help underweight patients regain weight as they may be challenged about their own eating habits and weight. Therapists who are overweight may find these patients hard to engage as some have a negative attitude toward people who are overweight. For example, we have encountered patients who cross the road to avoid passing someone with obesity or who will not sit in a chair vacated by someone who is overweight.

Another matter that merits thought is whether the therapist has an eating disorder or a recent history of one. Two perspectives should be taken: the well-being of the patient and the well-being of the therapist. With regard to the former, it makes little difference to the patient whether or not the therapist has, or has had, an eating disorder, as it would not be appropriate for therapists to disclose their psychiatric history. Nevertheless, such a history might render the therapist more attuned to the types of difficulty that the patient is facing, although a drawback can be loss of objectivity. As noted above, therapists who are visibly underweight can be at a disadvantage as patients may suspect that they have an eating disorder. The well-being of the therapist must also be considered, however. One of the distinctive characteristics of people with eating disorders is the level of interest they have in issues related to food, eating, shape and weight. The tendency of patients with anorexia nervosa to read recipe books and cook for others is well known, but similar behavior is seen across the eating disorder diagnoses and is, of course, an expression of the core psychopathology. This psychopathology can also influence career choice: For example, it may lead people with eating disorders, or histories of them, to work as personal trainers, beauty therapists or dieticians, or indeed as therapists for patients who have an eating disorder. If this applies, the therapist should consider whether it is in his or her best interests to engage in this type of work as doing so can maintain preoccupation with eating, shape and weight and serve as an obstacle to the broadening of horizons.

Significant Others

CBT-E is an individual, one-to-one, form of therapy. Despite this, it is our practice to see "significant others" if this is likely to facilitate treatment and the patient is willing for this to happen. We do this with the aim of creating the optimum environment to facilitate change in the patient. There are two specific indications for involving others:

1. If others could be of help to the patient in making changes
2. If others are making it difficult for the patient to change; for example, by commenting adversely on his or her appearance or eating.

The conduct of "Significant Other" sessions is described in Chapter 6 (page 87). We hold one or more such sessions with about three-quarters of our patients and have rather more such sessions with underweight patients (see Chapters 11). Topics outside the eating disorder are not usually addressed. With adolescent patients there is far greater involvement of significant others (see Chapters 14 and 15).

Implementing CBT-E

Five Notes of Caution

First, CBT-E is a complete treatment in its own right. It is not designed to be dismantled into segments to be used on their own. CBT-E is not merely a collection of techniques: The sum is more than its parts.

Second, CBT-E is not designed to be used in conjunction with other psychological treatments. It is especially important not to combine CBT-E with conceptually, or procedurally, incompatible treatments as this risks confusing the patient and undermining the treatment. (Readers will notice an exception to this general injunction in the "broad" version of CBT-E [see Chapter 13] in which CBT-E is combined with interpersonal psychotherapy [IPT].)

> **CBT-E is not merely a collection of techniques: The sum is more than its parts.**

Third, CBT-E is designed to be delivered by one therapist. It is not uncommon for patients with eating disorders to see multiple therapists at one time (e.g., a psychologist, dietician and physician). This is particularly common on inpatient units where it is inevitable to an extent, but it also occurs in outpatient settings, particularly those involving younger patients (see Chapter 14). This practice encourages patients to partition their problems and talk about specific topics with specific people. As a result there is the risk that no one sees and appraises the full clinical picture. In CBT-E just one therapist should be involved. This works well and is rewarding for therapists. It also means that CBT-E is more practicable (and therefore more disseminable) than multiple-therapist approaches. Access to other specialists is important, however. As stressed in Chapter 4, all therapists need to have access to a physician who can advise them on the management of any physical problems present in their cases, and each patient should have a named physician who will take responsibility for his or her physical health. Access to a specialist dietitian is also of value as it allows the discussion of nutritional issues and the dietary management of specific cases (most especially those who are underweight or overweight, and those who are adhering to vegetarian or vegan diets; see page 130).

Fourth, we have observed that some therapists are tempted to change therapeutic tack if progress is slow or difficult. We think that this is rarely appropriate. Although it might be tempting to switch to another therapeutic modality or try to integrate other techniques, we recommend that even under these circumstances the therapist persevere with CBT-E while trying to understand and address the basis for the lack of progress.

> **Experience can be a dangerous thing.**

Overcoming blocks to progress is often a turning point in treatment.

Fifth, experience can be a dangerous thing. We have noticed that more experienced therapists are tempted to deviate from the treatment protocol. This is not in the patient's interests. The protocol described in Chapters 5–13 provides a detailed description of the form of treatment that is empirically supported: Therapists' modifications are not. The wise therapist adheres to the protocol.

> **The wise therapist adheres to the protocol.**

Dependence on Treatment

Undue dependence on treatment, or the therapist, is not often a problem in CBT-E. This is in part because of the style of the treatment and in part because it is time-limited. Nevertheless, the occasional patient does show signs of becoming dependent. This dependence may be revealed by the patient's difficulty adjusting to the progressive decrease in the frequency of appointments or by attempts to make contact between sessions. Most at risk are patients with few social supports. If the therapist suspects that the patient is becoming dependent, this is probably the case. Under these circumstances the therapist should raise the topic with the patient and explain that some degree of dependence on treatment can happen and is not a concern. The therapist might say "*It is natural to become somewhat dependent upon treatment under the circumstances, but this will only be temporary.*" Patients should be told that as treatment progresses, they will feel more in control in general and more capable of functioning independently without the support of treatment. The therapist may add that most patients are pleased to end treatment by the time that it is due to finish.

Minimizing Non-Attendance and Dropping Out

More of a problem than dependence on treatment is stopping treatment early. This occurs commonly in routine clinical practice. In treatment trials dropout rates tend to be lower but are nevertheless unacceptably high.

Dropping out is rarely, if ever, a good sign. In some cases it is due to extraneous factors (e.g., having to relocate due a change of job), but more often it is attributable to the eating disorder itself or some problem with the treatment. Patients may not like the therapy or the therapist, or they may feel that they are failing at treatment.

As therapists it is important that we do our best to help patients complete their treatment. Some years ago we thought we could do better in this regard and so reviewed all our instances of dropping out looking for the likely explanation and possible early warning signs. We came to the conclusion that the risk of dropping out is increased under the following circumstances:

- If the therapist senses there is a problem with engagement (e.g., if the patient has a disinterested or scornful stance)
- If the patient misses an appointment or is repeatedly late for sessions
- If there are practical barriers to attending (e.g., a difficult or expensive journey; problems with child care)
- If significant others are skeptical about the value of treatment

We decided that the best strategy under such circumstances was to grasp the nettle and actively raise the subject with the patient. Thus we now say something along these lines: "*I am wondering how you are feeling about coming here. I am wondering whether you are having any misgivings about attending or continuing to attend.*" Our experience is that saying something like this is constructive as it tends to bring into the open problems that can often be successfully addressed. By doing this we have seen a steady decline in our drop-out rate from its previous level of 29% to 16% and on to its present level of 13%.

We have also evolved a protocol for dealing with late attendance or non-attendance. First, we try to prevent this from happening by encouraging patients to attend early and by engendering a sense of collective responsibility for the optimal use of our time. Thus the information sheet given to patients states:

> "*For everyone's sake it is important that appointments start and end on time. Your therapist will make sure he or she is ready at the due time and we request that you do the same. It is a very good idea to arrive a little time in advance — say 10 to 15 minutes beforehand. This will give you an opportunity to settle down and think over things.*
>
> "*If you are unable to attend a specific appointment, please let us know as soon as possible so that we can reschedule the appointment and offer someone else your slot.*"

If a patient is late for an appointment, we will call them after 15 minutes and express concern about their absence. Often the explanation is that they are feeling that they are not doing well enough. Alternatively, they may have slept in! Generally we try to reschedule the appointment as soon as possible.

Dealing with Breaks in Treatment

As explained in Chapters 5 and 6, we place great store on establishing and maintaining therapeutic momentum, and this is made clear to patients when deciding the best time for treatment to start. The need to avoid breaks in treatment is particularly stressed. Of course, this places an onus on therapists to ensure that they too are available. Therapists' absences are a problem.

To deal with therapists' absences, we employ an "understudying" system. We have an arrangement whereby our therapists serve as understudies for each other, an arrangement that is explained to patients in advance. Thus when a therapist is going to be away, another therapist will take his or her place so that the patient's treatment can continue virtually uninterrupted. The understudy is briefed by the patient's therapist as to the progress of the patient and the likely content of the next few sessions, and the understudy listens to the recording of the last session. In this way the understudy is reasonably in the picture. The understudy then undertakes the missed sessions, following the CBT-E protocol along the lines suggested by the primary therapist. Interestingly, patients report liking this arrangement and certainly preferring it to missing sessions.

Patients' absences are also a problem. As explained in Chapter 4, we ask patients not to be away for longer than 2 consecutive weeks during the course of treatment and not at all during the first 6 weeks. When they are away we try to straddle the gap by maintaining therapeutic contact. We may arrange weekly telephone sessions or we may use e-mail for this purpose. In both cases the patient will be asked to hold in advance a preplanned self-administered session following the usual session structure, barring the in-session weighing (see Chapter 5, page 62). The content of this review is then the subject of the telephone call or e-mail, and the therapist will respond with comments and suggestions. It is rarely appropriate to introduce new procedures while patients are away, but on the other hand the change in patients' circumstances may provide an opportunity for them to try new ways of behaving (e.g., in terms of food choice, eating pattern, clothing, ways of relating to others).

When to Provide Additional or Alternative Treatment

Under certain circumstances patients should be provided with additional or alternative treatment:

1. *When the patient is not benefiting at all from CBT-E.* This is unusual but it occasionally occurs with underweight patients. It is not appropriate to persist indefinitely with CBT-E under these circumstances. If there has been no progress by the mid-point in treatment, a more intensive treatment is indicated (see below).

2. *When the patient has benefited but is still significantly impaired.* This can be a reason to extend treatment. The main indication for doing so is the presence toward the end of Stage Three of eating disorder features that are significantly impairing the patient's functioning and are unlikely to resolve of their own accord. Under these circumstances Stage Three may be continued for some additional months with a detailed review of progress every 4 weeks to ensure that continuing is justified.

3. *When the patient has benefited from treatment but experiences a setback not long after treatment has finished.* In our experience setbacks can often be overcome with limited additional input. Although patients may feel "back to square one," in reality they have the knowledge and skills needed to get back on track. Often a little support and encouragement are all that is needed.

4. *When treatment has been disrupted* (e.g., by the development of a clinical depression or the occurrence of a life crisis — see Chapter 16 for a discussion of how to manage both problems). In such cases CBT-E should be extended to compensate for the disruption.

If a patient needs further full-scale treatment, what form should it take? There are no research findings to help answer this question. CBT-E is the latest version of the leading evidence-based treatment for eating disorders. There is no obvious trans-diagnostic alternative other than interpersonal psychotherapy (IPT), and the limited information available (from research on bulimia nervosa) suggests that IPT does not benefit those who do not respond to CBT. It is our view that patients who need further treatment should not be offered an alternative outpatient-based treatment: Rather, they should receive more intensive treatment. Intensive outpatient or inpatient CBT-E are two good options, as they are conceptually and procedurally compatible with conventional CBT-E. Both are described in Chapter 15.

Recommended Reading

Early Change in Treatment Predicting Outcome

Agras, W. S., Crow, S. J., Halmi, K. A., Mitchell, J. E., Wilson, G. T., & Kraemer, H. C. (2000). Outcome predictors for the cognitive behavior treatment of bulimia nervosa: Data from a multisite study. *American Journal of Psychiatry, 157,* 1302–1308.

Fairburn, C. G., Agras, W. S., Walsh, B. T., Wilson, G. T., & Stice, E. (2004). Prediction of outcome in bulimia nervosa by early change in treatment. *American Journal of Psychiatry, 161,* 2322–2324.

Grilo, C. M., Masheb, R. M., & Wilson, G. T. (2006). Rapid response to treatment for binge eating disorder. *Journal of Consulting and Clinical Psychology, 74,* 602–603.

Walsh, B. T., Sysko, R., & Parides, M. K. (2006). Early response to desipramine among women with bulimia nervosa. *International Journal of Eating Disorders, 39,* 72–75.

Guides to the Practice of CBT

See Chapter 1 (page 6).

Other Forms of CBT for Patients with Eating Disorders

Cooper, M. J., Todd, G., & Wells, A. (2000). *Bulimia nervosa: A cognitive therapy programme for clients.* London: Kingsley.

Garner, D. M., Vitousek, K. M., & Pike, K. M. (1997). Cognitive-behavioral therapy for anorexia nervosa. In D. M. Garner & P. E. Garfinkel (Eds.), *Handbook of treatment for eating disorders* (2nd ed., pp. 94–144). New York: Guilford Press.

Kleifield, E. I., Wagner, S., & Halmi, K. A. (1996). Cognitive-behavioral treatment of anorexia nervosa. *Psychiatric Clinics of North America, 19,* 715–737.

Waller, G., Cordery, H., Corstorphine, E., Hinrichsen, H., Lawson, R., Mountford, V., et al. (2007). *Cognitive behavioural therapy for eating disorders.* Cambridge: Cambridge University Press.

Other Articles of Relevance to Chapter 3

Johnston, C., Smethurst, N., & Gowers, S. (2005). Should people with a history of an eating disorder work as eating disorder therapists? *European Eating Disorder Review, 13,* 301–310.

Mitchell, J. E., Halmi, K., Wilson, G. T., Agras, W. S., Kraemer, H., & Crow, S. (2002). A randomized secondary treatment study of women with bulimia nervosa who fail to respond to CBT. *International Journal of Eating Disorders, 32,* 271–281.

Wilson, G. T. (2005). Psychological treatment of eating disorders. In S. Nolen-Hoeksema (Ed.), *Annual review of clinical psychology* (pp. 439–465). Palo Alto, CA: Annual Reviews.

Wilson, G. T., Grilo, C. M., & Vitousek, K. M. (2007). Psychological treatment of eating disorders. *American Psychologist, 62,* 199–216.

CHAPTER 4

The Patients:
Their Assessment,
Preparation for Treatment
and Medical Management

Christopher G. Fairburn, Zafra Cooper and Deborah Waller

This chapter discusses the assessment of patients and their preparation for CBT-E. It also addresses their medical management from the perspective of the non-medical therapist. It ends with a note on waiting lists, self-help and stepped care.

CBT-E is designed for patients with an eating disorder of clinical severity (i.e., the disturbance is persistent and is significantly interfering with the person's psychosocial functioning or physical health). As it is primarily an outpatient-based treatment it is essential that it is safe for the patient to be managed this way, both in physical terms and from the psychiatric point of view. In practice this means that the patients' physical state must be stable and they must not be at risk of suicide. The treatment has not been used with patients at the very extremes of the weight spectrum: Rather, it is designed for those with a BMI between 15.0 and 40.0. Although some patients with a BMI outside this range can be treated successfully using CBT-E, this is probably best left to therapists experienced at working with these particular groups. Throughout this chapter, and the ones describing the two main versions of the treatment (Chapters 5–13 inclusive), it is assumed that the patient is aged at least 18 years. The use of CBT-E with younger patients is described in Chapter 14.

Assessment and Preparation for Treatment

The essential first step in managing any psychiatric problem is an evaluation interview. Its goals are to engage the patient, establish the nature and severity of the problem, and decide how best to proceed. In the case of eating disorders, it may be that an apparent "eating disorder" is in fact an anxiety disorder (e.g., difficulty eating with others due to a social phobia), a presentation of a mood disorder (e.g., severe weight loss stemming from a clinical depression) or straightforward overeating in someone with obesity.

The Initial Evaluation Interview(s)

The initial interview has two interrelated goals. The first is to put the patient at ease and begin to forge a positive therapeutic relationship. This is important for a number of reasons. First, many patients referred with a possible eating disorder are highly ambivalent about treatment: Aspects of the psychopathology may be positively valued (especially dietary control and weight loss); there may be shame about other features (e.g., binge eating); and the patient may have had adverse treatment experiences in the past. The assessing clinician therefore needs to be sensitive to the patient's attitude to the referral and ask about it. The assessment process should be collaborative. First impressions are important and a positive first meeting can start to engage even the most ambivalent patient, whereas a negative encounter can have quite the opposite effect: Indeed, one may never see the patient again.

The other goal of the initial interview is to establish the nature of the eating problem, its severity, and the appropriate next step. Table 4.1 lists the topics that we routinely cover. It is not our practice to take an exhaustive personal history, nor do we attempt to provide patients with an account of their problem in theoretical terms (psychodynamic, cognitive behavioral, or other). Rather, we focus on our two goals and do our utmost to achieve them.

Patients are invited to bring others to the appointment if they wish. They may simply provide moral support (and stay in the waiting area) or they may be useful as informants. If serving as informants, we will see them together with the patient after we have conducted the one-to-one assessment, and we will see them only if the patient is willing for us to do so. One of our priorities is to ensure that the patient feels in control of the assessment process.

The perspective of informants is always of interest. Problems may be described that were not disclosed by the patient (e.g., that the patient takes an inordinate time to eat meals, will only eat on his or her own, or has extremely small portion sizes) or difficulties between the patient and the informant may become evident. With adults, it is not

---

TABLE 4.1. Topics Addressed in the Initial Evaluation Interview

---

 1. What the patient would like to be different
 2. Current problems with eating (as perceived by the patient or by others), including
    — Eating habits
    — Methods of shape and weight control
    — Views on shape and weight
 3. Impairment resulting from the eating problem
    — Psychosocial impairment
    — Physical impairment
 4. Development and evolution of the eating problem (including the patient's weight history and prior experience of treatment)
 5. Co-existing psychiatric and general medical problems (including any current treatment)
 6. Brief personal history
 7. Family psychiatric and general medical history
 8. Personal psychiatric and general medical history
 9. Current circumstances and plans
10. Attitude to attendance and treatment (and any ongoing treatment)

---

appropriate to insist upon the attendance of informants, as many patients will have kept their eating problem hidden from others and would not attend if disclosure were required from the outset. The situation is quite different with younger patients when an interview with the parents is integral to the assessment. Just as with the patients themselves, first impressions are relevant to one's encounter with informants. To obtain good information a positive atmosphere needs to be engendered, and it must not be forgotten that the informants might well have an influence over the patient's attitude to treatment and might play a role in it (see Chapters 6, 14 and 15).

Toward the end of the initial interview we weigh patients and measure their height. Weighing is an extremely sensitive matter for most patients and some are resistant to it. It is nevertheless essential if the assessment is to be complete. It is not appropriate to rely upon patients' self-reported weight, as this is sometimes inaccurate. We explain this to patients and say that we *have* to check their weight in order to complete the assessment and give them good advice. In our experience patients do not refuse. At this point we do not insist upon patients knowing their weight if they do not wish to do so.

We are not in favor of lengthy assessment appointments because they are exhausting for the patient and, in our view, unnecessary. Ninety minutes is our maximum. On the other hand we routinely see patients twice as part of the assessment process, as we often find that a second appointment, a week or two later, adds new information of value. On this second occasion patients are more relaxed, they may disclose information previously withheld, and we have an opportunity to pursue matters that require particularly careful exploration (e.g., the nature and extent of co-existing depressive features; see Chapter 16, page 246). The second appointment is also a good time to discuss the various treatment options in detail.

We routinely ask patients to complete certain questionnaires prior to the initial appointment. This is useful since it gives us standardized information on the nature and severity of the patient's eating problem. The two questionnaires we favor are the Eating Disorder Examination Questionnaire (EDE-Q 6.0; Fairburn & Beglin, 1994, 2008; see Appendix B) and the Clinical Impairment Assessment (CIA 3.0; Bohn & Fairburn, 2008; see Appendix C). The EDE-Q provides a measure of current eating disorder features and the CIA assesses the impact of this psychopathology on psychosocial functioning. Both questionnaires are short and easy to fill in, and both focus on the previous 28 days. In addition, we include one of the well-established measures of general psychiatric features.

For a thorough assessment of current eating disorder features most experts recommend the Eating Disorder Examination interview (EDE; Cooper & Fairburn, 1987), the latest version of which is in Appendix A. This is a semi-structured clinical interview, but it is too detailed and time-consuming to use on a routine clinical basis. Nevertheless readers may find the EDE schedule of interest since it provides widely accepted definitions of many eating disorder concepts (e.g., binge eating [or in EDE terms "objective bulimic episodes"]; driven exercising; over-evaluation of shape and weight). All these measures are available for use without charge.

Outcome of the Evaluation

By the end of the second appointment it should be possible to decide on the best treatment options. Generally these are as follows:

1. *"Do nothing."* This is appropriate with minor eating problems that are likely to be self-limiting.

2. *Observe.* This is appropriate if the nature or severity of the problem is not clear; for example, if it seems to be remitting. In our experience, this is sometimes the case in binge eating disorder.

3. *Recommend outpatient-based CBT-E.* This is appropriate for the vast majority of cases. We recommend CBT-E for virtually all patients with an eating disorder who have a BMI between 15.0 and 40.0. When doing so we take pains to inform patients about their prognosis, both with and without treatment. It is important that patients know that if they have an established eating disorder (other than binge eating disorder), the chances are low that it will resolve in the absence of treatment.

If CBT-E is to be recommended, it is important that it is accurately portrayed. Table 4.2 lists the main points that we make when describing the treatment to patients. Once it has been described (possibly with the aid of an information sheet) and patients have had an opportunity to ask questions and air concerns, it is our practice to suggest that they think over what has been proposed and let us know within a week what they have decided. In our experience the great majority say that they would like to proceed with CBT-E. Obstacles to starting CBT-E are discussed below.

4. *Recommend more intensive treatment for the eating disorder.* We recommend more intensive treatment for most patients whose body mass index is below 15.0 and for those whose physical state is not stable. Such treatment can be CBT-E-based (see Chapter 15) or it may be followed by CBT-E.

5. *Recommend referral elsewhere.* We refer elsewhere when the problem is not an eating disorder (e.g., an anxiety disorder or severe obesity [body mass index $\geq$ 40.0]).

If the patient reports having had CBT in the past, it merits thought whether it is appropriate to offer them the same treatment a second time. On the other hand, it is possible that the patient's current circumstances may now be more conducive to a good outcome; for example, the patient may be more motivated than before. It is also important to note that while the patient may appear to have had CBT in the past, it often turns out that it was quite different. Treatments referred to as "CBT" can differ remarkably from each other, either because they were different forms of CBT or because they were implemented idiosyncratically. It is always worth finding out exactly what the prior treatment involved.

Contraindications to Starting CBT-E Immediately

There are certain contraindications to embarking upon CBT-E straightaway. As mentioned earlier, it must be safe for the patient to be managed on an outpatient basis, both medically and from the psychiatric point of view. Other contraindications are listed below. They have in common the effect of substantially undermining the patient's concentration, motivation (which is a problem in many patients in any case) or their ability to work on treatment between sessions.

- *Compromised physical health.* Patients should be assessed by a physician if their physical state is of concern. This should happen before starting CBT-E. Features that are of particular note are listed later in the chapter (page 41).

TABLE 4.2. Main Points Made When Describing CBT-E to the Patient

Cognitive behavior therapy, or CBT, is the leading evidence-based treatment for adults with an eating disorder.

Our data indicate that about two-thirds of people who complete treatment make an excellent response.[a] There is no reason why you should not be in this group so long as you throw yourself into treatment and give it priority.

The treatment is a one-to-one talking-type of treatment that primarily focuses on what is keeping the eating problem going. It is therefore mainly concerned with the present and future. It addresses the origins of the problem as needed.

The treatment will be tailored to your specific eating problem and your needs. You and your therapist will need to become experts on your eating problem and what is keeping it going.

[*For patients with a body mass index over 17.5*] Treatment will involve 20 sessions over 20 weeks plus one initial assessment session, the first eight sessions being twice a week, the next 10 being weekly, and the last three being at 2-week intervals.

[*For patients with a body mass index between 15.0 and 17.5*] Treatment will involve about 40 sessions over approximately 40 weeks, the first 20 or so sessions being twice a week. Thereafter they will spread out.

It is important that there are as few breaks in treatment as possible because we want to establish what we call "momentum" in which we work from session to session to break into your eating problem. Breaks in treatment are very disruptive as momentum is lost. It is especially important that there are no breaks in the first 6 weeks and no longer than 2-week breaks thereafter. We need to take this into account when thinking when it would be best for your treatment to start.

Each appointment will last just under 1 hour, with the exception of the initial assessment session, which will take about an hour and a half.

For everyone's sake it is important that appointments start and end on time. Your therapist will make sure he or she is ready at the due time, and we request that you do the same. It is a very good idea to arrive a little time in advance — say 10–15 minutes beforehand. This will give you an opportunity to settle down and think over things.

If you are unable to attend a specific appointment, please let us know as soon as possible so that we can reschedule the appointment and offer someone else your slot.

You and your therapist will be working together as a team to help you overcome your eating problem.

You and your therapist will agree upon specific tasks (or "next steps") for you to undertake between each session. These tasks are very important and will need to be given priority. It is what you do between sessions that will govern, to a large extent, how much you benefit from treatment.

Since you have had the eating problem for quite a while, it is really important that you make the most of this opportunity to change, otherwise the problem is likely to persist.

Treatment will be hard work but it will be worth it. The more you put in, the more you will get out.

---

[a]This statement applies only to patients with a BMI over 17.5. Outcome is less good in patients with a lower BMI.

- *Suicide risk.* This risk is largely, but not exclusively, confined to patients who have a co-existing clinical depression, although heightened suicide risk is also present in patients who feel hopeless about the prospect of re-covery. All eating disorder therapists should be competent at assessing suicide risk.

> **All eating disorder therapists should be competent at assessing suicide risk.**

- *Severe clinical depression.* This is commonly missed or viewed as secondary to the eating disorder and not directly treated. Both are regrettable. The presence of a clinical depression interferes with psychological treatment in a number of ways. Depressive thinking results in patients being hopeless about the possibility of change, which undermines their ability to engage in treatment. The reduction in drive also has this effect. Concentration

> **Clinical depressions are commonly missed.**

impairment is a problem since it results in information not being retained. The identification and management of clinical depressions in patients with eating disorders are discussed in Chapter 16. Once the depression has been treated, CBT-E may be initiated.

- *Persistent substance misuse.* Intoxication in treatment sessions renders the sessions virtually worthless, and persistent intoxication outside sessions undermines the patient's ability to utilize treatment. The management of co-existing substance misuse is discussed in outline in Chapter 16. Once the substance misuse has been addressed, CBT-E may be initiated.

- *Major life events or crises.* These are distracting and so interfere with treatment. It may be that treatment should be delayed until the crisis has passed. The management of life events that occur before or during treatment is discussed in Chapter 16.

- *Inability to attend treatment.* As noted earlier, a central feature of CBT-E is establishing and maintaining therapeutic momentum (see Chapters 5 and 6). This requires that appointments be frequent (especially in the early stages) and regular. In our view it is essential that patients attend in this way, especially during the first 6 weeks. We ask patients to guarantee that they there will be no breaks in their attendance during these 6 weeks and no breaks of longer than 2 consecutive weeks throughout the rest of treatment. If this is impossible, for example, because of a pre-booked vacation, then we prefer to defer treatment. Patients generally understand and respect the rationale behind this firm stance. They can see that we are taking their treatment seriously and do not want to risk a "false start."

Some patients realize that their day-to-day commitments are such that they are likely to interfere with treatment. In such cases we explore with them the possibility that they might take 6 months or a year off from their current work so that they can fully devote themselves to overcoming their eating problem. Doing this is a major decision but one that few patients come to regret.

- *Absence of the therapist.* The need to establish and maintain therapeutic momentum places an obligation on the therapist as well as the patient. If the therapist is going to be away during the first 6 weeks of treatment, it is best to delay its start. Therapist absences later on in treatment are inevitable at times. Ways of minimizing their impact were discussed in Chapter 3 (see page 32).

Medical Management

The panoply of physical abnormalities seen in patients with eating disorders can cloud thinking about diagnosis and management. The situation is further complicated by the fact that much of the literature on eating disorders has been written by clinicians who work in highly specialized referral centers. As a result many of their recommendations are influenced by the challenges posed by severely ill patients whose health is markedly impaired. The problem is that one should not generalize from these patients to patients with an eating disorder as a whole. It must not be forgotten that most people with an eating disorder are not underweight and most are not seriously physically compromised.

The following account of the medical management of patients with eating disorders has been written with the non-medical therapist in mind, and it focuses on the types of patient typically seen in outpatient settings. It is presented in the form of bullet points for the sake of clarity. First, some general points need to be stressed:

- Patients' health and safety are of paramount importance and must never be neglected.
- Unlike most psychiatric disorders, eating disorders are associated with physical complications. Anyone with clinical responsibility for patients with eating disorders must be aware of these complications.
- Non-medical therapists need to have access to a physician who can advise them on the management of the medical problems of their patients.
- Therapists should ensure that each patient has a specific physician who will take responsibility for his or her medical management. The therapist should have the full contact details of each patient's physician.
- The physical abnormalities seen in patients with eating disorders are secondary to their disturbed eating habits (e.g., undereating, self-induced vomiting, misuse of laxatives or diuretics) and any abnormalities in body weight (either too low or too high).
- The great majority of these physical abnormalities are reversed by the restoration of healthy eating habits and an appropriate BMI. Exceptions are the dental damage that results from self-induced vomiting and possibly the osteoporosis seen in patients who have been significantly underweight.

> **Patients' health and safety are of paramount importance and must never be neglected.**

Physical Investigations and Diagnosis

- No physical investigations are required to make a diagnosis of an eating disorder. The diagnosis is made on positive grounds by detecting the characteristic behavioral and attitudinal features (see Chapter 2).

> **No physical investigations are required to make a diagnosis of an eating disorder.**

Features of Medical Concern

- If any of the features listed below are present at assessment, the therapist should ensure that patients see their physician for physical evaluation even though it is unlikely that medical treatment will be required. The same applies if these features develop or worsen during treatment.

Eating disorder features (if these features are present in combination, the level of concern is heightened):

- Marked undereating (e.g., not eating at all in the day) or under-drinking
- Frequent self-induced vomiting (two or more episodes a day)
- Frequent laxative or diuretic misuse (two or more episodes a day of modest doses, or less frequent consumption of higher doses)
- Heavy exercising when underweight
- Rapid weight loss ($\geq$ 1 kg per week for several weeks in succession)
- Low weight (BMI of 17.5 or below)

Physical symptoms or signs (if these features are present in combination, the level of concern is heightened):

- Episodes of feeling faint or collapsing
- Episodes of disorientation, confusion or memory loss
- Awareness of the heart beating unusually or chest pains
- Unusual muscle twitches or spasms
- Shortness of breath
- Swelling of the ankles, arms or face
- Weakness and exhaustion
- Difficulty climbing stairs or getting up from a chair without using the arms
- Blood-stained vomit

Physical Investigations That May Be Recommended

Note: Non-medical therapists should never interpret the results of physical investigations unless they have received the necessary training.

- *Blood tests.* A wide range of blood tests may be performed. What tests are recommended as a matter of routine varies from country to country. One is of particular note: the levels of electrolytes in the blood (especially potassium). These may be abnormal if the patient is vomiting or misusing laxatives or diuretics to a significant degree. Markedly disturbed electrolyte levels increase the risk of serious cardiac arrhythmias.
- *EKG (electrocardiogram).* Performed if there are concerns about the patient's heart function
- *Bone density scan.* Performed if there are concerns about the status of the patient's bones (generally patients with a history of having been significantly underweight)

Pharmacological Treatments That May Be Recommended

- *Potassium.* It may be recommended that patients take oral potassium supplements if their serum potassium level is very low (due to frequent purging). In general, however, the emphasis should be on helping patients to stop purging. If patients are taking potassium supplements, they will need intermittent blood tests to monitor their potassium level.

- *Vitamins.* A daily multivitamin preparation may be recommended for patients who have been undereating for a long time or are underweight.
- *Calcium.* Calcium supplements may be recommended for patients who have osteoporosis or osteopenia.

A Note on Waiting Lists

In some countries it is not uncommon for patients to have to wait a considerable time before starting treatment. It is nevertheless commonplace for patients to be offered an assessment appointment relatively quickly, have their eating problem thoroughly evaluated, be recommended treatment, and then be told that it will be many months (often 6–12) before treatment can start. This process can have adverse effects. Patients steel themselves for the assessment appointment, become engaged in the assessment process, and then are demoralized by the long wait, during which they may be offered nothing. This demoralization may make subsequent engagement in treatment even harder. It (almost) goes without saying that clinical services should do their utmost to minimize the waiting times of patients since doing so would not only decrease the duration of the patient's eating disorder but it might also improve treatment outcome.

If there has to be a significant gap between the initial assessment and starting CBT-E, we recommend that the patient be reassessed. This is because eating disorders evolve (see Chapter 2) as do life circumstances and psychiatric comorbidity. It needs to be determined whether any new obstacles to treatment have emerged (e.g., we have encountered the development of new episodes of clinical depression) and a fresh decision needs to be made as to precisely when would be the best time to start treatment.

Can anything useful be done while patients are waiting for treatment? This may be so in the case of binge eating disorder and possibly also bulimia nervosa. There is increasing, but inconsistent, evidence that "guided" self-help, using a cognitive behavioral self-help program, may help some of these patients overcome their eating disorder, and it certainly appears to do no harm. (Guided self-help generally involves following a self-help program, with support and encouragement from a non-specialist "facilitator.") The research is strongest with regard to binge eating disorder, for which emerging evidence suggests that guided self-help is reasonably effective. The findings are less clear with regard to bulimia nervosa. Overall, it would seem reasonable to provide this low-intensity treatment while such patients are waiting for treatment.

Similarly, there is good evidence that antidepressant medication has an "antibulimic" effect (i.e., it reduces the frequency of binge eating) in some patients with bulimia nervosa and binge eating disorder, whether or not they have a co-existing clinical depression. The effect is rapidly expressed (within 2 weeks), although it is often not sustained, but this is another intervention that can be tried while the patient is waiting for CBT-E. In our experience antidepressant medication rarely produces a complete resolution of the eating disorder: Rather, there is a suppression of binge eating with certain secondary benefits as a result. The over-evaluation of shape and weight tends to persist largely unchanged, as does the patient's weight-control behavior. Therefore CBT-E remains indicated.

Recommended Reading

Medical Management

Crow, S., & Swigart, S. (2005). Medical assessment. In J. E. Mitchell & C. B. Peterson (Eds.), *Assessment of eating disorders* (pp. 120–128). New York: Guilford Press.

Miller, K. K., Grinspoon, S. K., Ciampa, J., Hier, J., Herzog, D., & Klibanski, A. (2005). Medical findings in outpatients with anorexia nervosa. *Archives of Internal Medicine, 165,* 561–566.

Mitchell, J. E., & Crow, S. (2006). Medical complications of anorexia nervosa and bulimia nervosa. *Current Opinion in Psychiatry, 19,* 438–443.

Mitchell, J. E., Pomeroy, C., & Adson, D. E. (1997). Managing medical complications. In D. M. Garner & P. E. Garfinkel (Eds.), *Handbook of treatment for eating disorders* (2nd ed., pp. 383–393). New York: Guilford Press.

Self-Help for Bulimia Nervosa and Binge Eating Disorder

Grilo, C. M. (2007). Guided self-help for binge eating disorder. In J. D. Latner & G. T. Wilson (Eds.), *Self-help approaches for obesity and eating disorders* (pp. 73–91). New York: Guilford Press.

Sysko, R., & Walsh, B. T. (2007). Guided self-help for bulimia nervosa. In J. D. Latner & G. T. Wilson (Eds.), *Self-help approaches for obesity and eating disorders* (pp. 92–117). New York: Guilford Press.

Other Articles of Relevance to Chapter 4

Bohn, K., & Fairburn, C. G. (2008). Clinical Impairment Assessment Questionnaire (CIA 3.0). In C. G. Fairburn, *Cognitive behavior therapy and eating disorders* (pp. 315–317). New York: Guilford Press.

Cooper, Z., & Fairburn, C. (1987). The Eating Disorder Examination: A semistructured interview for the assessment of the specific psychopathology of eating disorders. *International Journal of Eating Disorders, 6,* 1–8.

Fairburn, C. G., & Beglin, S. J. (1994). The assessment of eating disorders: Interview or self-report questionnaire. *International Journal of Eating Disorders, 16,* 363–370.

Fairburn, C. G., & Beglin, S. J. (2008). Eating Disorder Examination Questionnaire (EDE-Q 6.0). In C. G. Fairburn, *Cognitive behavior therapy and eating disorders* (pp. 309–313). New York: Guilford Press.

Franko, D. L., & Keel, P. K. (2006). Suicidality in eating disorders: Occurrence, correlates, and clinical implications. *Clinical Psychology Review, 26,* 769–782.

Godart, N. T., Perdereau, F., Rein, Z., Berthoz, S., Wallier, J., Jeammet, P., et al. (2007). Comorbidity studies of eating disorders and mood disorders: Critical review of the literature. *Journal of Affective Disorders, 97,* 37–49.

Milos, G., Spindler, A., Hepp, U., & Schnyder, U. (2004). Suicide attempts and suicidal ideation: Links with psychiatric comorbidity in eating disorder subjects. *General Hospital Psychiatry, 26,* 129–135.

Peterson, C. (2005). Conducting the diagnostic interview. In J. E. Mitchell & C. B. Peterson (Eds.), *Assessment of eating disorders* (pp. 32–58). New York: Guilford Press.

ENHANCED COGNITIVE BEHAVIOR THERAPY FOR EATING DISORDERS: THE CORE PROTOCOL

Christopher G. Fairburn, Zafra Cooper, Roz Shafran,
Kristin Bohn, Deborah M. Hawker, Rebecca Murphy
and Suzanne Straebler

CHAPTER 5

Starting Well

It is crucial that treatment starts well.

When faced with a patient with an eating disorder, novice therapists can feel over-whelmed. There is generally a myriad of clinical features, marked psychosocial impairment (and perhaps physical impairment too), a long history, ambivalence and perhaps an account of prior failed attempts at treatment. Where does one start?

Where to Start

There is no doubt that engaging the patient is the top priority. Treatment stands little or no chance of succeeding

Engaging the patient is the top priority.

unless the patient is engaged. Therapists therefore need to become skilled at enticing patients into both treatment and the process of change. CBT-E is designed to do this, and doing so is of particular importance with patients who are underweight, as they tend to be especially ambivalent about change (see Chapter 11).

Assuming the patient is engaged, there is then the question of what to do next. Which of the multitude of clinical features should be addressed first? Fortunately, one does not need to tackle everything (for otherwise treatment would take years!). An analogy is useful here. The psychopathology of eating

The psychopathology of eating disorders may be likened to a house of cards.

disorders may be likened to a house of cards. If one wants to bring down the house, the key structural cards need to be identified and removed, and then the house will fall down. So it is with eating disorder psychopathology. The therapist does not need to address every clinical feature. Many are at the second or third tier of the "house" and so will resolve of their own accord if the key clinical features are addressed. Examples include the preoccupation with thoughts about food, eating, shape and weight; compensatory vomiting and laxative misuse; calorie-counting; and, in many cases, over-exercising. What therapists have to do is identify the clinical features that are maintaining (or "supporting") the patient's eating disorder and focus their efforts on removing them. This is now possible because over the past

30 years much has been learned about eating disorder psychopathology (see Chapter 2) and the modification of the processes that maintain it.

Practically speaking, it is crucial that treatment starts well. As mentioned in the previous chapters, across a range of disorders the amount of change that occurs in the first few weeks of treatment is a strong predictor of eventual outcome, and this is also true of bulimia nervosa and binge eating disorder. It is therefore important that the early weeks go especially well. The patient needs to be ready to start, as does the therapist. And, as described in the previous chapter, obvious impediments to treatment need to be addressed in advance if at all possible. "False starts" must be avoided, as it is difficult to make up lost ground.

This chapter is devoted to the first two sessions of CBT-E, the foundation upon which the rest of treatment is built.

The Initial Session (Session 0)

Depending upon the context within which one works, the person who conducts the initial interview or interviews with the patient (see Chapter 4) may or may not be the eventual therapist. In our context the therapist is often not the person who saw the patient first and so he or she will be meeting the patient for the first time at this initial session. This means that a second assessment needs to take place so that the therapist hears directly from the patient the nature of his or her problems. Inevitably this assessment overlaps to an extent with the one performed earlier. In our view the benefits of this second assessment in terms of engagement far outweigh the possible disadvantage of asking patients to repeat details of their history and present circumstances.

The initial session is atypical in a number of respects. It is longer than all the other sessions, often lasting in the region of an hour and a half, and its content is relatively fixed. The session has seven main components:

1. Engaging the patient in treatment and the prospect of change
2. Assessing the nature and severity of the psychopathology present
3. Jointly creating a formulation of the processes maintaining the eating problem
4. Explaining what treatment will involve
5. Establishing real-time self-monitoring
6. Confirming the homework assignments
7. Summarizing the session and arranging the next appointment

Engaging the Patient in Treatment and Change

A particular challenge when working with these patients is engaging them in treatment. There may be aspects of their disorder that they would like to change (e.g., binge eating), but generally there are other elements that they value and may even identify with (e.g., maintaining strict control over eating; losing weight). Many come to treatment with misgivings and varying degrees of reluctance. It is essential that the therapist understands and is sensitive to the patient's likely ambivalence.

The initial treatment session is especially important in this regard. The patient will be evaluating the therapist just as much as the therapist will be evaluating the patient. The therapist's manner and his or

> The patient will be evaluating the therapist just as much as the therapist will be evaluating the patient.

her apparent attitudes and choice of words will all be scrutinized. They therefore merit attention.

Much has been written about how to engage these patients in treatment. Although some have suggested that preparatory psychotherapeutic work is necessary, we do not agree. We prepare patients for treatment in the way described in Chapter 4, but do not view anything else as required. Competently administered CBT-E is inherently motivating and, most motivating of all, is experiencing the benefits of understanding one's prob-

> One success breeds further successes.

lem and beginning to change — something CBT-E strives to achieve from the outset. Also it must not be forgotten that one success breeds further successes. Minimizing the delay between the initial evaluation and the start of treatment (i.e., the waiting time) is also important.

Therapists can enhance engagement early on by following these guidelines:

- Be empathic and engaging in manner.
- Ask the patient what name he or she would like you to use, and state your name. It should not be assumed that all patients want the therapist to use their first name.
- Be professional but not intimidating. Convey understanding of eating problems and expertise in their assessment and treatment.
- Actively involve the patient in the assessment process and in the creation of the personalized formulation.
- Instill hope.
- Avoid being controlling or paternalistic.
- Repeatedly invite questions and check back that the patient is "on board."
- Enquire about any concerns that the patient might have.

Certain specific strategies and procedures may also be used. Because they are most often needed with underweight patients, they are described in Chapter 11 although they should be used with other patients if establishing or maintaining engagement is proving to be a problem.

Assessing the Nature and Severity of the Psychopathology Present

This second assessment is treatment-focused rather than diagnostic, so it differs somewhat from the one conducted initially when the patient first presented for help (see Chapter 4, page 35). A broad range of topics, listed in Table 5.1, needs to be covered. It may not be possible to cover them all, in which case some may be postponed until the next session. The primary focus should be on the patient's present state and what is maintaining it so that a personalized formulation may be created (see below). In the main an information-gathering style of interviewing should be adopted, with the thera-

TABLE 5.1. Topics to Cover When Assessing the Eating Problem

Current state of the eating problem (over the past 4 weeks and 3 months)
- Patient's account of the problem and what he or she would like to change
- Eating habits on a typical day (and, if applicable, a "good" and "bad" day)
- Dietary restraint (nature of attempts to restrict food intake): dietary rules; reaction to any breaking of these rules; calorie-counting; calorie limits; delayed eating (i.e., postponing eating for as long as possible)
- Dietary restriction (actual undereating)
- Other weight-control behavior (e.g., self-induced vomiting, laxative or diuretic misuse, over-exercising): frequency; relationship to perceived overeating
- Episodes of overeating (amount eaten and the context; whether or not there was a sense of loss of control at the time): frequency; triggers
- Other eating habits (picking, chewing and spitting, rumination, ritualistic eating)
- Drinking and smoking habits (consumption of water, coffee, tea, carbonated drinks and alcoholic beverages, and smoking habits — and their connection [if any] to the eating problem)
- Social eating: ability to eat with others; eating out
- Concerns about shape and weight
- Views on shape and weight
- Importance of shape and weight in self-evaluation
- Body checking (weighing, mirror use, other forms of checking); body avoidance
- Comparisons with others
- Feeling fat
- Impact of the eating problem on psychological and social functioning
- Effects on mood and concentration
- Effects on work
- Effects on other people (partner, family, friends, acquaintances)
- Effects on activities and interests
- Other effects

Development of the eating problem
- Details of onset and likely triggers
- Subsequent sequence of events (when the key forms of behavior started in relation to each other): evolution of the problem — first 6 months
- Weight history (before and since the eating problem started; true childhood obesity): lowest weight since present height; highest weight since present height
- Prior treatment (for an eating or weight problem): treatment-seeking; treatments offered; treatment experience and attitude to treatment; compliance with treatments and response to them

Personal and family history
- Where born and brought up
- Family during childhood (parents, siblings, atmosphere, disruptions and/or problems) and contact at present
- School, college and occupational history
- Interpersonal history — childhood/adolescent/adult interpersonal functioning
- Family psychiatric history (especially depression and alcohol abuse)
- Family eating disorder and obesity history
- Adverse events (including physical and sexual abuse, bereavements, accidents, bullying and teasing)
- Personal psychiatric history (especially anxiety disorders, depression, perfectionism, low self-esteem, self-harm, substance misuse): onset in relation to the onset of the eating problem; interactions

Current circumstances and functioning
- Living arrangements
- Occupation

TABLE 5.1 (*cont.*)

- Marital status, children
- Contact with family
- Interpersonal functioning (partner, family, confidantes, friends, gregariousness)
- Past interpersonal functioning (and since eating problem developed)
- Interests and aptitudes
- Past interests and aptitudes (and since the eating disorder developed)

Co-existing psychopathology

- Current psychiatric comorbidity (depression, anxiety disorders, substance misuse, self-harm, suicidal behavior, other)
- Current psychiatric treatment (psychological, pharmacological)

Physical health

- Current physical health (including menstruation)
- General medical history (including timing of puberty in relation to the eating problem)
- Current medication (including the contraceptive pill)

Attitude toward the eating problem and its treatment

- Views on what is keeping the eating problem going
- Attitude toward starting treatment
- Concerns about treatment and the prospect of change
- Goals

Anything else?

"Is there anything else that you would like to tell me, or anything else you think I should know?"

pist taking into account the patient's likely sensitivity about certain subjects (e.g., binge eating, self-induced vomiting).

Jointly Creating the Formulation

The next step is the creation of the "formulation"; that is, a personalized visual representation (a diagram) of the processes that appear to be maintaining the patient's eating problem. This is done in the initial session unless the patient is significantly underweight (see Chapter 11) or the eating disorder is unusual in form and difficult to understand. In such cases it is best to delay completing the formulation until the next session so that the therapist has ample time to think over its likely format.

The creation of the formulation has a number of purposes:

- It can help engage the patient in treatment.
- The process of creating the formulation distances the patient from his or her problems. Rather than simply having the eating problem, the patient is now being encouraged to step back and try to understand it and why it persists. The adoption of this "de-centered" stance is central to helping patients change,

> One wants to help patients be interested in, and intrigued by, their eating problem.

but at this stage one simply wants to help patients begin to be interested in, and intrigued by, their eating problem.

• The formulation conveys the notion that eating problems are understandable and are maintained by a variety of interacting self-perpetuating mechanisms. When discussing this, the therapist can point out (if applicable) that it is not surprising that the patient has found it difficult to change.

• By highlighting the main mechanisms that are maintaining the patient's eating problem, the formulation provides a guide as to what needs to be targeted in treatment (i.e., it identifies the "cards" that need to be removed). It is important to stress that the formulation is not an account of the reasons that the problem developed in the first place. If patients are puzzled by the fact that treatment does not appear to be addressing the origins of their eating problem, it should be explained that this is not generally necessary. The things that caused the problem to develop originally many years ago may be of no relevance now, but if they are, they will be addressed.[1] It is important to add that later in treatment the origins of the problem will be discussed (see page 117).

A composite transdiagnostic CBT-E formulation is shown in Figure 5.1. This should be used by therapists as a template from which personalized formulations can be derived that match each patient's eating problem. The more familiar the therapist becomes with the template formulation, the easier it is to create an individualized one to suit the patient concerned. We have not encountered any patients whose eating problems cannot be formulated in this way. Figure 5.2 shows the formulation of a patient with eating disorder NOS in which the patient's own terms have been used.

The creation of the formulation — best referred to as the *diagram* or *picture* — is a skill that is worth practicing because it is important that it is done well. The formulation should be created step-by-step in an unhurried manner, with the therapist taking the lead but with the patient being actively involved. It is best to start with something that the patient wants to change; for example, binge eating or feeling cold and sleeping poorly (both secondary effects of being underweight; see Chapter 11). Technical terms should be avoided and, whenever possible and appropriate, the patient's own words should be used. The formulation should focus only on the main mechanisms that appear to be maintaining the eating problem, as otherwise there is a risk that it will be over-detailed and confusing. As the formulation is based on information only just obtained, it should be made clear that it is provisional and will be modified as needed during treatment.

It is important that patients accept the formulation as a credible explanation of why their eating problem is self-perpetuating and resistant to change. Most will resonate with it. In those rare instances where patients remain unconvinced or hold a conflicting explanation (e.g., a psychodynamic or addiction-based one), the therapist should encourage them to reflect on the utility and validity of their current perspective (without making them defensive) while contrasting it with the present well-supported cognitive behavioral one. It is also important to explain that successfully addressing the processes that are maintaining the eating problem has many beneficial secondary effects: for

---

[1]On average, our patients have had their eating disorder for about 8 years and are in their mid-to-late 20s. It is therefore not surprising that the factors and processes that resulted in their eating problem developing are not necessarily still relevant. This does not apply to adolescent patients who have far shorter histories (see Chapter 14).

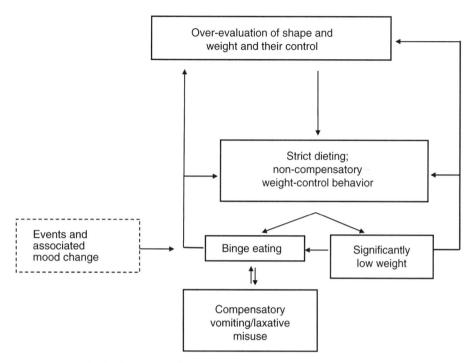

FIGURE 5.1. The composite transdiagnostic formulation.

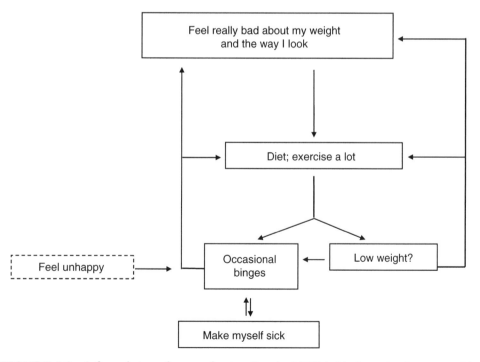

FIGURE 5.2. A formulation of a case of eating disorder NOS (with the patient's own words).

example, it generally enhances self-esteem and self-confidence and improves interpersonal functioning.

Once the formulation has been created, the therapist should discuss its implications. The main point to be made is that to overcome the eating problem, patients will need to address not only the things that they would like to change (e.g., loss of control over eating) but also the mechanisms that are responsible for maintaining them (the "vicious circles"). Thus, for example, with patients who binge eat, treatment commonly needs to focus on more than simply stopping the binge eating. It also needs to address their dieting, their ability to deal with adverse events and moods without binge eating, and their concerns about shape and weight. Not addressing these maintaining processes markedly increases the likelihood of relapse. The therapist might say something along these lines: *"The diagram shows the main things that are keeping your eating problem going. If we change these things — all of them — then you should get better. But we need to tackle all of them since otherwise you will be at risk of relapse."* The therapist should then relate the treatment plan to the formulation, perhaps by saying: *"I suggest we start by focusing largely on your eating habits, and then move on to addressing the other things shown on the diagram — for example, the way you feel about your shape and weight."*

At the end of the initial treatment session, patients should be given a copy of their formulation and asked to review it before the next appointment and modify it as seems necessary.

Explaining What Treatment Will Involve

It is important to explain to the patient what treatment will involve. Various topics need to be covered:

1. *Nature and style of the treatment.* Clearly patients need to be told the name, nature and style of the treatment. Generally much of the information provided in the context of the initial evalua-

> **The end of the treatment is as important as the beginning.**

tion bears repeating (see Table 4.2, page 39). It should be stressed that the end of the treatment is as important as the beginning, for it is at this stage that measures are put in place for minimizing the risk of relapse in the future (see Chapter 12). It is therefore most important that treatment is completed.

2. *Practicalities.* Patients should also be told the number, duration and frequency of the treatment sessions. It may be useful to arrive at an agreement about the time of day that sessions take place. We do our best to accommodate patients' commitments, the difficulties they face traveling and, in some cases, their desire for others not to know that they are in treatment. We give them the clinic phone number in case they need to contact us, and we take their phone number (cell phone is ideal) and e-mail address in case we need to contact them.

3. *Treatment sessions.* It is helpful for patients to know in outline how the sessions will be run. The therapist might say: *"We will start each session by reviewing how things have been going over the past week, and then we will set an agenda for the session to which both you and I will contribute."*

4. *In-session weighing.* We generally forewarn patients about the in-session weighing that will become an essential ingredient of treatment from the next session onward.

We are often asked whether patients ever refuse to be weighed. The answer is that the occasional patient is very reluctant, but in the context of an "engaging" initial session and the rationale being well-explained (see page 62), we find that refusal is not a problem. However, on occasions we do have to be quite insistent. Our experience is that if one accedes to patients' fears of in-session weighing, it is rarely, if ever, possible, to introduce the procedure later. This is unfortunate since in our view in-session weighing is one of the most valuable elements of CBT-E. This view is shared by patients, many of whom report at the end of treatment that the regular in-session weighing was extremely helpful. With patients who are extremely reluctant to be weighed, it can be helpful to say: *"Trying to get over your eating problem without knowing your weight is like having your hands tied behind your back. It is unlikely that you will be able to truly recover without facing up to your concerns about your weight and shape, and this requires that you know your weight."*

5. *Instillation of "ownership," enthusiasm and hope.* The notion that it is the patient's treatment, not the therapist's, needs to be conveyed. Throughout treatment, patients should feel clear about what is happening and why. They should be told that if they do not understand anything, they should ask. Similarly, should they disagree with anything, they should say so.

While many patients are keen to overcome their eating problem (including, in our experience, many of those who are underweight) and are eager for treatment to start, it is important to maximize enthusiasm and hope. Part of this involves conveying that one is knowledgeable about eating disorders in general and the patient's type of eating problem in particular. Not infrequently we come across patients who have been told that they will never recover. Rarely have we felt that such a statement was warranted. Unfortunately, a pronouncement such as this tends to become a self-fulfilling prophecy as it undermines any hope of recovery that the patient might have had. Research has failed to generate reliable predictors of outcome, and our clinical experience over the years has taught us that we do not have any either! We are continually surprised (usually favorably) by our patients' response to treatment.

6. *Dropping out from treatment.* It is worth raising the issue of dropping out. For example, the therapist might say: *"Some people drop out of treatment without completing it. This is always regrettable. It happens for various reasons. For example, some people stop attending because they think they are not doing well enough. Knowing yourself as you do, do you think you might be tempted to drop out?"*

Patients should be strongly encouraged to attend every session, and told that the final three appointments are perhaps the most important ones because they help prevent future setbacks. The therapist might add: *"If things are going badly and you feel like not attending a session, remember that this is the most important time to come. We can learn a lot from your difficulties. Most people who are thinking about not attending but then decide to turn up, say that they found it really helpful to talk though their problems and learned a lot from doing so."*

7. *Patients' questions and concerns.* As noted above, throughout treatment patients should be encouraged to ask questions and air their concerns. Common examples at this stage are listed below:

QUESTION: *"Is my eating problem bad enough to merit treatment?"*

— The therapist should respond by saying something along these lines:

"You have an eating problem that is interfering with your life and it has been going on for some time now. You have had a very thorough assessment, and Dr. _____, who has seen many people with eating disorders, thinks you would benefit from treatment. Remember, we are experts and we think that your problem merits treatment."

QUESTION: *"What happens if I am not better by the end of treatment?"*

— The therapist should respond by explaining that most patients are very much better by the end of treatment and do not feel in need of further treatment. It is also important to mention that it is common for patients to continue improving after treatment ends. Nevertheless, we state that if we thought that the patient did need further treatment, we would arrange this. Finally, it may be added that worrying unduly about the outcome of treatment can get in the way of getting *on* with treatment, and that it is best to focus on what needs to be done to overcome the problem.

QUESTION: *"Do you think I will get better?"*

— The therapist should respond by explaining that most patients are very much better by the end of treatment, and there is no reason why this should not happen in the patient's case. For example, the therapist might say: *"Based on what I know about you and your eating problem, I cannot see why you should not benefit from treatment. The best thing for you to do is to throw yourself into treatment and give it priority for 'The more you put in, the more you will get out.' "*

QUESTION: *"Will I gain weight?"*

— With patients who are unambiguously underweight (see Chapter 11), weight regain will be an explicit goal of treatment and so this question will not apply. With other patients the therapist should explain that since their eating habits will be changing during treatment, there may also be some changes in weight but, on average, there is little weight change. The therapist should go on to stress that the goal of treatment is that the patient overcomes the eating problem and as a result has control over his or her eating, and therefore, weight (at least as much as anyone has).

QUESTION: *"Who will I be if I don't have the eating problem? It's so much a part of me. I won't have an excuse for anything anymore."*

— Such concerns are not uncommon among those with longstanding eating problems. The main point to stress when responding is that the eating problem interferes with all aspects of functioning and that without the eating problem, the patient may be much more capable and effective than he or she assumes. It is usual for there to be major improvements in mood, interpersonal functioning and self-esteem. The patient may not need an "excuse" for things anymore. As for patients not knowing "who they will be" if they no longer have an eating problem, there is some basis for this concern as their true personality may have been masked by the eating problem. Our stance when faced with this worry is to reframe it positively by saying how exciting and interesting it will be to find out what their true personality is like and that they should look forward to discovering this. This topic is discussed in much greater detail in the chapter on underweight patients (see Chapter 11, page 164).

Establishing Real-Time Self-Monitoring

Real-time self-monitoring is the ongoing "in-the-moment" recording of relevant behavior, thoughts, feelings and events. It needs to be initiated from the outset of treatment and fine-tuned in session 1. It continues throughout treatment and is central to it. It should be explained along these lines:

"Self-monitoring is central to treatment. It is as important as attending our sessions. It is your tool for becoming an expert on your eating problem and overcoming it. It has two main purposes:

> **"Self-monitoring is central to treatment. It is as important as attending."**

"1. It will help you identify precisely what is happening on a moment-to-moment and day-to-day basis. We need to know exactly what you are doing, thinking and feeling, at the very time that you are doing, thinking and feeling things. We need to know the details, and then we can work out how you can make changes and thereby break into your eating problem. So you need to start to notice and record key things of importance. Self-monitoring is designed to help you do this.

"2. Second, self-monitoring will help you change. By becoming aware of what you are doing, thinking and feeling <u>at the very time that things are happening</u>, you will learn that you have choices, and that some things that you thought were automatic and outside your control (and perhaps awareness) can be changed with attention, effort and practice. But you can only achieve this with accurate real-time monitoring. Simply recalling how things were some hours ago won't, of course, work.

"I should forewarn you that self-monitoring will have a short-term negative effect. It will make you more preoccupied with your eating, but this only lasts a week or so and is worth it."

Note that this explanation emphasizes the fact that the recording is of thoughts, feelings and behavior and that it is designed to help patients change. Sometimes self-monitoring records are called "food diaries." This term is to be avoided because it conveys entirely the wrong impression about their purpose and use.

The monitoring record that we employ is simple to complete and use (see Figure 5.3). (A blank monitoring record is available online at www.psych.ox.ac.uk/credo/ cbt_and_eating_disorders.) What is difficult is recording in real time, yet this is of particular value because it helps patients observe, question and modify their thinking and behavior as they happen. Exactly what is recorded evolves during treatment and with occasional patients further columns are added as needed (e.g., to record exercising or alcohol intake). At the beginning the emphasis is largely on the patient's eating habits. When describing how to self-monitor, it is our practice to go over an example (created for this purpose) that roughly matches in form the eating habits of the patient in question, highlighting the following:

- The various columns
- How to note down food and drink using plain English descriptions

Day .....*Thursday*.........   **Date** .....*March 19th*....................

Time	Food and drink consumed	Place	*	V/L	Context and comments
7.30	Glass water	Kitchen			Thirsty after yesterday
8:10	Half banana ⎫ Black coffee ⎬	Cafe			Must be good and not binge today!
11:45	Smoked turkey on wheat bread ⎫ Light mayo Diet coke ⎬	Cafe			Usual lunch
6.40 to 7.30	Piece of apple pie 1/2 gallon ice cream 4 slices of toast with peanut butter Diet coke Raisin bagel 2 slices of toast with peanut butter Diet coke Peanut butter from jar Raisin bagel Snickers bar Diet coke – large	Kitchen	* * * * * * * *	V V	Help – I can't stop eating. I'm completely out of control. I hate myself. I am disgusting. Why do I do this? I started as soon as I got in. I've ruined another day.
9:30	Rice cake with fat-free cheese Diet coke	Kitchen			Really lonely. Feel fat and ugly. Feel like giving up.

FIGURE 5.3. A monitoring record (patient A; session 2). V = vomiting. L = laxative misuse. See Table 5.2 for a full description of self-monitoring and the abbreviations used.

A blank monitoring record is available online at www.psych.ox.ac.uk/credo/cbt_and_eating_disorders.

- The use of asterisks, brackets, V's and L's (see Table 5.2)
- How column 6 is used. At this stage it is simply used as a diary to record events that have influenced patients' eating and their concerns about eating, shape and weight. Each time patients weigh themselves, they should record doing so in column 6 as well as their weight.
- The level of detail required. All eating and drinking should be recorded with simple descriptions of the quantities involved. Patients should not weigh their food or record its energy (calorie) content.
- The records do not need to be neat, and patients should not worry about their spelling.

In addition, we discuss the process of recording, including how to record at work, at home and when socializing. We have not encountered any situation in which real-time recording was not possible. It helps if therapists try doing this themselves for a week or so in order to experience the difficulties it poses and share with patients ways of overcoming them. We routinely discuss the possibility that because of shame and embarrassment, the patient might be tempted to omit things from his or her monitoring records (usually episodes of perceived overeating). The point to make is that for treatment to have the best chance of succeeding, it is essential that the patient and therapist are aware of the full extent of the problem rather than discussing an expurgated version of it.

Patients should be asked how they feel about the prospect of recording, and they should be encouraged to raise any concerns and questions. The most common are listed below together with suggested responses.

QUESTION: *"I have done this before. It didn't help then, why would it help now?"*

— In our experience it is most unlikely that the patient will have monitored before in exactly this way and discussed his or her records in detail with a therapist. Some type of dietary record may have been kept, but real-time recording of behavior, thoughts and feelings is largely peculiar to CBT and in particular to this type of CBT. This should be explained while reiterating the two points made earlier about the purpose of monitoring.

QUESTION: *"Monitoring will make me even more preoccupied with eating than I am already."*

— It is true that starting to monitor in this way increases preoccupation with thoughts about eating, but this is a constructive and illuminating preoccupation. It increases patients' awareness of their behavior and the thoughts and feelings that accompany it. It is the beginning of their becoming an expert on their eating problem and starting to understand it. And the preoccupation fades after a few weeks.

QUESTION: *"Do I have to carry the records around with me all the time?"*

— Briefly, the answer is "Yes." This may be difficult under some circumstances but it should be possible. The day's record can be stuffed into a pocket or wallet, for example. We have yet to encounter a situation in which recording was truly impossible.

QUESTION: *"Can't I use a notebook instead of these forms?"*

— This is not to be recommended. Our experience over many years indicates that these particular monitoring records work well. They are large enough to allow the detailed recording of behavior, thoughts and feelings and they are capable of being used flexibly. Notebooks, etc., tend to restrict the quantity and quality of the information obtained.

QUESTION: *"What do I do if I am with others . . . say, in a restaurant or at work?"*

— The therapist should ask the patient to generate possible solutions. In many public situations it is possible to go to the bathroom at intervals and write things down there. The patient should record as soon as possible after eating if it is not possible to record while eating.

QUESTION: *"Do I let others see my records?"*

— We strongly discourage patients from letting others see their records, as this might affect what they write down. Rather, the records should be viewed as private documents (like a diary) and kept out of sight.

QUESTION: *"I'll be tempted to leave things off. It will be too embarrassing, won't it?"*

— This is a common temptation (especially for patients who binge eat), and if the patient does not raise it, the therapist should. The response is that the goal of treatment is to help the patient overcome his or her (entire) eating problem and to do this the whole problem needs to be examined, not just parts of it. The therapist might add (if applicable) that he or she has seen innumerable monitoring records and so will not be surprised or taken aback by anything that the patient reports. The therapist might say:

> *"Nothing you write down will shock or surprise me. Anyway, I am not here to judge you. I am here to help you, but I can't do that unless you are totally frank and open about things. Not recording accurately would get in the way of my being able to help you. So it is vital that you record things accurately and leave nothing off."*

Finally, we give the patient about 20 blank records together with written instructions for completing them (see Table 5.2). It is generally best for the patient to start recording straightaway or from the following morning onward.

Fundamental to establishing and maintaining accurate real-time recording is going over the patient's records in detail session by session, and especially in session 1 when the patient brings them back for the first time. It is our practice to file the records chronologically in a large ring folder so that earlier records can be reviewed easily if need be. For example, with patients who have difficulty recognizing the progress they are making, it can be helpful to go over past records to highlight the changes that have occurred, and when examining intermittent events (e.g., "residual binges" — see Chapter 10) it may be of value to refer back to previous instances of them.

Confirming the Homework Assignments

"Homework" is integral to CBT-E, and the patient's implementation of it is central to change. (Perhaps somewhat preciously, we do not use the term "homework" because of its connotations. Instead, we refer to the "Next Steps" and have a Next Steps sheet for patients to note down the agreed homework tasks.) There are two pieces of homework at this stage:

1. Starting real-time recording. As stated, this is best started immediately or from the beginning of the next day.
2. Reviewing the formulation. This involves the patient spending 15 minutes or so before the next session reviewing the written formulation and considering what seems most relevant, what may need to be added, and what should perhaps be dropped.

It is good practice to ensure that patients write down on a Next Steps sheet exactly what homework they have agreed to do.

TABLE 5.2. Instructions for Self-Monitoring

Instructions for Self-Monitoring

During treatment, it is important that you record *everything* that you eat or drink, and what is going on at the time. We call this "self-monitoring." Its purpose is two-fold: First, it provides a detailed picture of how you eat, thereby bringing to your attention and that of your therapist the exact nature of your eating problem; and second, by making you more aware of what you are doing at the very time that you are doing it, self-monitoring helps you change behavior that may previously have seemed automatic and beyond your control. Accurate "real-time" monitoring is central to treatment. It will help you change.

At first, writing down everything that you eat may be irritating and inconvenient, but soon it will become second nature and of obvious value. We have yet to encounter anyone whose lifestyle made it truly impossible to monitor. Regard it as a challenge.

Look at the sample monitoring record to see how to monitor. A new record (or records) should be started each day.

- The first column is for noting the time when you eat or drink anything, and the second is for recording the nature of the food and drink consumed. Calories should not be recorded: Instead, you should write down a simple (non-technical) description of what you ate or drank. Each item should be written down as soon as possible after it was consumed. Recalling what you ate or drank some hours afterward will not work since it will not help you change your behavior at the time. Obviously, if you are to record in this way, you will need to carry your monitoring sheets with you. It does not matter if your records become messy or if the writing or spelling is not good. The important thing is that you record *everything* you eat or drink, as soon as possible afterward.

- Episodes of eating that you view as meals should be identified with brackets. Snacks and other episodes of eating should not be bracketed.

- The third column should specify where the food or drink was consumed. If this was in your home, the room should be specified.

- Asterisks should be placed in the fourth column adjacent to any episodes of eating or drinking that you felt (at the time) were excessive. This is your judgment, regardless of what anyone else might think. It is essential to record all the food that you eat during "binges."

- The fifth column is for recording when you vomit (write *"V"*) or take laxatives (write *"L"* and the number taken) or diuretics (water tablets) (write *"D"* and the number taken).

- The last column will be used in various ways during treatment. For the moment it should be used as a diary to record events and feelings that have influenced your eating: For example, if an argument precipitated a binge or led you to not eat, you should note that down. Try to write a brief comment every time you eat, recording your thoughts and feelings about what you ate. You may want to record other important events or circumstances in this column, even if they had no effect on your eating. The last column should also be used to record your weight (and your thoughts about it) each time that you weigh yourself.

Every treatment session will include a detailed review of your latest monitoring sheets. You must therefore remember to bring them with you!

Summarizing the Session and Arranging the Next Appointment

In common with all subsequent sessions, the therapist should end this initial one by summarizing its content, restating the homework and booking the next appointment. Although it is often considered good practice to ask patients to take the lead in summarizing sessions, this can be unrealistic and inappropriate, and it risks making patients anxious that they will get it "wrong" or fail to remember. In our view the summarizing is best done collaboratively, thus avoiding patients feeling that they are being put on the spot. The goal is to help the patient remember the topics covered and place them within the context of their formulation and the overall treatment plan. It is usually best to end the session by booking a series of appointments. The next one will need to be in 3–4 days' time.

Session 1

The top priority in the second appointment, as in the first, is engagement. Therapists should do their best to cultivate enthusiasm, hope and drive, while addressing concerns, misgivings and pessimism. There are four other priorities that are similar, whatever the form of the eating disorder:

- Initiating in-session weighing
- Reviewing the recording
- Reviewing the formulation
- Educating about weight-checking (weighing) and weight

This appointment lasts about 50 minutes, as do all subsequent ones, but the structure of the session is idiosyncratic because of the need to go over the monitoring records in exceptional detail to establish and reinforce high-quality recording. As a result the session has the following format (with the *approximate* time allocation in parentheses):

1. Initiating in-session weighing (5 minutes)
2. Reviewing the recording (10–15 minutes)
3. Setting the agenda (3 minutes)
4. Working through the agenda (20–25 minutes)
   - Attitude toward treatment
   - The formulation and its implications
   - Education about weight checking and weight
   - Other items
5. Confirming the homework, summarizing the session and arranging the next appointment (3 minutes)

Each of these components will now be described in turn.

Initiating In-Session Weighing

The in-session weighing procedure has a number of purposes. First, it provides a good opportunity to educate patients about their weight and about body weight in general. Second, as patients' eating habits change in treatment, they are likely to feel anxious about any resulting change in their weight. In-session weighing provides them with good week-by-week data on their weight. Third, regular in-session weighing provides an opportunity for the therapist to help patients interpret the number on the scale, which otherwise they are prone to misinterpret. Fourth, in-session weighing addresses one form of body checking, namely weight checking. Many patients with eating disorders weigh themselves at frequent intervals, sometimes many times a day. As a result they become concerned with day-to-day weight fluctuations that would otherwise pass unnoticed. Others actively avoid knowing their weight while remaining highly concerned about it. Generally these patients weighed themselves frequently in the past but switched to avoidance because they found frequent weight checking too aversive. However, avoidance of weighing is as problematic as frequent weighing since it results in patients having no data to confirm or disconfirm their fears about their weight.

In-session weighing opens with what we term "collaborative weighing." This involves the therapist and patient together checking the patient's weight[2] (with the patient wearing indoor clothing and no shoes). This is done once a week except with underweight patients when it is done every session (see Chapter 11). The weighing should be as collaborative as possible with the therapist adopting a calm and matter-of-fact manner. The number obtained should be agreed upon and spoken out loud in units that the patient understands, thereby countering avoidance of knowledge of weight. The therapist and patient should then plot the number on to an individualized weight graph that the therapist has prepared in advance. Figures 5.4a, 5.4b and 5.5c show the format of the graphs that we use. Note that they differ depending upon whether the patient is underweight (Figure 5.4a), has a healthy weight (Figure 5.4b) or is overweight (Figure 5.4c). In subsequent sessions, but still at the outset of the session, the therapist and patient jointly interpret the emerging weight data. Obviously this cannot be done in session 1 as there is only one data point to consider.

Interpreting weight graphs is more complex than it might seem. Until quite a few weeks have passed it is difficult to work out what is happening because there are insufficient data. The goal is that patients learn that each reading is subject to error, mainly due to variation in their state of hydration, and that they need to focus on what has happened *over the past 4 weeks* to identify their current weight and what is happening to it, rather than concentrating on the latest single reading which is what they otherwise tend to do. Indeed, individual readings are almost impossible to interpret because of the uncertainty that surrounds them. For this reason therapists should repeatedly remind patients that *"One cannot interpret a single reading."*[3] To help patients identify what is happening to their weight, therapists should use a transparent ruler

"One cannot interpret a single reading."

---

[2]We favor medical beam balance scales as they are robust, accurate and give sufficient precision. We recommend avoiding scales that provide a digital readout since their apparent accuracy reinforces concern with trivial changes in weight.

[3]Clinicians also need to take note of the fact that *"One cannot interpret a single reading."* Sometimes one encounters clinical situations in which major management decisions have been based on a single reading on the scale. For example, this was true of old-fashioned behavioral weight restoration programs. The same considerations apply to behavioral experiments in which weight change is the outcome of interest.

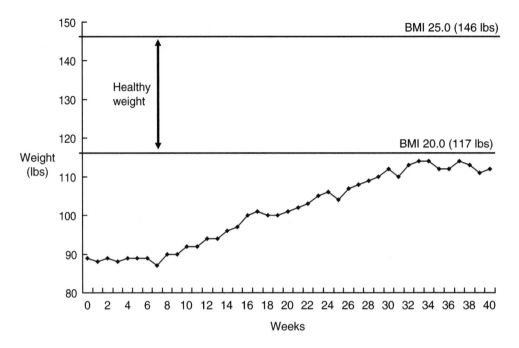

FIGURE 5.4a. A weight graph of an underweight patient.

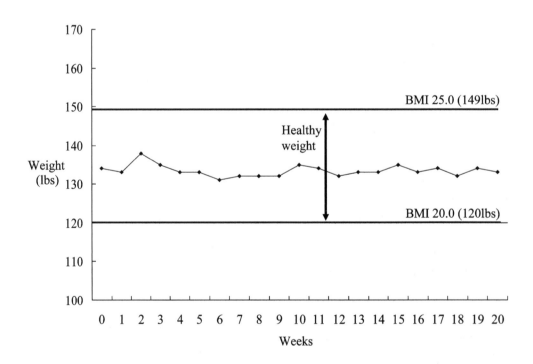

FIGURE 5.4b. A weight graph of a patient with a healthy weight.

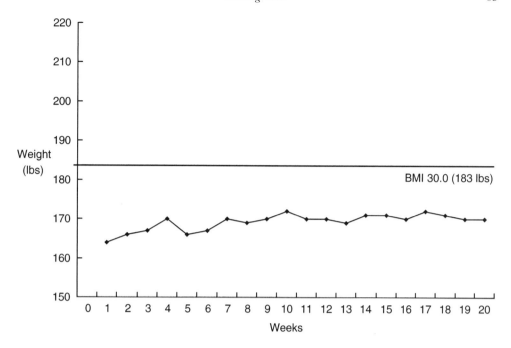

FIGURE 5.4c. A weight graph of an overweight patient.

to identify the emerging weight trend. Figures 5.5a and 5.5b show two schematic weight graphs, and the straight line crossing them identifies the underlying trend (i.e., the line represents where the ruler would be placed). It can be seen that the line does not necessarily intersect with the latest reading. Two tips are worth noting in this context. First, turning the weight graph through 90 degrees and looking at it again can highlight trends that were not obvious when the graph was inspected from the usual angle. Second, if patients are struggling to be objective about the interpretation of their graph, ask them to imagine that the graph is of something with less personal significance (e.g., weekly rainfall over several weeks) as this can help.

A crucial element of the in-session weighing intervention is that patients are asked not to weigh themselves between the weekly weigh-ins, but if they do, they should record this on their monitoring record. If they have a scale at home, they will find it helpful to make it inaccessible (and certainly they should put it out of sight).

Reviewing the Recording

As noted above, a major goal of session 1 is to establish and reinforce accurate real-time recording. This necessitates going over the patient's records in great detail with the patient taking the therapist through each day's record in turn. Even going through just 3 days' records may take 15 minutes.

There are two aspects to reviewing the records in session 1:

1. *Assessing the quality of monitoring.* This involves focusing on the process of recording. The therapist will want to know:

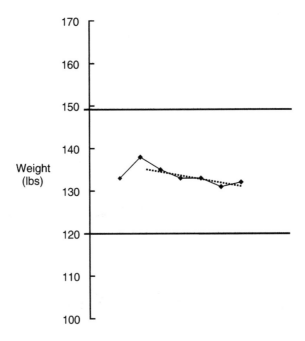

FIGURE 5.5a. Identifying weight trends.

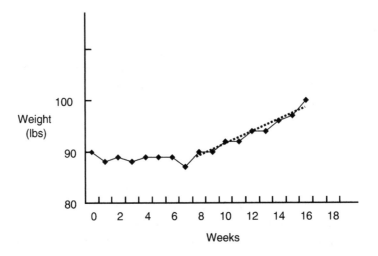

FIGURE 5.5b. Identifying weight trends.

- How the recording has been going from the patient's perspective
- The patient's attitude to the recording (see vignette below)
- How close in time to the eating and drinking the recording has taken place
- Whether meals have been identified with brackets, and whether asterisks have been used correctly
- Whether any episodes of eating or drinking were omitted or exaggerated
- If any particular difficulties were encountered

Vignette

"Tonight I started the recording and just in one evening I managed to use a whole sheet. I guess I can't keep going like this. When you first mentioned recording exactly what I ate (and where and when), I remember being quite horrified by it, but now I think I will be able to get used to it. I hadn't realized before that I was going to have to write down what I was drinking too, but that might be quite interesting. I drink a lot of hot drinks.

"I can see the importance of writing things down immediately because even just a short while later I wouldn't have bothered recording the same things, or perhaps even have noticed that I was thinking them. I feel slightly embarrassed by it all: If I had any time to think about it, I would rephrase things or avoid writing them down."

It is most important that patients are praised for their efforts at recording even if the records have shortcomings. For example, the therapist might say: *"That's a great start. We are going to learn so much about your eating problem and what is keeping it going. What we now need to do is get your recording even better so that we get the most out of it. With this in mind I suggest that you. . . . "*

Occasionally, but very rarely, a patient comes to session 1 having not recorded. Our stance in these circumstances is to react with perplexity and explore with the patient his or her reasons for not having recorded. A good tack is for the therapist to take some responsibility for the problem, perhaps by saying *"I think I can't have explained the reasons for recording clearly enough"* or *"I think I should have thought more carefully with you about the practicalities of doing this. Let's think about this together."* Then the therapist should address whatever problems emerge. Throughout it should be made clear that recording is absolutely integral to this treatment, and that treatment will not succeed without it. We never encounter patients who do not then start recording. This is not to say that we

> **Recording is integral to treatment. Treatment will not succeed without it.**

do not encounter problems with recording, nor is it to imply that once recording has been established it can be ignored. This is definitely not the case. Therapists should always keep in mind the process of recording, the accuracy of the records, and whether the records are being completed in real time.

2. *Assessing the information gained about the patient's eating habits.* The therapist will want to know whether the days were typical or atypical (and if so, in what respect). The therapist will also want to question the patient about any striking features. Figure 5.6 shows a sample monitoring record, and Table 5.3 lists some questions that the therapist might ask about it.

In subsequent sessions, the review of the records largely focuses on what has been recorded, although the therapist should intermittently ask the patient about the process of recording and the accuracy of the records. In these sessions the review should take generally no longer than 10 minutes. Therapists need to resist addressing any problems identified while doing this, but instead flag them for inclusion on the session agenda.

Setting the Agenda

In this session and all subsequent sessions the therapist should set the agenda for the main part of the appointment after reviewing the records and in conjunction with the patient. In principle, the agenda for every session (except the final one) includes elements from the following four sources:

1. *Homework assignments set in the previous session.* It should go almost without saying that one never sets homework without reviewing it in the next session. This review may be done in the context of going over the monitoring records, if doing so is relatively straightforward; otherwise it should be put on the agenda.

2. *Matters of significance identified during the review of the records.* The review of the records almost always identifies matters that need to be addressed in the main body of the session.

Day _Thursday_   **Date** _June 18th_

Time	Food and drink consumed	Place	*	V/L	Context and comments
6:30	Black coffee **A**	Bedroom			Had a sleepless night. Stomach doesn't feel good. **B**
11:45	Black coffee	Staff room			
2:15	1/2 can diet coke 1 Oreo cookie	Bedroom		S	Spat the cookie out – good! **C**
6:15	1 cup vegetables 1 tomato 1 apple 1 plum }	Bedroom			
8:00	Camomile tea	Bedroom			Feeling OK – haven't eaten a lot
9:30	4 Oreos 1 tbs peanut butter	Bedroom	*	V	I am SO disgusted with myself! Why did I do that? I felt like I couldn't stop myself **D**
10:00					500 sit-ups – I have to burn off those Oreos!
10:30				L	1 Dulcolax – needed this, my stomach is so fat

FIGURE 5.6. A monitoring record (patient B; session 2).

TABLE 5.3. Some Questions That the Therapist Might Ask about the Monitoring Record Shown in Figure 5.6.

Point A

- You didn't have breakfast — is that right?
- Do you never have breakfast? Why?

Point B

- What did you mean "Stomach doesn't feel good"?

Point C

- Why did you eat the Oreo at 2:15 P.M.?
- Did you know you were going to spit it out?
- Would you have eaten it if you were not going to spit it out?

Point D

- Why do you think you ate those Oreos and peanut butter? Was there a trigger?
- When did you know you were going to make yourself sick?
- How many Oreos would have been acceptable to you?

3. *Items that the patient wants to discuss.* Patients should always be invited to put items on the agenda. In the great majority of cases they are relevant and so are appropriate to discuss. Occasionally, they are not relevant (e.g., where to go on vacation) in which case the therapist should point this out in a sensitive manner.

4. *New topics based on the stage in treatment.* These items are introduced by the therapist and are dictated by the patient's progress and the point in treatment that has been reached. For example, the therapist may decide that it is time that body checking is addressed and will therefore put this topic on the agenda.

If there are too many potential items to cover, the therapist should determine the priorities and carry over additional items to the following session.

Working Through the Agenda

Attitude toward Treatment

Patients vary in their attitude toward treatment. Some are positive from the outset and remain so; others begin reluctantly or with ambivalence and are then won over; others remain ambivalent or reluctant; and yet others start with an enthusiasm that wanes over time. These changes are important as they may influence treatment outcome. Enthusiastic patients tend to throw themselves into treatment and the homework assignments, and often do well as a result, whereas those who have doubts are more likely to do their homework half-heartedly and make correspondingly fewer changes. They are also at greater risk of dropping out. For these reasons the patient's attitude toward treatment should always be on the therapist's mind and, intermittently, it should be formally assessed. Session 1 is one of these times.

Therapists should therefore inquire about the patient's view on treatment. Questions of the following sort may be asked:

"What do you feel about having started treatment?"
"Do you have any worries or concerns about treatment that you would like to discuss?"

It is also important to ask about practicalities, including the time it takes to get to and from sessions, the optimum time of day for appointments, difficulties with child care, etc. By paying attention to these very real issues, therapists can demonstrate that they are concerned about the patient's overall welfare and not just the state of the eating disorder. This broader focus helps to engage patients. It also brings to the therapist's attention difficulties that might otherwise lead the patient to drop out.

Reviewing the Formulation

An important element of this session is reviewing the patient's formulation: The patient's views on the diagram (e.g., Figure 5.2) should be sought and any misunderstandings resolved. Sometimes patients want to highlight processes that they think are particularly germane (e.g., binges triggered by breaking dietary rules) and sometimes new clinical features or processes will need to be added. Throughout, the diagram is described as provisional by saying something along these lines: *"This picture is our current understanding of what is keeping your eating problem going. We may need to change or embellish it as we get to understand your problem better, or if it changes."* The therapist should also restate the practical implications of the formulation; namely, that it highlights what needs to be targeted in treatment.

Education about Weight Checking

Patients need to learn how to interpret the number they obtain when they weigh themselves. They should be informed that *"the number on the scale"* fluctuates through the day, and from day to day, according to their state of hydration, the state of their bowels and bladder, their point in the menstrual cycle, and other factors as well. Frequent weighing results in preoccupation with inconsequential fluctuations in the number on the scale, and these tend to be misinterpreted — leading many patients to restrict their eating, whatever the reading: If it is "up" or "the same," they try to diet even harder; and if it is "down," their dieting is reinforced. This process can be illustrated by drawing a wiggly line on a piece of paper with regular vertical lines representing each episode of weighing (see Figure 5.7). The therapist should then identify a segment of the wiggly line (between two vertical lines) where there is apparent weight gain and project the line upward (see Line 1) pointing out that patients generally interpret any increase in the number on the scale as evidence that they are gaining weight and must therefore try harder to diet. The therapist should then identify a horizontal segment of the wiggly line suggestive of no weight change and point out that patients typically respond to no apparent weight change (see Line 2) by thinking that they must diet harder if they are to lose weight. Lastly, the therapist should identify a segment suggestive of weight loss and extend the line downwards (see Line 3) pointing out that patients generally respond to apparent weight loss with the thought that they must persist in dieting, now that it is beginning to work. The general point is that whatever the apparent weight change, patients tend to draw the conclusion that they must persist in dieting. This important maintaining process is disrupted by in-session weighing.

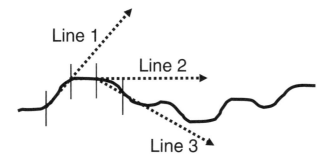

FIGURE 5.7. Interpreting fluctuations in weight.

Education about Weight, Weight Goals and Weight Change in Treatment

Patients should also be educated about body weight and their body mass index (BMI). The main points to stress are as follows:

- Body weight is under strong physiological control and is therefore difficult to influence in the long-term.
- The BMI is a convenient way of representing weight adjusted for height. It is weight (in kg) divided by height squared (in m) (i.e., Wt/Ht^2).

Below are recommended BMI thresholds for people with an eating disorder or a history of one. (For further information regarding these specific thresholds, see Table 2.3.) Therapists may want to adjust the terms used to label these categories to suit the individual patient.

Significantly underweight	17.5 or below
Underweight	17.6 to 18.9
Low weight	19.0 to 19.9
Healthy weight	20.0 to 24.9
(Somewhat) overweight	25.0 to 29.9
(Significantly overweight) obesity	30.0 or more

These thresholds apply to adults of either sex between the ages of 18 and 60 years, and they are based upon BMI levels known to be associated with adverse effects on health. With patients who have a BMI below 20.0 it can be helpful to point out that the average weight of people their age and gender is significantly higher than this.

Rather than having an exact desired weight patients should be advised to accept a weight range of approximately 6 pounds (or 3 kg) in magnitude to allow for natural weight fluctuations. The therapist might say something along these lines:

"Having an exact desired weight does not make much sense since it is impossible for the reading on the scale to remain exactly the same. It would be like having an exact desired pulse (heart rate). We are living organisms and just as one's pulse naturally fluctuates according to circumstances — for example, after walking up a flight of stairs — so does one's weight. The parallel with one's pulse extends further. People who repeatedly check their pulse tend to become concerned about changes that are of no significance. The same is true of frequent weighing: It brings to one's attention changes in weight that are trivial and of no importance.

Also, wanting your weight to be absolutely stable inevitably creates feelings of failure. It is impossible to have a perfectly stable weight."

Almost all patients are anxious about the effect treatment will have on their weight. Patients with bulimia nervosa or eating disorder NOS (other than those who are underweight) generally do not change much in weight. Nevertheless, there are some patients who gain weight and there are others who lose, and it is not possible to predict exactly what will happen to the individual patient. Patients should be told that one aim of treatment is to give them control over their eating and thus they will have as much control over their weight as is possible. It is best that patients postpone deciding upon a specific goal weight range until near the end of treatment when their eating habits have stabilized. Later in treatment patients are also advised against having a goal weight (range) that necessitates anything more than slight dietary restraint, as dietary restraint maintains preoccupation with food and eating and increases the risk of binge eating (see Chapter 10, page 125).

Confirming the Homework, Summarizing the Session and Arranging the Next Appointment

Generally two pieces of homework are given at the end of session 1:

1. Improving upon the recording
2. Resisting weighing at home

The therapist should end the session by summarizing its content, restating the homework and booking the next appointment. Below is a typical session summary.

> *"Let's summarize what we have done in this session. We started off with weighing, and then we reviewed in detail your records. You have made a great start with monitoring your eating. We then spent quite a lot of time discussing what it has been like monitoring. You told me that it was hard at first but you are beginning to get used to it. Is that right? What else did we do this session? . . . (Patient responds.) Yes, we talked about how pleased you were to be finally starting treatment, and how you thought the diagram was helpful, and you could see some of those vicious circles in your monitoring records.*
>
> *"We talked about your weight and what a healthy weight would be, and we worked out your body mass index. We thought that maybe part of what was keeping your problem going was how often you weighed yourself, and how you place a lot of importance on every single reading, despite weight fluctuating for all sorts of reasons. We thought that it would help you to restrict your weighing to once a week, something we will be doing here for the meantime.*
>
> *"Finally we agreed that you would keep on recording your food and drink intake and do your best not to weigh yourself at home."*

Recommended Reading

Recommended reading for Chapters 5–12 can be found at the end of Chapter 12.

CHAPTER 6

Achieving Early Change

The first few weeks of treatment are crucial as they have a great influence over treatment outcome. Engaging the patient is of particular importance, but it is not an end in of itself: It is simply a precondition for change. In this chapter and in most of the forthcoming ones, the focus is on the specific strategies and procedures needed to produce change, assuming that the patient is engaged. (The general strategy used to engage patients was described in the previous chapter. The engagement of highly ambivalent patients is discussed in detail in Chapter 11.)

Implementing the Rest of Stage One

Having completed the first two sessions of Stage One, as described in the previous chapter, most patients should:

- Be reasonably engaged in treatment and the prospect of change
- Understand and accept the provisional formulation
- Be getting adept at real-time recording
- Be accepting of weekly weighing and all that it involves

In this chapter, the remainder of Stage One is described; that is, the next 6 twice-weekly sessions (sessions 2–7).

From session 2 onward treatment sessions have a standard structure. Each lasts about 50 minutes and has the following elements (with their *approximate* time allocation in parentheses):

1. In-session weighing: collaborative weighing; updating and interpreting the weight graph (up to 5 minutes). This is done once a week (i.e., in one of the twice-weekly sessions).
2. Reviewing the latest monitoring records and any homework assignments (up to 10 minutes, no longer)
3. Collaboratively setting the agenda for the session (3 minutes)
4. Working through the agenda and agreeing on homework tasks (up to 30 minutes)
5. Summarizing the session, confirming the homework assignments and arranging the next appointment (3 minutes)

It is recommended that therapists adhere to this structure as not doing so results in far less being accomplished. It also helps one keep to time. The structure should be abandoned only if adhering to it is either impossible or doing so seems inappropriate (e.g., the patient is facing a major crisis; see Chapter 16, page 256, for a discussion of how to address crises within CBT-E). Note that at the beginning of each session patients are told the session number and how many sessions are left. This is to ensure that they (and the therapist) remain fully aware of the time-limited nature of the treatment.

Therapists not used to working this way might get the impression that CBT-E is rigid and formulaic. This conclusion would be to misunderstand the treatment and its implementation. What is being specified is how best to structure sessions to make them efficient and effective, as well as the optimum timing of two central features of CBT-E: in-session weighing and the review of the patient's records. The content of the main part of the session varies from patient to patient and is dictated by the patient's psychopathology, the strategies and procedures introduced so far, and the patient's progress to date.

The remaining sessions of Stage One have three new goals:

1. To educate the patient about eating problems (using a procedure we term "guided reading")
2. To establish a pattern of regular eating (eating style, purging, fullness, low weight and excessive exercising may also be addressed)
3. To involve significant others, if it would be helpful and the patient is willing

Generally both the guided reading and "regular eating" interventions are introduced in session 2 with the other interventions being implemented later in Stage One, if needed. Significant others are not generally involved until near the end of Stage One.

Educating the Patient about Eating Problems

Myths abound about eating and weight control. Patients with eating disorders are assiduous readers of popular articles, books and websites about diets and dieting and may acquire an idiosyncratic body of knowledge that is not well founded. Typically they are not well informed about some topics; for example, the effects of vomiting and laxative misuse on calorie absorption.

To ensure that patients have a reliable source of information, we recommend that they read one of the authoritative books on eating disorders written for the general public. We routinely use *Overcoming Binge Eating* (Fairburn, 1995) as it provides all the information needed (at this stage in treatment) for patients who are not underweight. Also, it is popular with patients. (CGF acknowledges the obvious conflict of interest.) Another advantage of the book is that it has a cognitive behavioral orientation and so is consistent with CBT-E. Part I is exclusively educational. With patients who are comfortable reading, the whole of Part I may be recommended. With patients who are less used to reading, certain chapters should be brought to their attention (especially Chapters 1, 4 and 5) and they should be asked to read one each week. It should be noted that *Overcoming Binge Eating* is relevant to all patients with an eating disorder, whether or not they binge eat, because it discusses eating disorder psychopathology in general and not just binge eating. If patients are dubious about its value, saying that it is not relevant as they do not binge eat, it should be explained that Part I is about eating problems in general and that in any case most people with eating problems are at high risk of binge eating, and the book explains why this is the case.

Table 6.1 lists the main topics that should be covered when educating patients. Note that some of this information will be relevant only to subsets of patients. The additional information needed by underweight patients is described in Chapter 11 (page 152).

It is our practice to provide patients with a copy of the book as in this way we can ensure that they read it at exactly the right point in treatment (generally week 2, although sometimes earlier). We ask them to annotate the book in the margins, putting ticks by sections that particularly apply to them, crosses by sections that do not, and question marks by sections that they do not understand or would like to discuss. Patients are asked to bring their book to the next session so that the therapist (in the main part of the session) can review which sections have ticks, crosses and

> **Guided reading allows patients to be educated in an efficient, thorough and personalized way.**

question marks. This review provides the therapist with useful additional information about the patient's psychopathology and allows any questions and concerns to be addressed. In this way guided reading allows patients to be educated in an efficient, thorough and personalized way. When doing this it is good practice to relate the information provided to the patient's formulation and embellish it if appropriate.

Establishing "Regular Eating"

The "regular eating" intervention is fundamental to successful treatment, whatever form the eating disorder takes. It is the foundation upon which other changes are built. For

> **The "regular eating" intervention is fundamental to successful treatment, whatever form the eating disorder takes.**

patients who binge eat, it reliably results in a rapid decrease in the frequency of binge eating, leaving what may be termed "residual binges," which can then become a focus of Stage Three (see Chapter 10). This reduction in binge eating is highly reinforcing for patients and is generally accompanied by a marked improvement in mood. (If there is no improvement in mood, therapists should consider whether there is a co-existing clinical depression. See pages 246–250 for a description of how to detect and treat such depressions within the context of CBT-E.) How the reduction in binge eating comes about is not entirely clear: It is likely to be through a variety of mechanisms. For patients who have unstructured and somewhat chaotic eating habits (e.g., a tendency to pick continuously at food rather than eat clear-cut meals or snacks), regular eating provides structure and control. For patients who have a high level of dietary restraint, regular eating addresses an important type of dieting, namely infrequent or delayed eating; that is, eating infrequently or putting off eating. And for patients who are underweight, the intervention introduces regular meals and snacks that can be subsequently increased in size. Regular eating also appears to facilitate reversal of the delay in gastric emptying seen in underweight patients, thereby reducing their propensity to feel full (see Chapter 11). With all patients

TABLE 6.1. Main Topics to Cover When Educating Patients about Eating Disorders

The Patient's Eating Disorder and Its Treatment

- The patient's eating disorder diagnosis
- Its prevalence and main characteristics
- Associated health risks
- Its course and prognosis without treatment
- The treatment options and their likely effects

Clinical Features of Eating Disorders

1. *Characteristic extreme concerns about shape and weight*
   - Judging of self-worth largely or even exclusively in terms of shape and weight and their control
   - Various secondary "expressions" that maintain the extreme concerns
     — Repeated body weight and shape checking (including unfavorable comparisons with others)
     — Body avoidance
     — Feeling fat
     — Marginalization of other aspects of life
   - Drives extreme weight-control behavior (dieting, self-induced vomiting, etc.; see below)
   - Highly impairing (e.g., distressing; preoccupation with thoughts about shape and weight; social sensitivity; difficulty with sexual relationships)

2. *Characteristic form of dieting*
   - Demanding dietary goals with multiple rigid rules
   - Markedly increases the risk of binge eating
   - May, or may not, lead to undereating and a very low weight
   - Highly impairing (e.g., difficulty eating with others and eating out; preoccupation with food and eating)

3. *Binge eating*
   - An episode of uncontrolled overeating (Clinicians tend to restrict the use of the term to episodes of eating in which an unusually large amount of food is eaten, given the circumstances, but many people's "binges" do not involve eating such large amounts.)
   - Usually experienced as highly aversive overall
   - Typically triggered by breaking a dietary rule or by the occurrence of an adverse event or negative mood
   - Highly impairing (e.g., secondary shame and guilt; requires secrecy and subterfuge; expensive)

4. *Self-induced vomiting*
   - Either to compensate for an episode of perceived or actual overeating or is a more routine form of weight control
   - Relatively ineffective. About half of what has been eaten cannot be retrieved.
   - If compensatory, belief in its effectiveness maintains binge eating because a psychological deterrent against further overeating is undermined
   - Adverse physical effects, especially electrolyte disturbance (which can be dangerous as it may result in cardiac arrhythmias), salivary gland enlargement, and erosion of the dental enamel of the inner surface of the front teeth
   - Highly impairing (e.g., secondary shame and guilt; requires secrecy and subterfuge)

5. *Laxative and diuretic misuse*
   - Either to compensate for an episode of perceived or actual overeating or is a more routine form of weight control
   - Ineffective. Laxatives have very little effect on food absorption and diuretics have none.
   - If compensatory, belief in their effectiveness maintains binge eating because a psychological deterrent against further overeating is undermined
   - Both have a short-lived effect on weight by causing dehydration (through loss of fluid in the form of diarrhea or urine respectively)

TABLE 6.1 (*cont.*)

- Adverse physical effects, especially electrolyte disturbance
- Highly impairing (e.g., secondary shame and guilt; require secrecy and subterfuge; expensive)

6. *Over-exercising*
   - Either follows an episode of perceived or actual overeating or is a more routine form of weight control
   - Relatively ineffective as a means of weight control
   - Can be "driven," in which case there is an inner compulsion to exercise, and exercising takes precedence over other activities
   - Physically dangerous if significantly underweight or in the presence of osteoporosis or electrolyte disturbance
   - Impairing if "driven" (e.g., takes up a great deal of time; socially disruptive)

7. *Being underweight* — see Chapter 11 (especially Table 11.2).

it tends to highlight thoughts, beliefs and values that may be contributing to the maintenance of the eating disorder.

The intervention is introduced around sessions 2 or 3, and it is the first time that patients are asked to change the way that they eat. It is difficult to give a simple and standard rationale for the intervention. Instead, we find that a pragmatic one works well: for example, the therapist might say:

> "*It is now time to begin making changes to your eating. The first one simply concerns when you eat, not what you eat. It has been found that eating at regular intervals through the day really helps people with eating problems. Doing this, and doing it well, is really important. It is the foundation upon which all other changes will be built.*"

There are two components to the intervention:

1. *Patients should eat three planned meals each day, plus two or three planned snacks.* A typical eating pattern would be as follows:

   - Breakfast
   - Lunch
   - Mid-afternoon snack
   - Evening meal
   - Evening snack

   If there is to be a third snack (e.g., with underweight patients; see Chapter 11) it would usually be mid-morning (i.e., between breakfast and lunch).

2. *Patients' eating should be confined to these meals and snacks.*

As establishing a pattern of regular eating is so important, detailed guidance for achieving it is given below:

- *Patients should choose what they eat in their planned meals and snacks.* The only condition is that the meals and snacks must not be followed by vomiting, spitting, laxative misuse, or any other form of compensatory behavior. Meals or snacks that are followed by purging do not "count." At this point in treatment patients should not be put under pressure to change what they eat as doing so tends to result in their being unable to adopt the pattern of regular eating. If they seek advice on what to eat, they should be told that the priority is their pattern of eating and not what they eat, but if they want some guidance it should be to adopt a varied diet with the minimum number of avoided foods. Patients should be discouraged from counting calories, and especially from any tendency to keep a running total.

- *Patients' definition of what constitutes a "meal" or "snack" should be accepted* so long as it is not nonsensical. A commonsense approach is called for (e.g., drinks do not count as "food," but soup does).

- *There should rarely be more than a 4-hour interval between the planned meals and snacks, and patients should not skip any of them.* If a meal or snack is skipped, this should be pointed out and the therapist should highlight the consequences of doing so (e.g., increased risk of overeating or binge eating later on; greater preoccupation with food and eating; perpetuation of the tendency to feel full).

- *The new eating pattern should take precedence over other activities* and be adhered to whatever the patient's circumstances or appetite. On the other hand, it should be adjusted to suit the patient's day-to-day commitments. Usually it will differ on workdays and days off.

- *Patients should plan ahead.* They should always know when they are going to have their next meal or snack, and what it will be. To emphasize this point we some-times say *"If I were to call you out of the blue, you should be able to tell me when and what you will next be eating,"* although we also make it clear that we will not being doing this! Each morning (or the evening before) patients should write out in outline their plan for the day on the top of the day's monitoring record. If the day is going to be unpredictable, they should plan ahead as far as possible and identify a time when they can take stock and plan the remainder of the day. Patients should be told that careful planning will help them gain more control over their eating and be less preoccupied with food at other times. Sometimes patients' plans will have to change because of unforeseen events. Under these circumstances patients should draw up and implement a revised plan (preferably written).

- *Patients should use the time and the behavior of others to govern when they eat, rather than feelings of hunger or fullness.* This is because these feelings of hunger or fullness are almost invariably disturbed as a result of the way that they have been eating. Once patients have been eating regularly for some months (without purging), they will experience a return of normal and appropriately timed sensations of hunger and fullness, but even then it is best not to use these sensations as guides to when to eat. Most people in Western societies eat because it is time to do so (e.g., lunch time) or because others are eating, regardless of how hungry they feel.

- *Patients' sensations of hunger and fullness should not be used to govern what they eat.* Instead, patients should consume no more than average-sized portions of food. The size of an average portion can be determined from the eating habits of friends or relatives, from recipes, and from the instructions on food packages.

- *Certain forms of social eating need particularly careful planning.* For example, if there is going to be limited choice (as at a dinner party) or if patients are going to an event where a wide range of foods will be laid out (as in a buffet), they should be advised to assess the situation and then take "time out" (perhaps by going to the bathroom) to plan what and how to eat, the goal being that they adhere to the regular eating pattern. With buffets, once patients have eaten, they should get rid of their plate(s) and cutlery. It is worth forewarning patients that drinking alcohol tends to undermine adherence to even the best-formulated plans.

• *Two rather different strategies may be used to help patients resist eating between the planned meals and snacks.* The second one is difficult for most patients, especially in the early stages of treatment. It is generally best left until later on, when urges to eat between meals and snacks are intermittent and less overwhelming.

  1. *Engaging in activities that are incompatible with eating or make it less likely.* This strategy needs to be applied for only 3 or 4 hours at most, by which time the urge to eat is likely to have waned and, in any case, the patient will be due to eat. Suitable activities include telephoning or visiting friends, going for a walk, exercising, e-mailing, surfing the Internet, or having a bath or shower. Patients who are stuck at home (perhaps because they have young children) may find that putting on certain types of music helps them resist eating. It seems that some music creates an "atmosphere" that is almost incompatible with binge eating, probably because it affects the patient's mood and displaces his or her mindset. (See Chapter 8 for a discussion of mindsets and how to manipulate them.) Music also has the advantage of permeating an entire living space.

  Creating in advance a list of possible incompatible activities is helpful so that when faced with a strong urge to eat, patients have at hand a variety of suitable strategies. The list can include involving others such as a close friend or partner. Again, patients should think ahead by trying to predict when difficulties are likely to arise and develop a plan for addressing them.

  2. *Focusing on the urge to eat and recognizing that it is a temporary phenomenon to which one does not have to succumb.* In this way patients learn to de-center from the urge, and observe it rather than try to eliminate it. As with feelings of fullness (see page 84), they will find that the urge generally dissipates within a few hours. "Riding out" urges to eat and discovering that they wane over time is sometimes referred to as "urge surfing."

• *Patients whose eating habits are chaotic and those whose eating is highly restrictive may need to introduce the pattern in steps.* At first these patients should focus on the part of the day when their eating is least problematic, usually the mornings, and once they have mastered this time period, they should extend the pattern in steps until it encompasses the entire day. This may take several weeks.

Six difficulties commonly arise when helping patients adopt this pattern of eating:

  1. *In response to perceived failures of dietary control, patients abandon their efforts for the rest of the day.* Even minor slips may be viewed as "failures" and the entire day regarded as ruined. This reaction is a good example of dichotomous (black-and-white) thinking with anything less than 100% success being classed as a failure. To counter this, the therapist should highlight the phenomenon and educate the patient about it, stressing that there are many degrees of compliance with the regular eating intervention. To demonstrate this the therapist and patient may make a rating (e.g., on a scale from 0 to 5) of the patient's degree of compliance each day based on his or her monitoring records.

2. *Patients may say that they have never eaten in this way* and nor do their family or friends. Therapists should respond that, while this may well be the case, adopting this pattern of eating will help them overcome their eating problem, and it will be the foundation upon which other important changes will be built. Once they have overcome their eating problem, it will be up to them to determine exactly how they eat, but for the meantime it is in their best interests to eat this way. It is also a healthy way of eating from a physiological point of view. Some patients are particularly reluctant to eat breakfast, fearing that if they start the day by eating they will not be able to stop. The regular eating intervention provides an opportunity to test, and disconfirm, this belief. Others are reluctant to have the evening snack, believing that eating in the evening makes one put on weight. Here education is required: What matters with regard to weight regulation is the overall amount of energy consumed in the day and not when it was consumed. Again the regular eating intervention provides an opportunity to test this belief.

3. *Some patients are reluctant to eat meals and snacks because they think that doing so will result in weight gain.* They can be reassured that this rarely occurs because they have not been asked to change the amount that they eat or what they eat. Also, with patients who binge eat, the therapist should point out that regular eating results in a decrease in the frequency of binge eating and, as a result, a significant reduction in their overall energy intake (even if they vomit they will absorb a significant amount of energy each time that they binge; see below). (Note that we use the term "energy" rather than "calories" because it is less emotive for these patients.) Despite such assurances, it is common for patients to select meals and snacks that are low in energy. There need be no objection to this, as the focus at this stage is on *when* patients eat and not on *what* they eat.

> **We use the term "energy" rather than calories because it is less emotive for patients.**

4. *A common problem is that some patients are liable to feel full after eating relatively little, and this feeling produces a desire to vomit or take laxatives afterward.* Feelings of fullness are especially prominent in patients who are underweight and can be attributed to the delay in gastric emptying that is a consequence of undereating. Patients should be reassured that feeling full generally subsides within an hour and that the propensity to feel full gradually declines with the adoption of the pattern of regular eating. Feeling full is discussed in detail later in this chapter.

5. *Some patients object in principle to the idea of planning.* These patients tend to value spontaneity and unpredictability. Unfortunately, such a lifestyle makes it difficult to overcome an eating disorder. This needs to be explained. They should be advised that for the next 20 weeks (i.e., during treatment) it is in their long-term interests to be more regular and predictable in their habits since otherwise the chances that they will overcome their eating problem will be diminished. They can always go back to their preferred lifestyle later.

6. *Some patients object to the use of distraction activities.* These patients think that distraction only delays the inevitable act of binge eating. This is not true. In such cases therapists should explain that what they are doing is learning to resist urges to eat (between the planned meals and snacks) and that every time that they do this, it is an achievement. They are "urge surfing." It is also worth pointing out that even if

they get another urge to binge later in the day, it does not discount their success at dealing with the earlier one. They should work from hour to hour, and from meal (or snack) to meal (or snack), as this way a stable pattern of eating will become established.

Implementing the regular eating intervention is a skill that all CBT-E therapists need to acquire. It involves conveying the rationale well, being persuasive, tackling objections and obstacles, and praising all signs of progress. A brief handout on regular eating is shown in Table 6.2. Some patients can adopt the entire pattern readily, whereas with others it can take 3 or more weeks. It is difficult to progress in treatment until it has been more or less successfully adopted. Therefore these Stage One sessions, and sometimes those in Stage Two, will have "regular eating" as a major item on the session agenda. If the patient is still having difficulty adopting this pattern of eating by the end of Stage Two and is someone who binge eats, a good strategy is to add "binge analysis" (see page 139), as this reinforces and extends the regular eating intervention.

Addressing the Patient's Style of Eating

Patients' "eating style" — that is, the way that they eat — does not need to be addressed unless there are obvious problems. Patients who have a tendency to overeat are an exception, however, as their eating style often contributes to their overeating. Below are some points worth highlighting. Further information may be found in Cooper, Fairburn and Hawker (2003).

TABLE 6.2. Patient Handout on Regular Eating

Regular Eating

Pattern of eating
- Breakfast
- (Mid-morning snack)
- Lunch
- Mid-afternoon snack
- Evening meal
- Evening snack

Points to note
- Eat these meals and snacks, but do not eat between them.
- Do not skip any meals or snacks.
- Do not go more than 4 hours without eating.
- Eat what you like in the meals and snacks, so long as you do not vomit or take laxatives to compensate.
- Always know when (and roughly what) you are next going to eat.

From *Cognitive Behavior Therapy and Eating Disorders* by Christopher G. Fairburn. Copyright 2008 by The Guilford Press. This table is available online at www.psych.ox.ac.uk/credo/cbt_and_eating_disorders.

- *Eating is best formalized.* Meals should have a clear beginning and end, and when at home patients should eat only when sitting down at a set place.
- *Eating directly from packages or pans is best avoided.* Instead patients should set out the food that they are going to eat and, before they start eating, put the remainder away. For the meantime it can be helpful to limit the supply of tempting foods available in the house.
- *It is best not to combine eating with other activities* (e.g., watching television or reading) as this can lead to inadvertent over-consumption. Instead, it is better to savor what is being eaten, as this is likely to lead to feelings of satisfaction and reduce the risk of subsequent overeating.
- *"Picking" at food should be avoided.* Some patients are prone to pick at food between meals or snacks or when cooking. One way to help break the habit is to chew gum at high-risk times. Underweight patients may pick at their food (or sometimes the food of others) rather than eating a full helping. This seems to be a way of pretending to themselves that they have not eaten. If prominent, this habit needs to be addressed as patients have to learn to eat in a normal fashion and accept that they are consuming food and eating meals and snacks.
- *Abnormalities in the speed of eating may need to be addressed.* The rapid eating that characteristically occurs during binge eating does not need to be tackled as the goal is to eliminate binge eating rather than modify the form that it takes. However, some patients eat rapidly outside episodes of binge eating, and this can lead to overeating. These patients generally find that slowing down their eating helps them control how much they eat. They should be encouraged to time their meals and try to spend at least 15 minutes on each one. This can be achieved by putting their cutlery down between mouthfuls; taking sips of water; engaging in conversation while eating; and deliberately eating at the same speed as others present.

The inordinately slow and ritualized eating seen in some patients who are underweight needs to be addressed if it is obstructing progress. Otherwise it can be ignored because it generally reverses as patients regain weight. If it does need to be tackled, this is easiest done in settings in which the patient's eating can be observed (see Chapter 15), but it can be addressed on an outpatient basis if the patient agrees that it is a problem (e.g., limits can be agreed on the time taken to eat meals).

Addressing Purging

Self-induced vomiting and the misuse of laxatives or diuretics ("purging") may serve various functions. As explained in Chapter 2, purging may be "compensatory" or "non-compensatory" with respect to weight control:

- *Compensatory purging* — This is when purging is used to compensate for specific episodes of perceived or actual overeating, in which case it follows these episodes and only occurs when they occur. If the patient's purging is exclusively compensatory, it generally does not need to be addressed in treatment because it will decline as the patient gains control over eating.
- *Non-compensatory purging* — This is when purging functions as a more "routine"

form of weight control, akin to dieting, in which case the link with episodes of overeating is not so close. Such purging generally needs to be tackled.

Whether the purging is compensatory or non-compensatory, all patients need to be educated about purging and its effects. The main points to stress are listed in Table 6.1 and detailed information (for the patient) may be found in *Overcoming Binge Eating*. These points should be highlighted when reviewing the patient's reading. It is especially important to stress the "ineffectiveness" of purging at controlling weight (and shape). Even vomiting only retrieves part of what has been eaten. In this context it can be salutary for patients who binge eat to calculate the calorie content of a typical binge and the likely number of calories that they will be absorbing on each occasion. This generally results in them becoming less enamored with vomiting as a means of compensating for overeating.

Patients who engage in non-compensatory purging (including spitting, with or without rumination) should be strongly advised to make the decision to cease doing so because persisting with this behavior undermines establishing and maintaining healthy eating habits. Therapists should try to help patients reach this decision and adhere to it. This is especially important in patients who are still engaging in non-compensatory purging toward the end of treatment (residual purging). If the purging takes the form of laxative or diuretic misuse, patients who take them intermittently should be able to stop in one go. Those who take them frequently are best advised to follow a planned withdrawal schedule during which the drugs are gradually phased out (e.g., each week the number taken per episode or day is halved). Some experience a week or so of weight gain due to rebound fluid retention. It is important to forewarn patients of this possibility to help them cope with any associated edema and, of course, the temporary increase in the number on the scale. Obviously patients should throw away their supplies. Some of the "regular eating" strategies used to help patients refrain from eating between meals and snacks may also be used to help them resist purging.

Purging serves additional functions for some patients in which case it can prove more resistant to change. Generally this will be evident by Stage Two and will necessitate the targeting of purging (and the mechanisms underlying it) in Stage Three. The main additional functions are as follows:

- *To avoid feeling full.* Some patients vomit in order to avoid feeling full (discussed in detail in the next section).
- *To empty the stomach or flatten the abdomen.* Some patients vomit in order to have a completely empty stomach. Of course, they are mistaken in this regard because vomiting does not totally empty the stomach. Some who take laxatives do this in part to empty out their gut and have a concave abdomen (when lying down). To achieve this, they usually need to induce a considerable amount of diarrhea. It is important that these patients understand that their laxative misuse has little or no effect on calorie absorption and thus no true effect on body shape. In other words a distinction needs to be drawn between having temporarily emptied out one's gut, thereby producing a concave abdomen, and influencing one's shape or "fatness."
- *To modulate mood.* Patients may discover that vomiting has a tension-relieving effect and that as a result it helps them cope with intense emotions. (Binge eating can have a somewhat similar effect.) Some of these patients have what may be termed "mood intolerance." Strategies for helping these patients are described in Chapter 10.

• *As a form of self-punishment.* Some patients induce diarrhea to punish themselves. Generally they have very low self-esteem although some are clinically depressed. It is important to assess these patients carefully and, if present, directly address the low self-esteem (see Chapter 13) or clinical depression (see Chapter 16) and the eating disorder.

Addressing Feelings of Fullness

Many patients with an eating disorder dislike feeling full and view it as evidence that they have overeaten or are fat. As a result they either restrict their eating to avoid feeling full or they vomit after having eaten. If feeling full, or patients' responses to feeling full, are proving a barrier to overcoming the eating problem, they need to be addressed.

"Feeling full" is a label for a number of different experiences, including the following:

> **"Feeling full" is a label for a number of different experiences.**

1. An internal physical sensation of feeling full (the sensation of having eaten or drunk a lot; the experience of there being a substantial amount of food or liquid inside one's stomach)
2. Thinking that one has eaten too much
3. Perceiving one's abdomen as sticking out excessively
4. Clothing feeling unduly tight
5. Feeling fat

Not infrequently several of these experiences co-exist.

The therapist needs to explain to patients that "feeling full" is a term used to refer to a variety of experiences so it is crucial to know exactly what they are experiencing at times when they feel full. Questioning the patient about the topic is best supplemented with a period of real-time recording of times when the patient feels full and the accompanying circumstances and sensations. The right-hand column of the monitoring record may be used for this purpose.

Once the nature of the experience has been identified, the therapist should address the experience directly along these lines:

• *Feeling full internally.* This is an unremarkable physical experience and is not indicative of having overeaten or gained weight. Patients who are, or have recently been, underweight are especially prone to feel full as a result of delayed gastric emptying (see Chapter 11). As noted above, neither fullness nor hunger should be used to guide eating, as both tend to be disrupted in people with eating disorders. It often takes some months of regular and healthy eating before these sensations start to normalize. In the meantime patients should follow the "regular eating" guidelines and over-ride any short-lived feelings of fullness that may result.

• *Thinking that one has eaten too much.* This is a cognitive phenomenon and is governed by patients' views about what is an appropriate amount to eat. A good clue as to the harshness of patients' standards for eating can be obtained from their use of asterisks on their monitoring records. Often patients need educating about daily energy requirements. We frequently meet patients who think that if they eat more than 1,200–1,500 kcal per day, they will gain weight and become fat.

- *Perceiving one's abdomen as sticking out excessively.* This is common, especially among patients who are underweight, and is markedly exaggerated by self-scrutiny. (It is an excellent example of a situation in which patients make harsh judgments about their own appearance yet have never seen anyone else's body from the same vantage point; see pages 111 and 178.) The apparent protuberance of the abdomen is exaggerated by certain clothing; by the consumption of a bulky high-fiber diet or large quantities of gaseous drinks; and it may be worse premenstrually. Discussion of this phenomenon should be focused on helping patients avoid equating the experience with having overeaten or with being fat. Commonsense measures can help reduce it, including choosing energy-dense foods rather than high-fiber ones, limiting the consumption of gaseous drinks, controlling scrutiny, and wearing clothes that do not exaggerate it. It may be worth asking patients whether they can see a difference in other people's shape (i.e., their abdomen) after they have eaten (e.g., at work when people come back from lunch). Patients often assume that everyone can see their abdomen sticking out after eating, whereas in reality it is most unlikely to be noticeable.

The educational and dietary aspects of this strategy should be combined with the regular eating intervention. The more shape-related aspects are best left until Stage Three when concerns about shape become a major focus of treatment (see Chapter 8).

- *Clothing feeling abnormally tight.* Addressing this aspect of feeling full involves education about the natural change in shape that may follow eating, and the fact that it passes and is not indicative of having overeaten or being "fat"; the effect of paying particular attention to sensations that would normally go unnoticed; and the potential value of avoiding wearing tight clothes when making changes to eating that could be perceived as eating more (i.e., the introduction of a pattern of regular eating in Stage One, and the tackling of other aspects of dieting in Stage Three). In some cases, and most especially in those who are regaining weight, the patient's clothes may be too small.

- *Feeling fat.* This experience and how to address it are discussed in Chapter 8 (pages 113–116). The topic is best left until Stage Three, although some of the educational points may be made at this point, especially the fact that *feeling* fat should not be equated with *being* fat.

Addressing Low Weight

Most patients with a BMI between 15.0 and 18.9 have to restrict their eating to stay at this weight (i.e., they are at a weight that is too low for them). Doing so maintains their eating disorder and they should be strongly encouraged to gain weight. How to help such patients address undereating and gaining weight is discussed in detail in Chapter 11. It generally necessitates treatment being extended in length.

Addressing Excessive Exercising

As discussed in Chapter 2, excessive exercising is not infrequent in patients with eating disorders. It is most commonly seen in underweight patients and thus is a particular problem in inpatient settings where patients tend to be cooped up and unable to be physically active.

Excessive exercising takes various forms, including:

- Excessive daily activity (e.g., standing rather than sitting; walking excessive amounts)
- Exercising in a normal manner but to an extreme extent (e.g., going to the gym three times every day)
- Exercising in an abnormal manner (e.g., doing extreme numbers of push-ups or sit-ups)

"Driven exercising" is a particular type of excessive exercising. It has the following characteristics:

- A subjective sense of being "driven" or "compelled" to exercise
- Giving exercise precedence over other activities (e.g., socializing)
- Exercising even when it might do one physical harm (e.g., after having been injured; when risking fractures if very underweight).

Like purging, excessive exercising may also be classified according to its function:

- *Compensatory exercising* — This is when exercising is used to compensate for specific episodes of perceived or actual overeating. Generally this type of exercising does not need to be addressed in treatment because it will decline as the patient gains control over eating. Some patients adjust their exercising to match their eating so if they think that they have overeaten they will try to "burn off" the excess number of calories. Others switch this around and try to burn off calories in advance of eating in order to be in "credit." This is referred to as "debting." A less extreme version of this is the view that it is only acceptable to eat if one has done some exercise beforehand.
- *Non-compensatory exercising* — This is when exercising is more like other "routine" forms of weight control (e.g., dieting), in which case the link with eating is not so close. Alternatively, exercising may serve an entirely different function; for example, it may be used to regulate mood (see Chapter 10).

Vignette

A patient was faced with the prospect of a dinner out with her work colleagues. She wanted to attend but was extremely concerned about the amount she would be obliged to eat. She therefore calculated the likely calorie content of the meal and took the preceding 3 days off work to "burn up" the requisite amount of energy.

If a patient's exercising seems excessive, its form and extent should be monitored using the right-hand column of the usual record. Then, assuming it is problematic, the patient should be educated about its potential adverse effects. The main points to stress are that excessive exercise takes up time that could be used in other, more positive ways (e.g., doing things with others); it may encourage overeating through being viewed as an effective means of weight control (whereas it is relatively ineffective); and it can result in over-use injuries. Underweight patients have to be particularly careful about exercising because they are at risk of fractures and adverse cardiac events. Furthermore, exercising can interfere with their weight regain (see Chapter 11).

Unless the exercising has other functions than weight control, it generally decreases during the course of CBT-E as patients become less concerned about their eating, shape and weight. An important exception is when exercising is being used to modulate mood, particularly feelings of tension and anger. Some patients come to rely on exercising to help them cope with their moods in much the same way as they may rely on purging as means of mood modulation. Specific strategies for helping such patients are described in Chapter 10.

It is important to note that CBT-E does not discourage exercising, even in underweight patients. Getting in "good shape" psychologically and physically is integral to CBT-E, but patients may need help in learning how to exercise in a different and less extreme way; for example, by taking up a team sport or by exercising with friends. Social exercising is of general benefit too as it may enhance patients' socializing, something that can be a problem, while also providing an opportunity for body exposure (see page 112). Breaking any link between eating and exercising is also important. Patients involved in high-level competitive sports are difficult to help because ongoing intense exercise tends to contribute to the maintenance of the eating disorder. It is sometimes necessary to advise them that they will have to discontinue the sport in question if they are to overcome the eating problem.

> **Getting in "good shape" psychologically and physically is integral to CBT-E.**

Involving Significant Others

CBT-E is an individual treatment for adults and hence it does not routinely involve others. Despite this, it is our practice to see "significant others" if doing so is likely to facilitate treatment and the patient is willing for this to happen. We include others with the aim of creating the optimum environment for the patient to change. There are two specific indications for involving others:

1. If others could be of help to the patient in making changes
2. If others are making it difficult for the patient to change; for example, by commenting adversely on their appearance or eating

There can be another benefit too. This is the removal of secrecy. Many patients with eating disorders have managed to keep their problem secret for years, and this secrecy has had the effect of making it easier for them to continue to engage in certain behavior (e.g., self-induced vomiting). For such patients "coming out" is tantamount to burning their boats as there is no going back. The benefit is that family and friends are generally supportive rather than critical, and doing so is evidence of the patient's commitment to change and desire to make a "fresh start."

Typically the sessions with others last about 45 minutes and take place immediately after a routine individual session (i.e., the whole appointment lasts about 95 minutes, the first 50 minutes being with just the patient and the therapist, with the significant other[s] joining the patient and therapist for the second half of the appointment). Preparation in advance is important and involves discussing with the patient the aim and format of the meeting and agreeing who will do what. Generally the meeting involves the following:

- An introduction by the therapist and a statement about the aims of the meeting
- The patient explaining something about treatment and its rationale, and what he or she is currently trying to do
- Listening to the point of view of the significant other(s), answering their questions and addressing their problems. For example, various aspects of eating disorder psychopathology can be extremely trying for those who live with the patient. These include undereating, slow eating, eating alone, and reluctance or refusal to eat out. Also difficult for partners is some patients' dislike of their body being seen or touched. All these problems are directly addressed in treatment. Another common complaint of significant others is patients' repeated reassurance-seeking (with regard to their eating or appearance). This can be very frustrating and may lead to arguments. The best strategy in such cases is the one used in the treatment of obsessive–compulsive disorder. This is to explain to the patient and significant other that providing such reassurance is not in the patient's interests because it only brings transitory relief, if that, and that instead it is better either to decline to provide reassurance altogether or to give it only once. Although difficult initially for the patient, this results in a progressive decline in his or her need for reassurance which is soon experienced as a relief.
- Discussing how the significant other(s) could be of practical help to the patient; for example:
    - By responding to requests for help, such as when the patient is having difficulty coping with urges to eat between planned meals or snacks
    - By helping underweight patients choose what to eat and how much and, later on, by stepping back and letting patients make these decisions themselves

We hold up to three such sessions with the significant others of about three-quarters of our patients. Sometimes we have more of these sessions with underweight patients (see Chapter 11). Topics outside the eating disorder are not usually addressed. With adolescent patients there is far greater involvement of others (see Chapters 14 and 15).

Moving to Stage Two

At the end of session 7, patients should be reminded that the appointments will now become weekly, and that part of the next session will be devoted to taking stock, the aim being to assess in detail the progress made so far.

Recommended Reading

Recommended reading for Chapters 5–12 can be found at the end of Chapter 12.

CHAPTER 7

Taking Stock and Designing the Rest of Treatment

This chapter is concerned with the second stage in treatment. This is a transitional stage and comprises one or two sessions. It has five aims:

1. To conduct a joint review of progress
2. To identify emerging barriers to change
3. To review the formulation
4. To decide whether to use the broad form of CBT-E
5. To design Stage Three

At the same time the therapist continues to implement the procedures introduced in Stage One. The sessions are now held once a week.

Conducting a Joint Review of Progress

As noted earlier, there is strong evidence across a variety of psychiatric disorders, including bulimia nervosa and binge eating disorder, that the magnitude of change during the first few weeks of treatment is a potent predictor of outcome. Thus it is crucial that the initial stages of treatment are implemented well. This finding also suggests that if progress is limited, this needs to be recognized early on, and the explanation sought, so that treatment can be adjusted to overcome any obstacles to change. This goal is achieved by conducting a formal review of progress early in treatment.

> If progress is limited, this needs to be recognized early on, and the explanation sought, so that treatment can be adjusted.

This review is best done systematically and jointly with the patient. It is a good idea to ask the patient to complete, once again, the EDE-Q, CIA and the measure of general psychiatric features used at the outset. In this way the patient and therapist can objectively assess the nature and extent of change.

Generally patients' views on their progress are unduly negative. It is important therefore that the therapist help the patient arrive at a balanced appraisal of what has changed and what has not. Typically there will have been an improvement in the pattern of eating and a decrease in the frequency of any binge eating and compensatory purging, whereas concerns about shape will not have changed (largely because they will not have been addressed). The aim is to identify what remains a problem and needs to be addressed while also highlighting the changes that have taken place. It can also be helpful to discuss with patients what has helped them so far. This tends to reinforce the therapeutic procedures already used. In addition, it is a good opportunity to praise patients and attribute change to them.

> **One important, and sometimes overlooked, reason for progress not being as great as might be expected is the presence of a clinical depression.**

One important, and sometimes overlooked, reason for progress not being as great as might be expected is the presence of a clinical depression. Ideally such depressions should be detected and treated before treatment starts, but inevitably some slip though the net and others develop afresh. Features suggestive of a clinical depression are described in Chapter 16 (page 246). Telltale signs in the context of treatment are a change in the patient's manner, typically characterized by increased self-criticism, reduced enthusiasm and drive, and decreased compliance with homework assignments (e.g., a deterioration in the quality of self-monitoring). If we conclude that there is a co-existing clinical depression, we treat it with antidepressant medication (following the guidelines on page 248) and often suspend CBT-E until the patient has responded, providing supportive depression-oriented sessions in the interim. Once the depression has resolved, we restart CBT-E with an initial catch-up session to re-orient the patient. In addition, we may extend treatment to compensate for the disrupting effect of the depression.

Identifying Barriers to Change

The second aspect of Stage Two is identifying barriers to change. This involves assessing the patient's attitude to treatment and use of its various procedures. This should be done overtly, with the therapist introducing the topic by saying something along these lines:

> *"This would be a good time to review not only your progress but also your feelings about treatment. Are you happy with what we are doing and how things are progressing? Are there any concerns that you would like to raise?*
>
> *"We should also review the extent to which you have been able to make use of treatment by making the changes that we have agreed. I have a table that lists the various elements of treatment so far. Let's go over the table together and consider how you have been getting on."*

The therapist then goes through the table with the patient, element by element (see Table 7.1).

If problems with engagement or the use of specific procedures are identified, the therapist needs to explore their origin. There are two sources: the eating disorder itself and other more general factors. With regard to the former, the mechanisms maintaining the eating disorder may be sufficiently potent to prevent patients from making the agreed changes despite their best efforts. For example, many patients continue to binge eat while eating regular meals and snacks. This can usually be ascribed in part to dietary restraint, which will not have yet been formally addressed, and in part to the influence of

TABLE 7.1. Elements of Stage One

Treatment elements	How treatment is going		
	Not going well	Going reasonably well	Going well
Attending sessions			
Being on time			
Recording (monitoring)			
Not weighing at home			
Reading *Overcoming Binge Eating*			
Eating regular meals and snacks			
Not eating between the meals and snacks			
Giving treatment priority			
Other elements			

mood and external events. Similarly, some patients may still be weighing themselves at home as a result of fears of weight gain, and underweight patients may not yet have decided to regain weight (see Chapter 11). Reviewing such barriers to change is best done with reference to the patient's formulation.

More general barriers to change include the following:

1. *Fear of change* (e.g., due to concerns about no longer having an excuse for not succeeding at things or no longer being "special")
   - The addressing of such fears is discussed in Chapters 5 (page 56) and 11 (page 164). Chapter 11 is especially relevant because it discusses in detail means of increasing the motivation of underweight patients, a notoriously ambivalent group. The strategies and procedures described there may be used with other patients who are ambivalent.

2. *Resistance to change in general* (i.e., rigidity)
   - In these cases the source of the resistance needs to be explored. Does it stem from fear of the consequences of change or is there more general resistance to any form of change? If the former, then the fear needs to be explored and addressed. If the latter, the resistance may be attributable to the psychological effects of being underweight (see Chapter 11) or the influence of clinical perfectionism (see Chapter 13).

3. *Competing commitments* (e.g., pressure of work, demands of children)
   - In these cases the importance of giving treatment priority needs to be stressed. A formal assessment of the pros and cons of change, adopting two time frames, is often helpful (see Chapter 11).

4. *External events and interpersonal difficulties*
   - Major life events invariably disrupt progress. The handling of life crises that occur during the course of treatment is discussed in Chapter 16. The broad version of CBT-E addresses interpersonal difficulties and so might be appropriate for such patients (see Chapter 13).

5. *Poor planning*
   - If this applies, the vital importance of planning needs to be re-emphasized (see Chapter 6) and the therapist needs to help the patient become more organized.

6. *Clinical depression*
   - As noted above, patients with a co-existing clinical depression tend to make limited progress as a result of their reduced drive and optimism. If a clinical depression is suspected, a full assessment needs to be made and the depression treated if necessary (see Chapter 16).

7. *Core low self-esteem*
   - Patients with severe low self-esteem tend not to believe that they are capable of making changes, nor do they think that they merit treatment. (These features may also been seen in those with a clinical depression.) The broad version of CBT-E addresses core low self-esteem (see Chapter 13).

8. *Clinical perfectionism*
   - Patients with clinical perfectionism apply their extreme standards to all aspects of life that they value. If they have an eating disorder they apply their high standards to their dieting, weight and appearance. This makes change especially difficult. They also apply their standards to treatment itself, which tends to complicate matters and slow progress. The broad version of CBT-E addresses clinical perfectionism (see Chapter 13).

9. *Substance misuse*
   - As noted earlier (see Chapter 4) persistent substance misuse undermines the patient's ability to utilize treatment. If it is proving to be a barrier to change, it needs to be addressed in its own right and CBT-E suspended or abandoned for the meantime. Intermittent substance misuse can often be addressed in the context of CBT-E.

10. *Dislike of CBT*
    - In our experience this is unusual. Occasionally patients who have received extensive prior exposure to other forms of therapy (e.g., psychodynamic psychotherapy or an addiction model-based treatment) have difficulty adjusting to the different rationale and mode of treatment. As noted in Chapter 4, under these circumstances we ask patients to try to suspend their skepticism and simply accept that this is an empirically supported treatment that has a good chance of helping them if they commit themselves to it.

11. *Poor implementation of the treatment by the therapist*
    - This situation is to be avoided if at all possible. We have weekly peer supervision meetings in the form of a "closed" group (i.e., it is restricted to our therapists). This arrangement is designed to provide a setting in which we can discuss our clinical work freely and at length. In addition, we are able lis-

ten to selected recordings of each others' treatment sessions. In this way we try to maintain a high standard of treatment implementation. As noted in Chapter 1, we recommend that all CBT-E therapists seek out training and ongoing peer supervision.

Reviewing the Formulation

It is important to review the formulation in light of what has been learned during Stage One and what has emerged during the review of progress and barriers to change. Often no modifications are required, but sometimes problems and processes are detected that were not obvious at the initial assessment when the formulation was originally created. For example, it may have emerged that non-compensatory purging is a far greater problem than had been thought. If so, the formulation needs to be revised.

Deciding Whether to Use the Broad Version of CBT-E

The decision whether or not to use the broad version of CBT-E is a major one because it governs the form and content of the treatment from this point onward. It is also likely to have an impact on the patient's outcome, either for the better or the worse. The basis for making this decision is described in detail in Chapter 13. Suffice it to say that the default form of CBT-E is the focused version. With most patients it is more effective than the broad version, and it is easier to implement. The following five chapters (Chapters 8–12) describe how to implement the focused form. Chapter 13 describes when and how to use the broad version.

Designing Stage Three

Stage Three is the main body of treatment during which the therapist addresses the key mechanisms that are maintaining the patient's eating disorder while continuing to implement the strategies and procedures introduced in Stage One. Thus, returning to the house of cards analogy (see page 47), this is the time when the key structural cards supporting the eating disorder are identified and removed. Precisely how this is done varies from patient to patient.

The Six Main Maintaining Mechanisms

A variety of mechanisms serve to maintain most eating disorders. These may be categorized under the following six headings:

1. The over-evaluation of shape and weight
2. The over-evaluation of control over eating
3. Dietary restraint
4. Dietary restriction
5. Being underweight
6. Event- or mood-triggered changes in eating

The relative contributions of these mechanisms vary from individual to individual. In some patients relatively few maintaining mechanisms operate, as in many cases of binge eating disorder, whereas in others the opposite is the case, as in the binge eating/purging form of anorexia nervosa.

The Over-Evaluation of Shape and Weight

Most adults with an eating disorder have the characteristic over-evaluation of shape and weight, the so-called "core psychopathology" (see Chapters 2 and 8). This will have been detected at the initial assessment and will occupy a central place in the patient's formulation. It is likely to have proved a barrier to change in Stage One.

The Over-Evaluation of Control Over Eating

In a subgroup of patients there is over-evaluation of control over eating per se rather than a desire to control eating in order to influence shape and weight (see Chapter 9), although the two may co-exist. Such patients tend to be especially concerned about the details of their eating (e.g., their exact calorie intake, their food choice and when they eat) and they show relatively little body checking, body avoidance or feeling fat. This type of presentation is most common in young patients, especially those with a short history. It is also seen in non-Western cases.

Dietary Restraint

The term "dietary restraint" refers to attempts to restrict eating. As noted in Chapter 2, this may or may not result in actual undereating in the physiological sense (dietary restriction). In most patients with an eating disorder there is a particularly rigid form of dietary restraint with multiple extreme dietary rules. Although dietary restraint is almost always maintained by the over-evaluation of shape and weight, or the over-evaluation of controlling eating per se, it generally needs to be tackled in its own right.

Dietary Restriction

Dietary restriction refers to true undereating in the physiological sense. It results in weight loss or the maintenance of an unduly low weight. If either is present, the dietary restriction needs to be addressed (see Chapter 11).

Being Underweight

There is no single BMI threshold that satisfactorily defines being underweight in all cases, but the thresholds specified earlier (see page 15) make clinical sense and work well in practice. They are as follows:

Significantly underweight	BMI 17.5 or below
Underweight	BMI 17.6–18.9
Low weight	BMI 19.0–19.9

With a BMI below 19.0 most people experience some adverse physical and psycho-social effects of being underweight, and few people in Western societies (other than some of Asian origin) can maintain a BMI at this level without actively restricting what they eat. At a BMI of 17.5 or below people are subject to marked adverse physical and psychosocial effects (see Chapter 11).

Event- or Mood-Triggered Changes in Eating

In some patients the eating disorder is seemingly autonomous and more or less impervious to outside events and circumstances. More commonly, events, circumstances and moods influence the patient's eating.

If the eating disorder is very reactive, in the sense that its state appears to be particularly sensitive to outside events or moods, it may be that certain of its features are serving the function of helping the patient cope with adverse thoughts and feelings. This is often the case with binge eating and vomiting, and exercising may serve this purpose too.

Choosing Which Mechanisms to Address and in What Order

To design Stage Three the therapist needs to consider the relative contributions of these maintaining processes. Next, the order in which they are addressed needs to be decided. Below are some guidelines to help therapists make this decision.

- If the patient is underweight, this is the top priority because being underweight is physically harmful and the psychosocial consequences of starvation powerfully maintain the eating disorder. The treatment of underweight patients is described in Chapter 11.
- If there is over-evaluation of shape or weight, or of controlling eating, it is best to open Stage Three by starting to address this because it is one of the most difficult and time-consuming of the mechanisms to tackle (see Chapters 8 and 9).
- In patients who are not underweight, dietary restraint and dietary restriction may be dealt with together (see Chapters 9 and 11 respectively). It is best to start doing this a week or two after beginning to address the "over-evaluation" mechanisms. In patients who are underweight dietary restriction is tackled in the course of addressing the low weight.
- In patients in whom the eating disorder is clearly sensitive to outside events and moods, this is best addressed a week or two after starting to tackle dietary restraint, assuming that restraint is present. On the other hand, if the phenomenon is particularly prominent (e.g., if there are frequent event- or mood-triggered episodes of binge eating), it is best to reverse this sequence.

Thus the plan for Stage Three is determined by the formulation and these guidelines. However, the plan should not be inflexible: It may need to be adjusted in light of circumstances and changes in the form of the eating disorder. Throughout, therapists should try to maintain the therapeutic momentum established in Stage One.

Recommended Reading

Recommended reading for Chapters 5–12 can be found at the end of Chapter 12.

CHAPTER 8

Shape Concern, Shape Checking, Feeling Fat and Mindsets

At the heart of most eating disorders is the distinctive "core psychopathology," the over-evaluation of shape and weight and their control; that is, the judging of self-worth largely, or even exclusively, in terms of shape and weight and the ability to control them. As described in Chapter 2, most other features of these disorders appear to be secondary to this psychopathology and its consequences (e.g., under-eating leading to low weight; rigid and extreme dietary restraint leading to binge eating). It is for this reason that this psychopathology occupies a central place in most patients' formulation and is a major target of treatment. Clinical experience and research evidence suggest that unless it is successfully addressed, patients are at substantial risk of relapse.

> **Most features appear to be secondary to the core psychopathology.**

In this chapter strategies and procedures for addressing the concerns about shape and weight are described. This aspect of treatment takes time to deliver and change is gradual. Therefore, when designing Stage Three it is best to ensure that it is started early. It has six main elements:

1. Identifying the over-evaluation and its consequences
2. Enhancing the importance of other domains for self-evaluation
3. Addressing shape checking and avoidance. Weight checking and avoidance were addressed in Stage One
4. Addressing "feeling fat"
5. Exploring the origins of the over-evaluation
6. Learning to control the eating disorder mindset

Generally the first four elements are introduced in this order, and early on, as they take time to implement and have their effect. The last two are best left until near the end of

Stage Three. Once this psychopathology has begun to be addressed, it should remain a permanent item on the session agenda.

Identifying the Over-Evaluation and Its Consequences

The starting point is educating the patient about the rather complex and abstract topic of self-evaluation. The therapist then helps the patient identify his or her particular scheme for self-evaluation. Finally the implications of this scheme are discussed and a plan for addressing the over-evaluation is devised.

As therapists are often unsure about how to broach the subject of self-evaluation, an illustrative dialogue is provided below.

THERAPIST: *We've decided that today we are going to focus primarily on your concerns about your shape and appearance. I'd like to go back to why we are doing this. If we look back at the diagram that shows the things that you and I have identified as driving your eating problem [the therapist refers to the patient's formulation], you can see that your concerns about your shape and weight occupy a central position. Clearly we need to focus on them in addition to your eating as they seem important in keeping your eating problem going and they really worry you.*

PATIENT: *Yes, my shape is the main thing I worry about. It really bothers me . . . the fact that I am always worrying about my shape . . . and the fact that it is so awful. I hate it.*

THERAPIST: *Well, to start with we need to talk about the way we all evaluate or judge ourselves — something most of us don't even think about. All of us have a system, or way, of judging ourselves. If we are meeting our personal standards in the areas of life we value, we feel reasonably good about ourselves, but if we are not we feel bad. Typically people judge themselves according to various things; for example, relationships with others are often important . . . say, how one is doing in one's relationships with one's parents (and children, if one has any) and one's relationships with friends. Other things that may be important are how one is getting on at work and at important pastimes . . . say, sports, singing, music, cooking, or whatever. And one's appearance too may be important. Now, if things are going well in these various areas of life, one feels fine, but if they are not, one feels bad. Indeed, feeling bad is the best clue as to an individual area's importance. If one feels really bad if an aspect of life is not going well, this strongly suggests that this aspect is very important to one's self-evaluation. Does this make sense?*

PATIENT: *Yes, I think so. The way I look, for example, it makes me feel really bad. I won't go out some days.*

THERAPIST: *Exactly. So this indicates that your shape or appearance is very important in how you see, or judge, yourself. Now a good way of representing all this is to draw a pie chart, with the various slices representing the various aspects of life that are important to you in terms of how you judge yourself as a person, and the bigger the slice the more important it is. Now what I would like us to do is to try to draw your pie chart.*

What we first need to do is list the things that are important in the way you judge, or evaluate, yourself. What might they be?

The therapist then helps the patient generate a list of areas of life that are important to his or her self-evaluation. Sometimes it is necessary to help patients distinguish things in their life that they regard as "important" in general (i.e., because they are widely regarded as such; e.g., work) but do not in practice influence the way they view themselves, and things that truly have an impact on the patient's self-evaluation. If the patient finds it difficult to generate such a list, the therapist should provide typical examples, perhaps by saying *"Some people judge themselves in terms of the quality of their relationship with their partner, what they manage to achieve at work, their musical accomplishments, their appearance, etc."* In the great majority of cases the list will include shape (i.e., appearance) and weight, and the ability to control them, but as mentioned earlier in a minority of cases there is over-evaluation of controlling eating for its own sake and not for the sake of controlling shape or weight. If shape, weight or controlling eating are not mentioned by the patient, the therapist should mention them, perhaps along these lines: *"And what about your appearance, your shape and weight and controlling your eating, are they important? Should we include them?"*

Having generated a list, the therapist should go on to explore with the patient the relative importance of the identified domains of self-evaluation, the best clue to their relative importance being the magnitude (in terms of intensity and duration) of the patient's response to things going badly in each area. In this way the various areas can be ranked. Therapists should ensure that they establish how patients really evaluate themselves, not how they think they ought to evaluate themselves. If the patient seems hesitant, the therapist might add: *"Most people with eating problems are not happy with their means of self-evaluation, but it is important that we characterize it accurately so that we can understand it and its effects."* Finally, the therapist and patient draw out a tentative pie chart, the size of each slice representing the relative importance of that area of life in the patient's self-evaluative scheme. A representative pie chart is shown in Figure 8.1, the pie charts of patients with eating disorders typically being dominated by a large slice representing the over-evaluation of shape and weight and their control. This is quite unlike the type of pie chart drawn by healthy young people without an eating disorder (illustrated in

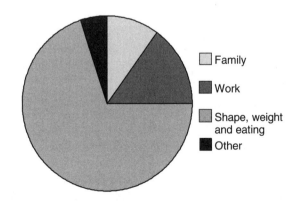

FIGURE 8.1. The pie chart of patient A.

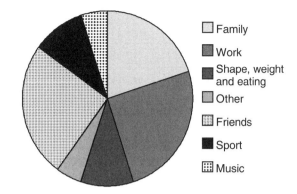

FIGURE 8.2. A pie chart of a young woman without an eating problem.

Figure 8.2). Finally, the therapist should ask for the patient's view on his or her pie chart. Many patients are embarrassed and ashamed about the importance they place on their shape and weight. They should be reassured that this over-evaluation is typical of people with eating problems and is something that they can change.

As homework, patients should be asked to review their pie chart and think whether it accurately represents the true state of affairs based on their day-to-day attitudes and behavior. To this end it can be helpful for patients to redraw their pie chart at intervals (on the back of the day's monitoring record). At the next session the pie chart should be discussed further and the size of the slices adjusted as needed. Generally, any revision takes the form of expanding the size of the slice representing the importance of shape and weight.

Next, the patient should be asked to consider the implications of his or her scheme for self-evaluation (as represented by the pie chart) and think whether there might be any problems inherent to it. This discussion should lead to the identification of the main adverse consequences of over-evaluating shape and weight and their control:

1. *Having a pie chart with a dominant slice is "risky."* In this context the therapist might say:

> *"It is like having all your eggs in one basket. This is fine so long as everything is going well in this regard, but if it isn't, one is in trouble. A parallel can be drawn with top athletes who also tend to have a dominant slice in their pie chart, one concerned with their athletic performance. If, unexpectedly, they can no longer compete, say as a result of injury or illness, they tend to have great trouble adjusting to this change in their circumstances because all their self-evaluative 'eggs' have been in one single basket."*

2. *Having a pie chart with a dominant slice narrows one's life and is self-perpetuating.* It results in the marginalization of other aspects of life. Nothing else much matters. It leads to life being seen from this perspective only. As a result interests, aptitudes and relationships can get ignored and life gets reduced to controlling shape, weight and eating. In this regard it can be helpful to ask patients to take a long-term perspective on the consequences of having such a dominant slice. They can be asked what they would like to

have achieved by the time they reach old age. They may not wish to have attained a flat stomach to the detriment of other aspects of their life (see following vignette).

Vignette

A contributor to *Overcoming Binge Eating* (Fairburn, 1995) wrote:

"As I grow into middle age I realize with great sadness how much energy I have directed toward controlling my weight and eating and the misery of the regular and consequent binges. I could be doing something productive with my energy — building relationships, reading, writing. I don't know what I might do, but I don't want my epitaph to be 'Jane wished she was thin.'" (p. 132)

---

3.   Judging oneself on the basis of appearance and weight, and one's ability to control them, is inherently problematic. The therapist might say:

"In your case the problem is not only one of having most of your eggs in one basket, it also lies in the nature of the basket itself. It is not a good one. This is because success in this area of life is elusive and apparent failure ever present. This is for a number of reasons, some of which we will discuss in great detail later, but briefly, it is problematic basing one's self-evaluation on one's appearance and weight because:

"a.   One's shape, weight and eating are not fully under one's control. We only have a limited ability to control our eating (and hence our shape and weight), because it is under strong physiological control. One can manipulate it in the short-term but to do so on a long-term basis requires considerable and sustained effort, and one pays a price as a result [see below]. Similarly, one's overall body shape or physique is only partially under one's influence. It is mainly something one just has to accept.

"b.   There will always be lots of people who seem more attractive (i.e., successful in your eyes) than you. In part this is because of the way people with eating problems judge their appearance, which is prone to make them see themselves as unattractive; and in part it is because of the way they compare themselves with others, which has the same negative effect. We will discuss both these topics later. The result of these two processes is that people with eating problems repeatedly feel that they are failing.

"c.   Judging yourself in this way leads you to do things that harm you, such as . . . [the therapist lists applicable examples, such as undereating, binge eating, self-induced vomiting, laxative misuse, etc.], *and it maintains your eating problem. And doing these things also impairs the quality of your day-to-day life."* [The therapist may highlight the main sources of impairment detected on the CIA questionnaire completed in Stage Two.]

This discussion leads naturally to the final step in the consideration of self-evaluation, namely the creation of an "extended formulation" that includes the consequences of the over-evaluation. The therapist starts this process by asking the patient what he or she does, or experiences, as a result of the importance he or she places on shape, weight and appearance. The goal is to derive a figure resembling that shown in Figure 8.3, with the therapist adding and emphasizing the feedback arrows, saying something along these lines:

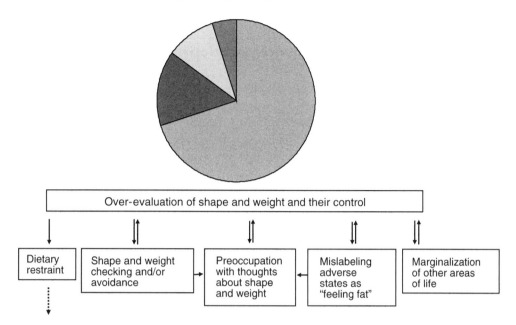

FIGURE 8.3. The over-evaluation of control over shape and weight: an "extended form-ulation."

From *Cognitive Behavior Therapy and Eating Disorders* by Christopher G. Fairburn. Copyright 2008 by The Guilford Press. This figure is available online at www.psych.ox.ac.uk/credo/cbt_and_eating_disorders.

"These things that you do, or that happen, as a result of your concerns about your shape and weight, and your wish to control them, are themselves likely to maintain your concerns. For example, repeatedly checking your body will intensify your dissatisfaction with your shape. Similarly, avoiding seeing parts of your body or avoiding knowing your weight will result in your fears and concerns persisting unquestioned. We haven't yet discussed 'feeling fat,' but it tends to be equated with 'being fat' and so keeps one unhappy with one's appearance. The point is that it is vital that we tackle these consequences of your concerns because they main-tain your dissatisfaction with your shape and weight. As you can see there is a set of vicious circles here, and tackling these things is the best way of breaking into them."

Finally, in collaboration with the patient, the therapist devises a plan for addressing the concerns about shape and weight and their control. This involves employing two complementary strategies, both of which are important:

1. *Enhancing the importance of other domains for self-evaluation* (i.e., increasing the size and number of other slices in the patient's pie chart)

2. *Reducing the importance attached to shape and weight and their control* (i.e., decreasing the size of the shape and weight slice). The most potent way of doing this is to tackle the expressions of the over-evaluation. In terms of shape, they are shape checking, shape avoidance and feeling fat. With respect to weight, they are frequent weighing and the avoidance of knowing one's weight, both of which were addressed in Stage One. In terms of control over eating, they are dietary restraint and dietary restriction (see Chap-ters 9 and 11 respectively).

Enhancing the Importance of Other Domains
for Self-Evaluation

> **The over-evaluation of shape and weight results in the marginalization of areas of life that might contribute positively to self-evaluation.**

The over-evaluation of shape and weight results in the marginalization of areas of life that might contribute positively to self-evaluation. There are two aspects to the marginalization: First, the other areas are few in number (i.e., there are few other slices in the patient's pie chart); and second, they are of limited importance (i.e., the slices are small in size). The goal therefore is that patients begin to engage in other areas of life, and that these areas become more important in their self-evaluation.

Enhancing the importance of other domains has an additional benefit. Eating disorders generally begin in mid-to-late adolescence. Those cases that persist into adulthood will have generally been present for many years. During this time the patient's life will have been dominated by the eating disorder while other interests, activities and aptitudes will have fallen by the wayside. While the patient's life has been

> **Patients with eating disorders miss out on important normative age-related experiences and develop secondary interpersonal deficits as a result.**

taken up with dieting, exercising and concerns about shape and weight, his or her contemporaries will have been doing the many things that people their age do. Thus patients with eating disorders miss out on important normative age-related experiences and develop secondary interpersonal deficits as a result. Assisting them to develop previously marginalized domains for self-evaluation often has the added benefit of helping them catch up developmentally.

There are five steps in helping patients engage in, and begin to value, other aspects of life:

1. *Explain the rationale for doing this.* For example, the therapist might say:

> *"You have said that you are unhappy with the way your current pie chart looks. In particular you have said that you would like the eating, shape and weight slices to be smaller. One way of achieving this is by engaging in other aspects of life, areas that have been pushed aside. Investing time doing this will result in these other areas becoming more important and more relevant to how you judge yourself as a person."*

2. *Identify new activities in which the patient might become involved.* A clue may come from activities or interests that the patient had prior to developing the eating disorder. The patient might have been a tennis player or painter, or been interested in hiking or acting. It does not matter what the activity was or how good the patient was at it, it is simply valuable to consider previous interests and activities. A "brainstorming" approach is best here with all possibilities being listed even if they seem (to the patient) silly or intimidating. Some patients are hesitant and so rule out quite promising possibilities, and many have difficulty thinking of activities, having spent so much time preoccupied with thoughts about eating, shape and weight. Sometimes good ideas can come from patients' considering what their friends or work colleagues do in their spare time.

3. *Agree on one, or possibly two, activities that the patient will try.* These can be anything so long as they are feasible and not single one-off events. It is best if they involve others as they are more likely to become self-perpetuating. Furthermore, contact with others can help patients "catch up" interpersonally.

4. *Ensure that the patient actually does start to engage in the activity identified.* The therapist should ask the patient to record the activity in the last column of his or her monitoring record, and barriers to engaging in it should be reviewed and solutions sought. A problem-solving approach is often best. (With some patients problem-solving will have been taught in the context of addressing event-triggered changes in eating [see Chapter 10]. In others the technique will need to be introduced at this point.) Therapists should not refrain from being active in helping hesitant patients get started. For example, if the patient is considering joining some type of dance class, it would be quite appropriate for the therapist to help the patient work out ways of identifying suitable classes and the steps involved in joining them. This is because the priority is to get the patient started. Thereafter the therapist should step back.

5. *Review progress week by week* (as a permanent item on the session agenda). The therapist should be encouraging and facilitative. Patients should be helped to use problem-solving to overcome any difficulties they encounter. Over the course of treatment additional new activities may be identified and adopted, while others may be dropped. Toward the end of treatment it is worth asking patients to draw their pie chart again, as doing so provides an opportunity to review progress and praise patients for the changes that they have made. What is usually found is that the "slice" representing shape and weight has shrunk in size and new slices have appeared.

Addressing Shape Checking and Avoidance

At the same time as enhancing the importance of other domains for self-evaluation, the therapist should target the patient's over-evaluation of shape and weight. Often it is best to begin by addressing shape checking, as this tends to be particularly influential in maintaining dissatisfaction with shape, but before doing so it is worth noting with the patient that one form of body checking has already been addressed, namely weight checking. This was tackled in Stage One in the context of "in-session weighing" (see page 62). Almost invariably patients will have found in-session weighing helpful because (after a few weeks) it will have decreased their level of concern about weight (i.e., the number on the scale). They should be told that equivalent benefits will result from addressing shape checking.

The importance of tackling shape checking and shape avoidance has only recently been appreciated. The reason is quite simple: Few clinicians were aware of these phenomena. This lack of awareness was due in part to patients' not disclosing the behavior unless directly asked; indeed, many patients are not even aware that they do it. Strangely, the behavior has been right under our nose, as it were, as it is not uncommon for patients to check their shape during treatment sessions. (This will become apparent if therapists observe carefully what patients are doing with their hands. Some repeatedly touch their arms, shoulders or collar bones to check that they can feel their bones, and many do this without being aware of it.)

Educating Patients about Shape Checking and Avoidance

The initial step is to educate the patient about shape checking and shape avoidance and their effects, stressing the following four general points:

1. Everyone checks their body to some extent, but many people with eating problems repeatedly check their bodies and often in a way that is unusual. Such checking can become so "second nature" that they may not be fully aware that they are doing it; for example, when taking a shower some people are also shape checking. In people with eating problems such shape checking needs to be addressed, as it tends to maintain their dissatisfaction with their body and appearance.

2. Some people with eating problems avoid seeing their bodies and dislike other people seeing them too. Often these people engaged in repeated shape checking in the past but switched over to avoidance because the checking became too distressing. Shape avoidance may take the form of avoiding looking in the mirror, not wearing tight clothes, covering the stomach (e.g., with the arms), and not looking at photographs. It is problematic because it allows concerns and fears about shape and appearance to persist in the absence of knowledge about what one actually looks like. Therefore it too needs to be tackled.

3. Shape checking and avoidance can co-exist. Some patients repeatedly check parts of their body and avoid others, or switch from checking to avoidance and back.

4. Comparing oneself with others is a special form of shape checking. People with eating problems do this repeatedly and in a way that makes them seem unattractive relative to other people. This too must be addressed.

Assessing Shape Checking

Next, the therapist needs to assess the patient's shape checking. Although there are various standard body checking questionnaires (see Recommended Reading, page 192), we find that asking patients to record each time they check their body (using an adaptation of the usual monitoring record; see Figure 8.4) is more informative clinically, not least because some forms of shape checking become so second nature that patients are not fully aware that they do them. For this reason scores on questionnaires can be spurious. As recording shape checking can be very distressing, it is best to ask patients to do it for just two 24-hour periods, one (if the patient works) being a working day and the other being a day off work. The therapist may say something along these lines:

> "To find out what shape checking you are doing, please record every time you check your body or compare someone else's body with your own. It is best to do this recording on one workday and on one day when you are not working, as they may differ. Here is an adaptation of our usual record for doing this. You may find that you have a lot to write down. Don't worry about this. It may also be quite upsetting: Indeed, you may feel like leaving some things off. Try to write everything down as we need to know exactly what you are doing."

To help patients record their shape checking it is best to discuss the types of behavior that should be recorded. Common examples include looking in the mirror (or at reflective surfaces) at particular body parts, measuring body parts with a tape measure or the hands, pinching or touching body parts, assessing the tightness of particular items of

Time	Food and drink consumed	Place	*	V/L	Checking (what done, time taken)	Place	Context and comments
6:30	Glass water	Kitchen			Looked at reflection in mirror (2 mins.)	Kitchen	My face looks really fat
7:00					Looked in mirror while getting dressed – stood sideways (2 mins.) Pinched my fat rolls (5 mins.)	Bedroom	Ughh my stomach is so gross
7:10	Banana, bowl of cheerios	Kitchen					Fine
8:30					Checked to see if my backside looks big in this skirt (5 mins.)	Bathroom at work	How can I be so fat already? I have only eaten breakfast!
10:00	Cereal bar	At desk	*		Looked down at stomach while having snack (2 mins.)	Desk	Cannot believe that my stomach is so big – it is making me grossed out to look at it – why can't I just be skinny?
1:15	Peanut butter and jelly on whole wheat (2 slices of bread)	Park			Watched thin runners in the park (15 mins.)	Park	Shouldn't have had peanut butter, it is so fattening. I SHOULD be running during lunch like all of those other people!
3:00	Apple	Desk					At least I was able to just have an apple and not eat the cake in the office kitchen
6:30	Veggies (large plate) and tuna fish	Kitchen				Living room	Good dinner – feeling in control
7:30					Read US Weekly about latest celeb diet (15 mins.)		I am so jealous of these women – if only I had a personal trainer and more willpower.
9:00	One small pot of yogurt	Living room			Looked at my thighs as they spread out when sitting down (1 min.)	Living room	I am so sick of this! I hate myself.

FIGURE 8.4. A body checking monitoring record (patient A).

clothing (e.g., waistbands of pants) and accessories (e.g., watches or rings), and looking down at one's body (e.g., at one's thighs or stomach when sitting). Some patients may also do these things in an unusual way so it is important to ask for details of what is done, how it is done (e.g., looking in the mirror sideways) and for how long. Patients should also record their thoughts and feelings during and after checking. All this should be recorded "live" as far as possible. Male patients tend to be especially concerned about their build and muscularity but less concerned about their weight.

At the next session the therapist should review in detail what has been recorded, asking the patient if the selected days were typical ones to ensure that most forms of checking have been identified. It is common for patients to be shocked at how often they check their shape.

Questioning Shape Checking

Having identified the various forms of body checking, patients should be asked to consider why they check themselves in this way and what the consequences are.

QUESTION 1: *"What are you trying to find out when you check your body? Do you think you can find it out this way?"*

— Most patients have not really considered what they are trying to find out from their shape checking but will have some ideas. They may say that they check their shape in order *"To find out what my shape is like."* If this is the case it is helpful to explain that scrutiny is prone to magnify apparent defects (see page 107). Given this, they are unlikely to be able to discover more about their true shape by repeatedly looking at their body. Education may also need to be provided regarding aspects of shape that are normal (e.g., having a slightly protruding abdomen) as patients may have picked up inaccuracies from media images.

Other patients say that they are checking *"To see if my shape is changing"* (or *"To see if I am getting fat"*). In this case it is helpful to discuss how most forms of body checking do not generate sufficiently reliable quantitative information to detect change. Instead they simply provide an impression about shape. Checking oneself in the mirror is a good example. We cannot with any accuracy compare one "look" say first thing in the morning with another "look" a few hours later because we do not have a photographic memory of the type that would enable us to contrast the first image with the second.

QUESTION 2: *"Why are you checking yourself so frequently? Do you think you might be checking yourself too often?*

— Usually patients have difficulty answering this question and eventually come up with a reply along the lines that *"To check that my shape hasn't changed."* The therapist should respond by asking whether the patient thinks that his or her shape is changing so rapidly as to justify their frequency of body checking (often in the absence of any weight change), which clearly he or she does not. In this way patients can be helped to arrive at the conclusion that it does not make sense to check their shape so often. Occasionally patients express the concern that their abdomen changes in shape through the day. It is helpful to point out that this is an example of a normal fluctuation in shape that is *not* indicative of weight gain nor is it perceptible to others. To illustrate this point, patients may be asked if they have ever met a friend and noticed that the person has just eaten a large meal. Patients should be told that the only way of determining whether their body is likely to be changing in size is to examine how their weight is changing over time. (See page 63 for guidance on how to interpret weight data.)

QUESTION 3: *"Do you ever look at parts of your body that you like?"*

— Almost invariably the answer is *"No."* This leads naturally to asking patients whether their checking makes them feel better about themselves.

QUESTION 4: *"Do you feel better after checking your body?"*

— Again, almost invariably the answer is *"No."* Occasionally patients (usually those who are underweight) say that it is reassuring to check their body because it reminds them of how "thin" they are. Even if this is the case, they will usually agree that it is unhelpful because it keeps them preoccupied with their shape.

QUESTION 5: *"Do you think your body checking has any adverse effects?"*

— In discussing the patient's answer to this question, the therapist will want to emphasize the following points:

• The shape checking of people with eating problems generally involves the repeated studying of aspects of appearance that are disliked. This is bound to maintain body dissatisfaction as it involves a negatively biased appraisal of one's shape and it keeps concerns about appearance at the front of one's mind (at the expense of thoughts about other aspects of life). Few patients feel better about their appearance after shape checking.

• As with all forms of shape checking, what one discovers depends to a large extent upon how one looks. If one studies in detail certain aspects of one's appearance, apparent "flaws" that would normally go unnoticed become prominent and, once noticed, they are hard to forget or ignore. Even the most attractive person would find flaws if he or she looked for them.

• Scrutiny is prone to magnify apparent defects. For example, people with a phobia of spiders tend to think spiders are larger than they really are. This is because when looking at spiders they tend to focus down on them and their unpleasant characteristics while not looking at the surrounding environment. As a result they have no reference points for scale or size. Another example is what happens when one stares at a blemish on one's skin. The more one looks at it, the more prominent it becomes. In the same way scrutinizing aspects of one's body that one dislikes is prone to make them seem "worse." In short, if you look for fatness, you will find it.

Scrutiny is prone to magnify apparent defects.

"If you look for fatness you will find it."

Addressing Shape Checking

The therapist and patient should then go on to categorize the identified forms of checking into two groups: behavior that is probably best stopped, and behavior that needs to be adjusted. The strategies used to achieve these goals differ. In addition, the therapist will want to discuss two particularly common forms of shape checking: mirror use and comparison-making.

Examples of behavior that is best stopped include using a tape measure to check the circumference of the thighs; checking that there is a gap between the thighs when standing with the knees placed together; and, when lying down, placing a ruler across the ileac crests (pelvis) to check that the surface of the abdomen does not touch it. Such behavior tends to undermine self-respect and, after a few weeks, stopping it is experienced as a relief. Patients are usually able to do this if the rationale is well explained and they are provided with support. There is generally no need to phase out the behavior.

Other forms of behavior that are worth stopping include pinching parts of the body to assess their "fatness"; repeatedly touching the abdomen, thighs and arms; feeling bones; checking the tightness of rings and watch straps; and looking down when sitting to assess the extent to which one's abdomen bulges out over the waistband of one's pants or the degree to which one's thighs splay out. Generally these forms of behavior have to be phased out. To do so, patients need to become aware of doing them in real time and then learn to question themselves before doing so (i.e. "think first"), the goal being to gain control over the behavior and become better at interpreting what they find. As with reducing the frequency of weight checking in Stage One, the modification of habitual shape checking results in a short-lived increase in preoccupation with thoughts about shape, but this is subsequently followed by a marked reduction in these thoughts and the associated concerns. Some patients are concerned that if they reduce their frequency of body checking, they will not notice themselves getting "fatter" because they will no longer be keeping an eye on their shape. These patients need to appreciate that they have not been getting accurate information from what they have been doing, and that (as discussed above) the only way of determining whether their body is likely to be changing is to examine changes in their weight over time.

For many patients simply recognizing how unhelpful body checking is can be sufficient to help them curb or stop the behavior. However, other patients struggle to do this. In these cases it can be helpful to ask them to identify the situations in which they are most prone to body check (e.g., when undressing, when sitting down, after eating, during an aerobics class) and then help them identify and practice means of resisting the urge to do so (e.g., by undressing away from mirrors).

A different strategy needs to be used with more normative forms of shape checking, such as looking in mirrors.

Addressing Mirror Use

Looking at oneself in the mirror is a particular form of shape checking that has the potential to provide highly credible, but misleading, information about appearance. We all tend to believe what we see in the mirror, yet assessing oneself in the mirror is a far more complex act than is generally realized. To illustrate this point, consider the size of your image when you look at your-

> **Mirrors have the potential to provide highly credible, but misleading, information about appearance.**

self in a full-length mirror. Is its height the same as your true height? If not, what height is it? And what about the width of the image? (To find out the answer, ask a friend to mark the top and bottom of your reflection as you see it on your mirror [when standing back so that you can see your head and feet] and measure how far apart they are. You will find that your image in the mirror is half your size in all dimensions, yet you have probably not noticed this before.) The fact that you have not noticed this remarkable discrepancy should help to persuade you (and your patients) that mirror reflections are not quite what they seem and that a lot of mental processing is involved "behind the scenes."

To a large extent what one "sees" depends upon how one looks. This point is well illustrated by asking patients whether they have ever had the experience of accidentally catching sight of themselves in a reflection (e.g., a shop window). Many will acknowledge that, at first glance, they saw themselves as they really are and that, only once they realized who it was, did they view themselves nega-

What one sees depends upon how one looks.

tively. In addition, many patients will acknowledge that how they are feeling emotionally seems to influence what they look like in the mirror.

Problematic mirror use, especially scrutiny, is likely to play a major role in the maintenance of many patients' body dissatisfaction. The addressing of mirror use is therefore of great importance. As always, the first step is to find out exactly what patients are doing. Below are the key questions to ask:

- How often do you look in the mirror?
- How long do you take?
- What exactly do you do?
- What are you trying to find out?
- Can you find it out this way?
- How many different mirrors do you use?

Patients then need to be educated about mirrors and how to interpret what they "see." The key questions (and answers) are listed below:

QUESTION: *"What are good reasons to look in the mirror?"*

— To check one's hair and clothing.
— Women may need a mirror to apply or remove make-up, and men need a mirror to shave.

QUESTION: *"Is there any other good reason to look in the mirror?"*

— No. For people with an eating problem there are no reasons to look in the mirror other than those listed above.
— Mirrors are "risky" things for people with an eating problem. They are best used judiciously.

QUESTION: *"How many mirrors does one need at home?"*

— One for the face and another full-length one.
— It is best to get rid of the rest unless they are purely decorative. It is difficult to avoid excessive mirror use if there are a large number of mirrors at home.

QUESTION: *"How can one avoid the 'magnification' that comes from scrutiny?"*

— Ensure that one does not focus on body parts that one dislikes. Look at the rest of your body, including more neutral areas (e.g., hands, feet, knees, hair). In addition, look at the background environment as this helps give a sense of scale.

QUESTION: *"Is it ever necessary to study oneself naked in the mirror?"*

— Not really, unless one is going to admire oneself!

— People with eating problems are most unlikely to admire themselves. Rather they are at risk of focusing on disliked parts and scrutinizing them.

As with the other forms of shape checking, patients need to become aware of their mirror use in real time and question themselves before doing it, the goal being that they modify the behavior and become better at interpreting what they find. This is not to say that total avoidance is to be recommended; rather, the advice is (for the meantime) to restrict the use of mirrors to the purposes listed above.

Addressing mirror use takes, at a minimum, several sessions. It can have a remarkable effect, as illustrated by the vignette below.

Vignette

A quotation from a patient whose mirror use had been extreme:

> *"I'm feeling more positive about my appearance generally. It feels quite odd because sometimes I look in the mirror and . . . it's almost like re-recognizing myself. Although I haven't lost any weight or tried to lose any weight, I feel smaller. I don't feel like a tiny person — I just think that I've lost the image I was carrying around in my head . . . that of an overweight person."*

In the context of addressing mirror use, it is worth asking patients whether they have difficulty choosing what to wear if they are going out. Some spend an inordinate amount of time doing this and will try on three or more outfits in front of a mirror. This is typically accompanied by a progressive decrease in mood, increase in shape dissatisfaction and drop in self-confidence (with every outfit). Sometimes it will result in them abandoning the whole enterprise and staying at home. In such cases patients should be advised to choose their outfit before trying it on (e.g., by laying outfits out on the bed) and to commit themselves to the decision. It is also important to encourage patients not to get dressed in front of the mirror.

Addressing Comparison-Making

A particular form of shape checking that actively maintains concerns about shape is making repeated comparisons with other people. This is seen mainly in patients who are of average or low weight. The nature of these comparisons typically results in patients concluding that their body is unattractive relative to that of others.

The general points about body checking also apply to comparison-making, but there are some additional points that need emphasizing. As noted above, patients' appraisal of their shape often involves scrutiny and selective attention to body parts that are disliked. The scrutiny is liable to result in the magnification of perceived defects and the selective attention increases overall dissatisfaction with shape. In contrast, patients' assessment of other people is very different. They tend to make superficial and often uncritical judgments about them. Furthermore, when making these comparisons they tend to choose biased reference groups composed of people of the same gender and age (or younger) who are thin and good-looking. These people are selected from those they encounter in their day-to-day life and from people in the media (e.g., as seen in magazines, newspapers, television, films, Internet). When making these comparisons they fail to notice others who are less thin and good-looking. Thus the playing field is uneven with there being an inherent bias (unfavorable to the patient) in the way that shape is being assessed and in the subject of the comparison.

There are eight steps involved in addressing comparison-making:

1. *Explain the rationale for doing this.* See above.

2. *Identify when and how the patient makes comparisons.* The monitoring records can be used for this purpose. Information of the following type is needed:

- Who was the subject of the comparison? How were they selected? Were they representative of people of the patient's age and gender, or were they a select and atypical subgroup?
- How was the person assessed? What body parts were the focus of the comparison and how were they evaluated?

3. *Help the patient consider whether the comparison was inherently biased in terms of both the person chosen and how his or her shape was evaluated.* Two points are worth highlighting:

- Comparing oneself with people portrayed in the media is problematic since they are an unusual subgroup and their images may well have been manipulated.
- Most ways of assessing one's body are idiosyncratic: It is difficult, if not impossible, to get the same perspective on someone else's body. For example, looking down at how much one's thighs splay out when sitting down is a view one has only of oneself: One never sees another person's thighs from this vantage point. The same applies to looking in the mirror, feeling one's stomach, touching one's bones, and pinching one's flesh. It is also not possible to study other people in the same amount of detail as one can study oneself.

4. *Design homework tasks to explore any bias in comparison-making.* For example, patients may be asked:

- To be more scientific when choosing someone with whom to compare themselves. Instead of selecting thin people, the therapist may ask them to select every third person (of their age and gender) whom they encounter. What they will discover is that people's bodies vary a great deal and that attractiveness is not directly related to thinness.
- To scrutinize other people's bodies. The goal is to demonstrate the point that *"What you see depends (to an extent) upon how you look."* One way of doing this is for the patient to go to a changing room (e.g., of a swimming pool or gym), select someone nearby of about the same age who is reasonably attractive, and

then (unobtrusively) scrutinize his or her body focusing exclusively on the parts that the patient is most sensitive about. The longer the scrutiny, the better. What patients will discover is that even attractive people have apparent flaws, be they dimpled thighs or buttocks ("cellulite"), a protruding stomach, or wobbling flesh.

5. *Explore the implications of any detected bias* in terms of the validity of the patient's views about his or her appearance relative to others. The goal is that patients become aware in real-time that their comparison-making is yielding misleading information about other peoples' bodies in relation to their own.

6. *Discuss how patients are comparing themselves with others in terms of a single domain (i.e., appearance)* rather than personality, intelligence, aptitudes, etc. It may be worth considering why the patient neglects these attributes, possibly in the context of the historical review (see page 117). The distinction between appearance and attractiveness should also be explored (see page 166).

7. *Explore the consequences of the comparison-making.* For example, does the patient consider this to be a good use of his or her time and helpful in terms of getting over the eating disorder? Also, spending a significant amount of time looking at other peoples' bodies (either in person or in the media) is likely to maintain preoccupation with shape and weight. In addition, it encourages the marginalization of other aspects of life. Some forms of this behavior are best stopped altogether (e.g., looking at pro-anorexia websites) or stopped for the meantime (e.g., buying fashion magazines; watching fashion TV channels).

8. *Modify comparison-making.* The goal is to reduce its frequency, heighten real-time awareness of any inherent bias, and broaden patients' focus of attention so that when they look at other people, they do not focus exclusively on their shape but also observe shape-neutral features (e.g., the person's hair and shoes) and other characteristics (e.g., the person's behavior, sense of humor). A further goal is to heighten awareness of the diversity of people's shapes.

Generally addressing comparison-making is relatively straightforward. One complication that can crop up stems from patients comparing their shape with that of the therapist. This does not occur if the therapist is older than the patient or of the opposite gender, but it does happen if the patient and therapist are the same gender and similar in age. Such comparison-making tends not to be mentioned, but it may be observable from the way that the patient looks at the therapist. Occasionally it is spoken out loud. For example, a patient said to one of us, *"It is not appropriate for you to tell me to gain weight when you are underweight yourself."* After giving the matter careful thought, the therapist decided to disclose her BMI, which was about 22, whereas the patient had thought it was below 18. (See page 29 for a discussion of the body shape of therapists.)

Addressing Shape Avoidance

Shape avoidance can be profoundly impairing. As well as maintaining dissatisfaction with shape (through assumptions not being challenged), it may result in patients not being able to socialize or be physically intimate with their partner, and in not being able to go swimming, use public changing rooms, or buy new clothes.

"Exposure" in its technical and literal sense is the strategy here. Patients need to get used to the sight and feel of their body and to learn to make even-handed comparisons with the bodies of others. They need to get used to others seeing their body too. Dressing and undressing in the dark will need to be stopped; they will need to be able to use mirrors (following the guidelines above); and they will need to abandon wearing baggy, formless clothes. Participation in activities that involve a degree of body exposure can be helpful too, for example, swimming. Other activities that require body awareness and acceptance are of value, including applying body lotion (see the following vignette; one patient referred to this as "positive touching"), having a massage and yoga.

Vignette

A patient was unable to touch or look at any part of her body. Her avoidance was so extreme that she could not properly wash herself.

The therapist and patient decided that she would start to address the problem by beginning to wash an area of her body that she felt was just about "bearable." At first she was only able to do this with a sponge. Gradually she was able to wash her entire body with a sponge. Then she was encouraged to use her hands. When she felt that she could fully wash herself, she moved on to applying body lotion in a "conscious" way, saying out loud the name of each body part and looking at it. Over a few months the patient became more comfortable touching and seeing her body. She came to realize that it was nothing like she had imagined it.

Depending upon the extent of the problem, tackling body avoidance may take many successive sessions. As there is a risk that patients will switch over to repeated body checking, they need help establishing normative forms and levels of body checking.

Addressing "Feeling Fat"

"Feeling fat" is an experience reported by many women, but the intensity and frequency of this feeling appear to be far greater among people with eating disorders. Feeling fat is an important target for treatment since it tends to be equated with being fat, whatever the patient's true shape or weight. Hence feeling fat is not only an expression of over-concern with shape and weight but it also

> **Feeling fat tends to be equated with being fat.**

maintains it. It is important to stress that some people with obesity have this experience too, but many do not despite being dissatisfied with their shape. (See Cooper, Fairburn, & Hawker [2003] for detailed information on addressing the shape concerns of people with obesity.) Whatever the patient's BMI, feeling fat should be addressed if it is a prominent feature.

There has been very little research on feeling fat: Indeed, remarkably little has been written about it. What is noteworthy is that the experience fluctuates in intensity from day to day and even within a day. This is quite unlike most other aspects of the core psychopathology (including body dissatisfaction), which tend to be relatively stable as is

> **In patients with eating disorders feeling fat is often the result of mislabeling of certain emotions and bodily experiences.**

body weight and true "fatness." It is our view that in patients with eating disorders feeling fat is often the result of the mislabeling of certain emotions and bodily experiences. Why this occurs is not clear, but it could be a consequence of these patients' longstanding and profound preoccupation with shape.

In general the addressing of feeling fat is best left until inroads have been made into shape checking and avoidance, but this is not invariably the right strategy. With patients in whom feeling fat is particularly prominent or distressing, the therapist should reverse the order and address it first.

There are six steps in addressing feeling fat:

1. *Establish whether patients feel fat at times* (explaining that one is not talking about whether they believe they *are* objectively fat, but whether they *feel* fat) and ask whether this is a problem. It is almost invariably seen as such. Explain that it would be useful to learn more about their experience of feeling fat. To encourage their curiosity it can be helpful to highlight the fact that the term is "feeling" fat, although obviously "fat" is not an emotion.

2. *Educate patients about feeling fat.* It should be stressed that the experience of feeling fat may be masking other feelings or sensations that are occurring at the same time, and that it is important not to equate feeling fat with being fat (i.e., the shape of one's body) as the two are quite different. Even very thin people can feel fat while many people who are objectively overweight do not feel fat — although they may well say that they are "fat" and are dissatisfied with their weight (i.e., they do not have fluctuating feeling of fatness). Patients should be asked whether there are times when they have particularly intense feelings of fatness and other times when they are less aware of feeling fat. If this is the case (which is likely), the therapist should point out that while feelings of fatness fluctuate from day to day and within each day, one's body shape barely changes within such a short time frame. (It can be useful to illustrate this point with a simple schematic diagram; see Figure 8.5.) Therefore something else must be responsible for the fluctuations in the feelings of fatness.

3. *Ask patients to monitor when they have particularly intense feelings of fatness.* Asking them to monitor every time they feel fat does not work as the feeling tends to be ever present in the background. This monitoring of intense feelings of fatness can be done as part of the normal recording process with the right-hand column of the monitoring record being used for the purpose. When patients record feeling fat, they should also think (and record) what else they are feeling at the time. They should ask themselves questions such as *"How am I feeling mentally and physically? Has something just happened that might have triggered this feeling?"*

4. *In the next session, review each occurrence of feeling fat in terms of the context in which it occurred and the presence of any possible masked feelings or sensations.* Over the following week patients should be asked to record in greater detail the context in which subsequent feelings of fatness occur, the goal being to improve their identification of masked feelings and their triggers.

By the following session it should be clear that the patient's experience of feeling fat tends to be triggered either:

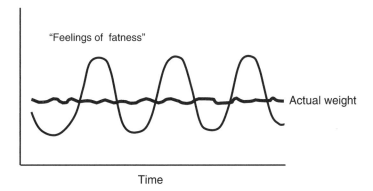

FIGURE 8.5. A schematic diagram illustrating fluctuating "feelings of fatness."

From *Cognitive Behavior Therapy and Eating Disorders* by Christopher G. Fairburn. Copyright 2008 by The Guilford Press. This figure is available online at www.psychiatry.ox.ac.uk/credo/christopher_fairburn.

  i. by the occurrence of certain negative mood states, or
 ii. by forms of behavior or physical sensations that heighten body awareness.

Examples of these types of stimulus include:

- Feeling bored, depressed, lonely or hungover
- Body checking and comparison-making
- Feeling full, bloated, hot or sweaty; feeling one's stomach bulge over one's pants; feeling one's body wobble or thighs rub together; feeling that clothes are tight.

Note that these are normal body sensations that are heightened under certain circumstances.

5. *Thereafter patients should practice:*
  i. Identifying when they have intense feelings of fatness.
 ii. Asking themselves the question *"What am I* really *feeling right now, and why?"* In this way common triggers may be identified and noted down on the monitoring record.
iii. Addressing the triggers, generally using the problem-solving approach described in Chapter 10.

Vignette

A patient tended to feel fat if she felt full when eating out with friends. It emerged that she thought that after eating her stomach protruded to such an extent that it was visible to others. The therapist suggested that she try sticking out her stomach on purpose and, after a while, ask her friends if they had noticed anything unusual. It emerged that they hadn't.

---

6. *With regard to body sensations, therapists should help patients appreciate that the problem is their negative interpretation of these sensations, rather than the sensations per se.* It can be help-

ful to ask patients to record in real time the occurrence of these sensations and practice re-labeling them correctly. (See also "Feeling Full," page 85.)

Vignette

A patient reported profound feelings of fatness (and revulsion) during a journey on the London Underground. The therapist and patient concluded that it might have been either due to the patient's body wobbling or it being extremely hot. The patient was asked to monitor her subsequent feelings of fatness and the circumstances under which they arose. It emerged that they occurred when she was hot. In hot weather she became more aware of her body, and the heightened body awareness led her to feel fat. It was agreed that it was important for her to correctly identify triggers for feeling fat, and that feeling fat should not be viewed as being indicative of *being* fat; rather, it suggested that she was too hot. This reinterpretation of the experience proved to be a turning point in her treatment.

Addressing "feeling fat" often takes many successive weeks and, once begun, it needs to be a recurring item on the session agenda. Generally the frequency and intensity of "feeling fat" progressively declines and patients' "relationship" to the experience changes such that it is no longer equated with being fat. This change is important since once it has happened "feeling fat" tends to lose its significance and as a result no longer maintains the patient's shape concerns.

Vignette

Below is a quote from a patient describing a change in her "relationship" to feeling fat:

> *"It's as if I suddenly saw the absurdity and ridiculousness of it all. It's not as if the thoughts have gone away, but I find I simply don't engage with them anymore. It's as if I can suddenly see myself as I am, and I'm not fat. It's as if feeling fat has suddenly evaporated. So I am laughing at these feeling fat moments, and not feeling fat. Something's really shifted."*

Effects of These and Other
Cognitive Behavioral Interventions

This complex set of inter-related and complementary strategies and procedures results in the progressive erosion of the main expressions of the over-evaluation of shape (i.e., shape checking, shape avoidance and feeling fat) and weight (i.e., weight checking and avoidance). By removing their reinforcing effect on the core psychopathology (i.e., the feedback pathways shown in Figure 8.3) this in turn has a gradual but profound impact on the core psychopathology, an effect that continues even after treatment has ended. This effect is augmented by the increase in the importance of other domains of life, by the addressing of dietary restraint and restriction (see Chapters 9 and 11 respectively), and by tackling event-related changes in eating (see Chapter 10).

It is most important that therapists appreciate that the effects of these interventions take time to be fully expressed. As part of our research we follow patients over time, and doing so has made it clear that the over-evaluation of shape and weight slowly, but progressively, declines over 6–9 months post-treatment so long as patients continue to *"Do the right thing"*; that is, continue to behave in line with the ways identified during treatment (and specified in their maintenance plan; see Chapter 12). It is as if the mind needs time to catch up with the change in the patient's behavior and adjust to its implications. Therapists can say to patients *"If you continue to 'Do the right thing', your thinking will slowly catch up."*

> **It is most important that therapists appreciate that the effects of these interventions take time to be fully expressed.**

As always in CBT-E, this work is supplemented with generic cognitive behavioral interventions (such as the addressing of prominent cognitive biases). Later in Stage Three two additional strategies complement this work:

1. Exploring the origins of the over-evaluation
2. Learning to control the eating disorder mindset

Exploring the Origins of Over-Evaluation

Toward the end of treatment it is helpful to explore the origins of the patient's sensitivity to shape, weight and eating. This can help make sense of how the eating problem developed and evolved. In addition, it can highlight how it might have served a useful function in its early stages and the fact that it may no longer do so.

To help patients review the past (termed in CBT-E the "historical review"), they should be asked to consider four periods in their life:

1. Prior to the onset of the eating disorder (which may be defined as their life up to 12 months before the onset of sustained attempts to restrict eating or the regular occurrence of binge eating or purging)
2. The 12 months immediately prior to its onset
3. The 12 months after its onset
4. Since then

Within each time period patients should consider whether any events or circumstances might have sensitized them to their shape, weight or eating, or reinforced existing concerns. These may then be tabulated in a life chart (see Figure 8.6). In this way hypotheses can be built up about why the eating problem developed and evolved in the way that it did. Typically the events in the first period are of a type that might increase the salience of shape, weight and eating, whereas those in the second (the 12 months leading to the onset) tend to be disruptive triggers but non-specific in nature. Often the patient will have been unhappy and may have had difficulty adjusting to a change in circumstances (e.g., moving from one city to another and changing school; parental separation or death). The third period, if it was characterized by dieting, is often described in posi-

Time period	Events and circumstances (that might have sensitized me to my shape, weight and eating)
Before onset of eating problem (up to age 16)	• *Mother very anxious about eating throughout my childhood* • *A bit overweight age 9* • *Always have been on the tall side and a bit clumsy (have felt too "big")* • *Friend developed anorexia; slightly jealous*
The 12 months before onset (when I was 16)	• *Moved to new city and house* • *New school* • *Unhappy; no friends*
The 12 months after onset (when I was 17)	• *Started to cut back on my eating* • *Felt good and in control* • *Fights with my mom* • *Lost weight rapidly for a while*
Since then (17 – 26)	• *Started purging (18)* • *Binge eating (18/19)* • *Went to college (19)* • *Regained weight (19); out of control; awful* • *Eating problem just as it is now (20 to present)* • *Dropped out of college (23)* • *Psychotherapy and antidepressants (24)*

FIGURE 8.6. A life chart (patient A).

tive terms and frequently there is reference to having felt "in control." The fourth period is generally the one during which the eating disorder became self-perpetuating and the processes outlined in the formulation began to operate. It is at this point that the eating disorder became more or less autonomous.

Very occasionally specific events are identified that appear to have played a critical role in sensitizing patients. Commonly these involve patients having been humiliated about their appearance. In these instances the therapist should help the patient reappraise the critical event from the vantage point of the present.

This review of the past needs to be done sensitively and under the guidance of the therapist. It is best if it takes place in-session as a major item on one session agenda, and is followed up with a detailed review at the next session. Between the two sessions patients should be asked to think over what has been discussed.

Obviously it would be naïve to assume that the factors and processes identified in the historical review necessarily operated in the way specified or could constitute anything like a full explanation for the eating disorder. Nevertheless, reviewing the past in this way seems to benefit patients, and particularly so in the later stages of treatment when they can see that their eating problem is beginning to die away. It serves to distance them still further from the problem; it tends to enhance their understanding of the processes currently operating; and it has a valuable "depathologizing" function.

Learning to Control the Eating Disorder Mindset

The task of psychological treatments is to change the "mind" that gets automatically switched on by particular contexts, and, ultimately, to give individuals, themselves, greater control over the switching in and out of different minds-in-place. (Teasdale, 1997, p. 91)

The core psychopathology of eating disorders may be viewed as a "mindset" or a frame of mind that has multiple effects. For example:

- It leads patients to filter external and internal stimuli in a distinctive way (e.g., preferentially noticing thin people; interpreting clothing being tight as evidence of fatness).

> The core psychopathology of eating disorders may be viewed as a "mindset" or a frame of mind.

- It results in the characteristic forms of behavior seen in people with eating disorders (e.g., rigid and extreme dietary restraint; self-induced vomiting; laxative misuse; driven exercising).
- It results in the mislabeling of various physical and emotional experiences as "feeling fat."

These consequences of the eating disorder mindset tend to reinforce it through the mechanisms described in the composite transdiagnostic cognitive behavioral formulation (see Figure 5.1, page 53) and in its extended form (see Figure 8.3, page 101). As a result the mindset becomes locked in place. Similar processes appear to occur in depression:

> Normally, the mind-in-place changes over time, old minds being "wheeled out" and new minds being "wheeled in" as circumstances change. In contrast, in mood disorders, such as depression, patients seem to get stuck in one mind, so that their thinking seems to be dominated by a limited number of recurring themes. (Teasdale, 1997, p. 101)

The cognitive behavioral strategies used in CBT-E are designed to address the key features of the eating disorder and the processes that are maintaining them. As a result the mechanisms that have been holding the eating disorder mindset in place are gradually eroded. This has the effect of allowing healthier and more situationally appropriate mindsets to move into its place. At first this happens only transitorily, but as the maintaining mechanisms are further eroded it happens more and more often. In patients who are making good progress such shifts in mindset typically become evident in the last third of treatment. The first signs are often reported spontaneously: For example, patients may describe (sometimes with surprise) that they were not preoccupied with food and eating on one particular day; that they were able to eat out with no difficulty; that they could watch a film without worrying about what they had eaten; or that they went out without worrying about their appearance. Such reports are evidence that the mindset is slipping out of place.

It is at this point that patients should learn about mindsets and how to control them. When introducing the topic, an analogy that we find useful is to compare the mind to a DVD player, saying something along these lines:

"Think of your mind as a DVD player and that it has a variety of DVDs that it can play. It can play one titled 'Work' and when playing it you will be in a work frame of mind. You will be seeing the world from that perspective and will be thinking mainly about work-related matters. You will have other DVDs too . . . we all have. You will have a 'Friends' one for when you are with your friends, and it will process information quite differently. You will have a 'Parents' one that will come into place when you are with your parents, and again it will result in your thinking differently and behaving differently too. We all have a range of DVDs to suit different occasions. All this is perfectly normal.

"The trouble is that if one has an eating problem one also has an 'eating disorder' DVD and, unlike the others, once it has fully developed it tends to get locked into place so that it keeps playing whatever the circumstances. As a result, wherever you are, you think eating disorder thoughts and you engage in eating disorder behavior (e.g., body checking, avoiding eating). With effort you can force the right mind (or DVD) into place to suit the circumstances (e.g., the 'Work' one when trying to work), but the eating disorder one is liable to keep popping back and displacing it. Does this account of things fit your experience in any way?"

Most patients relate to this type of explanation: It matches their experience. This is especially so in the later stages of treatment when their eating disorder mindset is less firmly in place and as a result is liable to be displaced at times. Indeed, this possibility may be raised along these lines:

"In the later stages of treatment, once the main things that have been keeping the eating problem going have been disrupted, most people notice that there are times when they are not 'playing' their eating disorder DVD . . . that they are able to focus on other things; that they are not thinking eating disorder thoughts; that they are (for a while) not doing eating disorder things. Are you experiencing anything like this?"

Another rather easier way to raise the topic is to capitalize on a recent setback if there has been one. For example, a patient may have had an episode of binge eating after a gap of a few weeks. Typically the binge will have activated the eating disorder mindset and put it firmly back in place. In fact, it is likely that the "DVD" was activated a day or so prior to the binge (perhaps by an adverse shape-related event) resulting in the patient's resumption of rigid dieting and so becoming vulnerable to binge eat. Patients notice setbacks of this type and can see the contrast between the period prior to the setback, when their eating disorder DVD was not in place, and their state during the setback, which they often experience as being *"Back to square one."* At these times their DVD will be "playing" just as it did prior to treatment.

Having introduced the topic of minds-in-place, the therapist should explain that now their eating disorder mindset (DVD) is no longer locked in place by the eating disorder maintaining mechanisms, they are in a position to influence whether or not they play it. More specifically, they can learn:

1. To identify stimuli that are likely to put the eating disorder mindset or DVD back in place
2. To recognize the first signs that their eating disorder mindset is coming back into place (i.e., to recognize the first "track" of the eating disorder DVD)
3. To displace the mindset (i.e., press the "eject" button)

It is not possible for patients to do these things early in treatment, as at that point their eating disorder mindset is firmly locked in place and they have no other state with which to contrast it.

Identifying Stimuli That Put the Mindset Back in Place

At first, when patients have only recently begun to experience periods when they are not "playing" their eating disorder DVD, they are vulnerable to have it triggered by a wide variety of stimuli. These tend to be of the following nature:

- Shape or weight-related events (especially those that are adverse)
  — E.g., an increase or decrease in weight; an apparent increase in "fatness" (e.g., due to clothing feeling tight or mirror scrutiny); feeling fat; critical comments from others
- Adverse eating-related events
  — E.g., breaking a dietary rule (e.g., eating an avoided food, exceeding a calorie limit); binge eating; feeling full
- Other personally salient adverse events
  — Negative events in general, especially those that threaten self-esteem
- Persistent negative mood states
  — These may be secondary to adverse circumstances or an expression of a clinical depression

This propensity of the eating disorder mindset to be reactivated should be discussed with patients. They can be assured that their mindset will become less likely to be triggered the longer it has not been "in place" (i.e., the eating disorder DVD will move down their stack of DVDs and become less accessible), but for the meantime they are at risk. It is therefore useful for them to learn what types of stimuli are most likely to serve as triggers and to be on the lookout for them in real time. Such in-the-moment awareness can be sufficient to inoculate them against the influence of these stimuli, although it can be supplemented with help countering them (e.g., help reinterpreting feeling fat or feeling full).

Recognizing the Mindset Coming Back into Place

However good the patient is at identifying potential triggers of his or her eating disorder mindset, there will invariably be circumstances when it comes back into place. Once this happens the eating disorder becomes activated and the patient starts to have eating disorder thoughts and feelings and begins to engage in eating disorder behavior. Within a day or two, eating disorder maintaining mechanisms will start to lock the mindset in place, and as time passes it will become progressively more difficult for the patient to dislodge it.

Therefore patients need to learn to spot the eating disorder mindset coming into place, and the earlier this can be done the easier it is to displace. Essentially they need to recognize what comes up on the "screen" when they start to play their eating disorder DVD. In the case of disorders such as depression, this is difficult because the initial changes are not readily observed. The case of eating disorders is quite different because these patients' behavior changes quickly and in distinctive and recognizable ways.

It is the therapist's task to help patients identify these early changes (their so-called "relapse signature") and to recognize that such changes are early warning signs of their eating disorder mindset coming back into place. One good way of doing this is to review the details of a recent setback.

Vignette

A patient reported a recurrence of binge eating after a break of some weeks. The therapist reviewed in detail the context in which this occurred. It emerged that the morning before the setback began the patient had an extended shape-related conversation with an old friend. After this she ate a very small lunch, spent twice the normal time in the gym and engaged in some old forms of body checking while there. She omitted her afternoon snack, ate an evening meal of diet food and had no evening snack. As a result she was set up to binge the following day.

By going over this course of events in some detail the therapist and patient decided that future early warning signs were likely to be a change in her food choice, skipping snacks, an increase in her exercising and reversion to old forms of body checking.

Displacing the Mindset

As noted above, displacing the eating disorder mindset is relatively straightforward if it is done soon after it has been activated, but it becomes progressively more difficult as more maintaining mechanisms start to operate and begin to lock it in. In principle, the patient needs to do two things:

1. *"Do the right thing"* (generally the opposite of the behavior driven by the eating disorder mindset).
2. Engage in distracting interpersonal activities.

"Do the right thing" refers to following what has been learned in treatment about overcoming the eating disorder. In the case of the patient described in the vignette, if she had recognized her eating disorder mindset while at the gym (by this time she had changed her food choice, reverted to old forms of body checking, and increased her exercising), she could have paid particular attention over the following few days to sticking to a pattern of regular eating (i.e., not skipping the afternoon and evening snacks), eating an evening meal not composed of diet food, and avoiding problematic forms of body checking. This would have prevented the eating disorder maintaining mechanisms from starting to operate.

At the same time patients should seek out ways of getting involved in activities that are engaging and likely to displace the eating disorder mindset. The best activities are interpersonal in nature. They might include arranging to see a friend, going out to a party, or having someone round. Doing this is likely to be difficult as it may well run counter to what the patient feels like doing, but it is important if the mindset is to be firmly dislodged.

Practicing spotting the mindset coming back into place and dealing with it effectively is of great value: it is less useful to simply think about these things in the abstract. It is therefore helpful if patients experience occasional setbacks later in treatment as this gives them an opportunity to utilize these strategies and procedures and subsequently review their efforts with the therapist.

Recommended Reading

Recommended reading for Chapters 5–12 can be found at the end of Chapter 12.

CHAPTER 9

Dietary Restraint, Dietary Rules and Controlling Eating

Dieting is one of the most prominent characteristics of people with eating disorders. With the exception of those with binge eating disorder, patients with eating disorders engage in a persistent and highly distinctive form of dieting. Rather than adopting general guidelines about how they should eat, they set themselves multiple demanding, and highly specific, dietary rules, their goal being to limit what they eat. This dieting is motivated either by a desire to lose weight or prevent weight gain and fatness, or by a wish to maintain strict control over eating. The dietary rules are varied in nature but typically concern when they should eat (e.g., not after 6 P.M.), how much they should eat (e.g., less than 600 kcals per day) and, most especially, what they should eat, with most patients attempting to avoid eating a large number of foods ("food avoidance"). As a result, these patients' eating becomes stereotyped and inflexible.

> **Rigid and extreme dieting is profoundly impairing.**

As stressed in Chapter 2, rigid and extreme dieting of this type is profoundly impairing. It can make everyday eating an anxiety-provoking and guilt-ridden experience. Even deciding which sandwich to have for lunch can involve protracted agonizing, and for people who live with the patient meals may become a nightmare. Social eating is markedly affected and events that involve eating (e.g., going out with friends, visiting relatives) may be avoided altogether. As a result patients' lives become severely curtailed.

As noted earlier, the attempts to restrict eating ("dietary restraint") may or may not be successful. Thus it is far from inevitable that they result in true undereating in physiological terms ("dietary restriction"). The focus of this chapter is on addressing dietary restraint and dietary rules, and the over-evaluation of control over eating. The tackling of dietary restriction is addressed in the chapter on underweight patients (see Chapter 11).

There is a two-fold strategy for addressing dietary restraint. The first is to focus on the motives driving it, especially the concerns about shape and weight (see Chapter 8). In most cases this work begins early in Stage Three. Typically, a few sessions later (and assuming a pattern of regular eating has been established), dietary rules also become a focus of treatment, the starting point generally being food avoidance. Prior to tackling dietary rules, however, there is a need to help patients see that their dieting is a "problem."

Addressing Dietary Restraint

Helping Patients View Their Dieting as a "Problem"

There is one major obstacle to the addressing of the dieting of these patients which is that they do not view it as a problem. This is for a number of reasons:

- Some patients see themselves as good at dieting. They see it as a measure of their strength and will-power, and therefore identify with it. It is valued.
- Even if patients see themselves as failing at dieting, they believe that their failure is because they are weak, rather than viewing their dietary rules as being too rigid and extreme (i.e., they see themselves as the problem, not their dieting).
- Dieting provides them with a strong sense of being in control.
- Dieting is their main method of weight control.
- In those who binge eat (objective or subjective episodes), dieting is generally one of their main means of compensating for the binge eating.
- Dieting is seen as appropriate in patients who have been, or are, overweight. It is especially difficult for these patients to moderate their dieting. (The management of patients who have both an eating disorder and co-existing obesity is discussed in Chapter 16, page 253.)

The therapist's first task is therefore to help patients see that their dieting is indeed a problem. There are two inter-related lines of argument. First, their type of dieting plays a central role in the maintenance of their eating problem and so has to be addressed if they are to overcome it. Second, their dieting has major adverse effects, including the following:

> **The first task is to help patients see that their dieting is a problem.**

- *It is a major cause of preoccupation with thoughts about food and eating.* This preoccupation interferes with concentration and many aspects of day-to-day life (e.g., patients may find it difficult to read, follow conversations, or keep their mind on the plot of TV programs or films; they may even find themselves dreaming about eating). This preoccupation is generally experienced as aversive.
- *It is anxiety-provoking.* Dieting makes eating an emotive and aversive experience. It engenders anticipatory anxiety and distress. Any episode of rule-breaking is a source of considerable regret (generally referred to as "guilt") and is viewed as evidence of weakness and lack of will-power.
- *It restricts the ways in which patients can eat.* As noted above, patients' eating becomes stereotyped and inflexible. They can eat only a limited range of foods and may find it impossible to eat food of uncertain composition. Some cannot tolerate being seen eating in front of others for fear that this will be interpreted as a sign of weakness or indulgence. As a result social eating becomes difficult, if not impossible.

> **Generally dietary restraint leads to binge eating through cognitive mechanisms rather than physiological ones.**

- *It is a major contributory factor to binge eating (objective or subjective).* It is most important that patients understand this point as many view their restraint as an understandable response to binge eating and as a means of preventing future episodes. Generally dietary restraint leads to binge eating through cognitive mechanisms rather than physiological ones (i.e., not from dietary restriction or true undereating), although both mechanisms may contribute in some instances. The basis of the cognitive mechanism is the presence of rigid dietary rules rather than flexible dietary guidelines coupled with a tendency to react in an extreme and negative fashion to the (almost inevitable) intermittent breaking of these rules. Even minor dietary slips tend to be viewed as evidence of a complete failure of dietary control and, as a consequence, patients respond by temporarily abandoning their dietary restraint and giving in to the drive to eat that arises from it. The resulting period of uncontrolled eating (i.e., subjective or objective binge eating) is followed by the resumption of dietary restraint later the same day or the next morning. Most patients who binge eat recognize this sequence when it is described. They may even have terms for aspects of it; avoided foods may be described as "trigger foods" or "danger foods" as the patient knows that eating these foods triggers binge eating (through rule-breaking). One patient described her cognitive response to rule-breaking as her "screw it" reaction.

It is also worth helping patients see that a major factor influencing what they eat during binges is what foods they are attempting to exclude from their diet. People tend to binge on those foods that they are otherwise trying not to eat. If they reintroduce these foods into their diet this tends to reduce the craving to eat them that is unleashed by rule-breaking.

Patients who do not binge (especially those who are underweight) may dismiss this potential adverse effect of dieting as being of no relevance to them. They need to know that this stance is not wise because they are actually at considerable risk of binge eating through the very same mechanisms.

• *Dietary restraint may result in dietary restriction, which may lead to weight loss or the maintenance of an unduly low weight.* While this is exactly what most patients want, it has many major adverse consequences (described in Chapter 11).

Vignette

A patient did not view her dieting as a problem until the therapist helped her see how it restricted her life. For months prior to her birthday she was dreading having to eat a slice of birthday cake with her work colleagues. She even contemplated not going into work that day to avoid having to do so. Eating out with friends was another problem. She had to know in advance where they were going to eat so that she could look at the menu on the Internet to decide what she could possibly eat. She knew she would not be able to make the decision at the time.

By highlighting the impairment that resulted from the dieting, the therapist was able to help the patient see that her dieting did indeed need to be tackled.

Educating Patients about Dietary Restraint and Dietary Rules

Helping patients see that their dietary restraint is a problem is best accompanied by education about dieting. The main points to stress are as follows:

1. Dietary restraint is a problem if it is "rigid": that is, it is characterized by the presence of highly specific dietary rules that must be followed for eating to be viewed as being in "control." It is this type of dieting that encourages binge eating.
2. Dietary restraint is also a problem if it is "extreme" in either of the two following ways:
   - There are many dietary rules.
   - These rules are demanding in nature.
3. This type of extreme dietary restraint has negative consequences whether or not patients are successful at following their rules:
   - If successful, there will be many adverse effects, particularly with regard to psychosocial functioning and physical health.
   - If unsuccessful, patients will feel they have failed and perhaps extend this to viewing themselves as failures. They will also be at increased risk of binge eating.
4. Successfully addressing dietary restraint is essential in order to remove the array of adverse consequences that stem from it and to overcome the eating problem.

Identifying Dietary Rules

The next step involves identifying the patient's dietary rules. This is not necessarily straightforward, as some patients deny having them or the rules have become so second nature that they are not aware of them. Clues to their presence come from the use of asterisks on the monitoring records and from descriptions of having "broken" something. Triggers of binges (of any size) are particularly revealing. Patients should be asked to try to detect their rules on an ongoing basis. This can be done "live" by noting them down as they are spotted on the back of the day's monitoring record.

If there appear to be no rules, it is worth asking patients how they would feel about going out to a new restaurant or having a meal at someone's house, as this typically unearths them. Would this concern them and, if so, why?

Dietary rules vary in content. Commonly they concern:

- What to eat (or rather, what not to eat)
- When to eat (or rather, when not to eat)
- How much to eat (or rather, the setting of a limit in terms of calories, fat intake, portion size, numbers of items [e.g., number of cookies])
- Not eating . . . more than anyone else present
- Not eating . . . until one has earned it (e.g., by exercising or doing a certain amount of work)
- Not eating . . . unless one is hungry
- Not eating . . . unless it is "necessary"
- Not eating . . . food of uncertain composition (in terms of calorie content)
- Not "wasting" calories

Addressing Dietary Rules

The principles underlying the addressing of dietary rules are as follows:

1. *Identify a specific rule and what is motivating it.* A good clue to the latter is what concerns would be activated if the patient broke the rule in question. Generally dietary rules are driven by the desire to lose weight or by a fear of weight gain and fatness, but patients who binge eat (objective or subjective) may also be motivated by the fear that breaking the rule will result in an episode of binge eating.

2. *Explore with the patient the likely consequences of breaking the rule.* For example, breaking most dietary rules will not necessarily result in weight gain or fatness or the cessation of weight loss. This depends upon how much is eaten. Also, breaking a dietary rule will not invariably result in binge eating. It may have done so in the past, but the patient can be reassured that this need not happen in the future (see "Food Avoidance" below).

3. *Devise a plan with the patient for breaking the rule in question in order to explore the consequences of doing so, and help the patient do this.*

4. *Analyze the implications of the planned rule-break* both in terms of the patient's beliefs about what would happen and the potential advantages of freeing himself or herself from such rules.

5. *Plan further episodes of breaking the same rule* and help the patient continue to do this until breaking the rule has no particular significance for him or her.

Food Avoidance

Most patients with eating disorders attempt to exclude a range of foods from their diet ("food avoidance"). This is generally the best type of rule to address first as it is simple in form and reasonably easy to detect. The strategy for addressing food avoidance is as follows:

• Patients with food avoidance tend to believe that eating certain foods (e.g., chocolate) will inevitably lead to weight gain and fatness, and perhaps also to an episode of binge eating. This latter belief can be disconfirmed by asking patients to introduce an avoided food into one of their planned meals or snacks on a day when they are feeling in control and capable of resisting binge eating. They need to plan ahead how much of it they will eat and, if relevant, what they will do with the remainder (e.g., with the other half of the chocolate bar). Patients do not need to eat much of the avoided food, as eating even a small quantity will break the rule in question. By doing this time after time patients learn that the feared consequence (binge eating) that had been driving the dietary rule is not an inevitable result of breaking it. It is as if eating the food repeatedly "inoculates" the patient against its triggering effect on binge eating.

• It is not possible to disconfirm the belief that breaking the rule will result in weight gain or fatness (or cessation of weight loss) as these would be longer-term consequences if they were indeed to happen. In this regard simple nutritional education should be sufficient focusing on how much has been eaten (in caloric terms) in relation to the patient's overall daily energy needs. A major point that needs to be stressed in this context is that *"There are no inherently fattening foods. It all depends upon how much of them one eats (in terms of energy or calories)."*

• The repeated consumption of avoided food and the analysis of the implications of doing so have the effect of gradually undermining and eroding the basis for the food avoidance, thereby allowing the patient's eating to become progressively more varied in content.

As food avoidance generally affects a wide range of foods, the first step in addressing it is to identify all the kinds of food being avoided. A good way of doing this is to ask patients to visit a local supermarket and list all the foods that they would be reluctant to eat because of their possible effect on their shape or weight or because they fear that eating them might trigger a binge. Having done this they should divide these foods (often comprising 40 or more items) into groups that they would find increasingly difficult to eat; usually four or five groups are sufficient (see Figure 9.1). Then, over the following weeks, patients should introduce these foods into their diet, starting with the easiest group and moving on to the most difficult. As always, they should record what they are doing on their monitoring records. Figure 9.2 shows a monitoring record that illustrates the tackling of food avoidance (see "NEW" in column 2).

Therapists should not be concerned if the avoided foods list is dauntingly long. When selecting foods for the patient to tackle, the therapist should identify ones that are likely to be representative of a class of foods as their successful consumption will address the whole class rather than a single item. As noted above, the amount eaten need not be large although the eventual goal is that the patient should be capable of eating normal quantities without difficulty.

The systematic introduction of avoided foods should continue until patients are no

Group 1 — I would never eat	*Group 2*
Nuts	*Potato chips*
Butter	*Pastries & croissants*
Cream	*Jelly, honey*
Peanut butter	*Sugar in coffee*
Chocolate bars	*Cake*
French fries	*Cookies*
Pie	*Hard candies*
Dips	*Fried chicken*
Ice cream	*Mexican food*
Doughnuts	
Group 3	*Group 4 — I would consider eating but it would be really hard*
Pasta	*Wheat bread*
Noodles	*Bagels*
Burgers	*Some cheeses*
Potatoes	*Greek yogurt*
Coconut	*Some cereal bars*
Avocado	*Sushi*

FIGURE 9.1. An avoided food list (patient B).

Day .... *Monday* ....   **Date** ...... *April 7th* ....

Time	Food and drink consumed	Place	*	V/L	Context and comments
6:30	Glass water	Kitchen			Feeling good and a little worried about adding in new food
7:10	Banana Bowl Cheerios Skim milk Black coffee	Cafe			Normal breakfast PROBLEM! ⟶
10:00	Apple Cereal bar	Desk at work			Didn't want to have this as having big lunch, but wanted to stick to plan.
1:00	Greek salad with feta cheese and dressing (NEW!) Roll Water	Cafe			Decided that I would eat 3/4 of salad beforehand. Was pretty nervous the whole time, but was able to eat it and keep it down!
3:00	Yogurt	Desk at work			Thought about not eating this, but didn't want a huge gap.
6:30	Salmon (small piece) Rice (1/2 cup) Spinach	Kitchen			Realized this could be a problem earlier today – PS worked!
9:30	Ice cream cone with hot fudge (NEW!)	Ice cream parlor with friends			Planned to have 2 scoops and was fine! Really enjoyed getting this with my friends, as I usually don't go.

FIGURE 9.2. A monitoring record showing the introduction of avoided foods (patient A).

longer anxious about eating them. Sometimes patients say that they do not want to get used to eating these foods because doing so would be unhealthy. It is important to point out that the goal is not to encourage patients to eat an "unhealthy diet," but rather to address their fears about eating certain foods so that afterwards they can freely choose what to eat (which they cannot do at present). They should be capable of eating any foods on the list without feeling guilty or anxious about weight gain or binge eating afterward.

Patients who are adhering to a vegetarian or vegan diet require special consideration. It is important to establish the basis for the vegetarianism or veganism because both can be expressions of eating disorder psychopathology and be essentially diets in disguise. If this is the case, the core psychopathology and resultant dieting should be addressed in the usual way. On the other hand, if the vegetarianism or veganism is for moral reasons, the therapist needs to work within the resulting constraints. Neither poses much difficulty unless the patient is underweight. If this is the case, regaining weight can be even more difficult than usual, and most especially for those following a vegan diet. In these cases the therapist might want to seek advice from a specialist dietitian. It is also worth asking patients to consider suspending their vegetarianism or veganism for some months to give themselves a better chance of overcoming their eating disorder. In our experience many are willing to do so.

Other Dietary Rules

Other dietary rules should be tackled in a similar fashion with the focus being both on the belief that is maintaining the rule and on practicing breaking it and analyzing the implications of so doing. Throughout, the therapist should stress how liberating it is to free oneself from the restrictions imposed by dietary rules. With this in mind it is especially important to address rules that interfere with social eating.

> **Throughout, the therapist should stress how liberating it is to free oneself from the restrictions imposed by dietary rules.**

Often some simple discussion needs to take place to prepare patients for rule-breaking. Below are some key points listed by types of rules:

Rules concerning what to eat (or rather what not to eat):

- As noted above, there is no food that is inherently fattening. It all depends upon how much of it one eats.
- Avoiding eating foods of uncertain composition is likely to impair social life, as it almost invariably precludes eating out. Knowledge of exactly what one is eating (e.g., usually in terms of calorie or fat content) is not needed for successful weight control.

Rules concerning when to eat (or rather when not to eat):

- There is no "right" or "wrong" time to eat and no significant difference in energy absorption through the day.
- "Delayed eating" — that is, having some form of rule concerning putting off eating as long as possible — may be associated with a type of asceticism that sometimes accompanies the over-evaluation of control over eating. This value system needs to be questioned, as there is nothing inherently worthy about resisting eating.
- Eating at regular intervals addresses rules about when to eat (see Stage One, page 75).

Rule concerning how much to eat:

- The "right" amount to eat overall, and of any particular foodstuff, is the amount that is consistent with maintaining a stable healthy weight and follows accepted nutritional guidelines. A good source of reliable information is www.health.gov.

Rules concerning not eating in front of others:

- These greatly impair social functioning.
- They generally stem from the assumption that others will notice how one eats and will view one's eating as evidence of "weakness," "lack of will-power" or "greediness." This view is particularly common among underweight patients.
- As noted in Chapter 11 (see page 165), this type of rule involves the assumption that the patient's own views are shared by others. This is most unlikely to be the correct. Others are unlikely to notice the patient's eating, and it is almost inconceivable that they would think about it in this way.

Rules concerning not eating more than anyone else present:

- This is a bizarre rule. Imagine if we all had it! And it makes no more sense than trying to breathe less often than everyone else!
- The rule takes no account of what others have eaten beforehand (or will eat afterward), or their energy needs in relation to their recent activity level, or their weight or height.

Rules concerning not eating unless one is hungry or not eating until one has earned it:

- As with delayed eating, this type of rule may stem from asceticism. Again, it is important to note that there is nothing inherently "good" about resisting eating.

Vignette

A patient who was highly calorie conscious had the rule that she should eat only foods of known calorie content. For this reason, she insisted on preparing all her own food so that she knew its exact composition. She would not allow her mother to cook for her (even if the patient watched her mother making the food) because she was afraid that her mother would not measure the quantities correctly.

The therapist encouraged the patient to practice eating in a wide variety of circumstances (e.g., restaurants, dinner parties, picnics) and to eat as varied a diet as possible. The patient was helped to view this as an experiment that tested what happened to her anxiety and preoccupation with eating if she repeatedly ate food of uncertain calorie content. Within weeks there was a decrease in her fears and preoccupation with thoughts about eating. Soon afterward she was able to eat with the family and eat out.

Some Tips and Problems

- Typically it is several weeks into Stage Three before dietary restraint begins to be addressed. It is certainly best left until a pattern of regular eating has been established and binge eating is intermittent. Explaining the rationale and principles behind rule-breaking occupies much of the initial session, but thereafter it can be just one item on the session agenda.

- Therapists should be very specific when agreeing on homework. For example, the patient and therapist should agree which foods will be introduced over the following week and on how many occasions they will be consumed.

- If patients have an unusually strong reaction to breaking a dietary rule, they should be told that this is a good sign because it means that the rule has particular significance for them.

- There should be sustained emphasis on enhancing social eating. The goal is that patients are able to eat with others and in a wide a range of circumstances.

- A small number of patients find it extremely difficult to break their dietary rules: For example, they may be highly reluctant to introduce "banned foods." With such patients some form of therapist-assisted eating may be helpful. This is probably best done in specialist settings (see Chapter 15, pages 235 and 241).

- With patients who are underweight (see Chapter 11), it is best to leave the addressing of dietary rules until their weight is close to the healthy range, although weight regain will invariably involve the breaking of some rules.

- The treatment of patients with co-existing obesity is discussed in Chapter 16 (see page 253). Generally the emphasis of treatment should be on addressing the eating disorder rather than the weight problem. Nevertheless patients need guidance on weight management, a major part of which will concern dieting. In this context patients need to learn about "binge-proof dieting," a type of dieting that is not prone to encourage binge eating. It is characterized by setting modest achievable goals and encouraging adherence to dietary guidelines rather than dietary rules, the distinction being that guidelines are flexible and bend whereas rules are inflexible and break.

Addressing Patients' Reaction to Rule-Breaking

With patients who respond to rule-breaking by temporarily abandoning control over eating, it is also important to address the underlying cognitive mechanisms so that they are not prone to react this way. Standard cognitive behavioral procedures are used to this end. As noted above, the basis for the patient's response is the presence of rigid dietary rules rather than flexible dietary guidelines, coupled with a tendency to react in an extreme and negative fashion to the breaking of these rules. The problems inherent in having dietary rules rather than guidelines will have been discussed in the context of addressing dietary restraint, but what also needs to be emphasized is the dichotomous (black-and-white) nature of the patient's rules. However minor the instance of rule-breaking (see the following vignette), patients interpret it as evidence that they have lost control (*"I've broken my diet"*) and lack will-power (*"I've failed"*). It should therefore be stressed that there are many degrees of dietary control and that even people who are quite careful about what they eat "let their hair down" at times and relax their eating.

Vignette

A patient who had particularly extreme dietary rules and pronounced dichotomous thinking set herself a limit of five grapes per snack. On one occasion she ate six. This was sufficient to trigger a binge.

In addition, patients' response to rule-breaking needs to be examined because it involves them temporarily abandoning their attempts to control their eating with binge eating being the result. This abandonment of control (due to thinking *"There's no point, I might as well give up"*) is a further example of dichotomous thinking.

The therapist's goal is that patients spot this type of thinking as it happens in real time, question it, and respond accordingly so that they do not end up criticizing themselves and reacting by binge eating.

Further strategies are sometimes needed to tackle rigidity surrounding eating. Many patients (especially those who are underweight) have difficulty coping with any change to their way of eating, especially if there is a degree of unpredictability (e.g., if it is not clear when or where the next meal will take place). Some cannot tolerate such uncertainty and either have to stick to their usual way of eating or not eat at all. Therapists can help such patients practice tolerating a degree of uncertainty by having them plan three or more eating options for each evening and then letting the roll of a dice dictate which option is followed.

Addressing the Over-Evaluation of Control Over Eating

As noted earlier, in a subgroup of patients there is over-evaluation of control over eating per se rather than a desire to control eating with the aim of influencing shape and weight. These patients tend to have an especially high level of dietary restraint and a large number of dietary rules. They tend to be particularly concerned about checking the details of their eating because this is their way of assessing their degree of control over eating. Thus they tend to count calories (i.e., keep a running total of their calorie intake), monitor other aspects of their nutrient intake and weigh their food too. Some also try to assess their energy expenditure. We recently saw a patient who had a detailed spreadsheet documenting her energy intake and expenditure over many years. As noted earlier, a few practice "debting" whereby before they allow themselves to eat, they have to burn up the equivalent number of calories in the form of exercise.

To address the over-evaluation of control over eating the therapist should follow the principles specified above and in Chapter 8. The optimal sequence of procedures is as follows:

1. *Identify the over-evaluation and its consequences.* This involves adopting the strategy used to address the over-evaluation of shape and weight (see Chapter 8, page 97) but adapting the content so that it matches the over-evaluation of control over eating per se. The extended formulation differs from the typical one in that the expressions of the over-evaluation are not body checking, etc., but exclusively concern dietary control (see Figure 9.3).

2. *Enhance the importance of other domains for self-evaluation.* This involves the same strategies and procedures as those described in Chapter 8 (page 102).

3. *Reduce the importance attached to the control of eating.* The most potent way of doing this is to tackle the expressions of the over-evaluation. This involves following the guidelines described in the present chapter. Food checking needs to be discouraged (e.g., checking food packets, weighing food, calorie-counting) because it maintains pre-

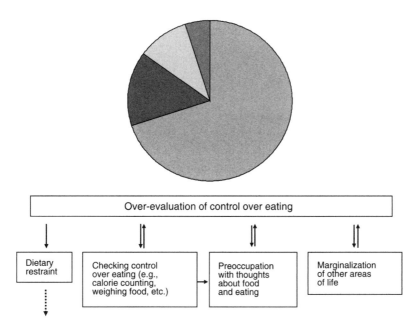

FIGURE 9.3. The over-evaluation of control over eating: an "extended formulation."

From *Cognitive Behavior Therapy and Eating Disorders* by Christopher G. Fairburn. Copyright 2008 by The Guilford Press. This figure is available online at www.psych.ox.ac.uk/credo/cbt_and_eating_disorders.

occupation with food, eating and calories. Patients should also be discouraged from reading cookery books and recipes, and from visiting websites concerned about food and eating.

4. *Explore the origins of the over-evaluation.* As described in Chapter 8 (see page 117).

5. *Learn to manipulate the eating disorder mindset.* Also as described in Chapter 8 (see page 119).

Recommended Reading

Recommended reading for Chapters 5–12 can be found at the end of Chapter 12.

CHAPTER 10

Events, Moods and Eating

As would be expected, the eating habits of patients with eating disorders are responsive to outside events and changes in mood. This is to a variable extent. It is sometimes least obvious in the severest cases where the eating disorder may appear almost autonomous, whereas it may be prominent in milder cases. It generally becomes more evident as treatment progresses and the mechanisms that have been maintaining the eating disorder start to break down. The changes in eating may take the form of eating less, stopping eating altogether, overeating or frank binge eating (subjective or objective), or there may be a change in the frequency of purging or over-exercising. A variety of mechanisms are responsible, including:

- Eating less to gain a sense of personal control when external events feel outside the patient's control. This is most often seen in underweight patients: For example, arguments will often result in these patients stopping eating.
- Eating less to influence others; for example, to demonstrate feelings of distress, defiance or anger.
- Overeating as a "treat." This is most characteristic of overweight patients.
- Binge eating or vomiting, or both, to cope with negative events or adverse moods. Binge eating has two relevant properties in this regard: First, it is distracting and so it can take the patient's mind off troubling thoughts; and second, it has a direct mood-modulatory effect in that it dampens down intense mood states. This latter property is also true of vomiting and intense exercising.

If in Stage Three events and moods appear to be contributing to the maintenance of the eating disorder, this connection needs to be assessed, and in all likelihood addressed, the goal being to help patients deal with events and moods directly and effectively without their influencing their eating.

As a preliminary step patients should be asked to identify examples of event-related changes in eating from their pervious monitoring records. Then the therapist and patient should review these in detail with the aim of identifying what seem to have been the main processes involved. After this, and depending upon what appear to be the main mechanisms operating, the therapist should introduce the first, or both, of the following two strategies:

- Proactive problem-solving to address triggering events
- The development of functional methods of mood modulation to address mood-related changes in eating

Addressing Event-Related Changes in Eating

To help patients address events that trigger changes in eating, cognitive behavioral treatments for eating disorders have long used training in problem-solving. Although it may seem prosaic as a technique, it is remarkably effective in most cases and is

> **Problem-solving is remarkably effective as a technique and is liked by patients.**

liked by patients. However, the training in problem-solving needs to be done well if it is to be effective. It involves seven steps.

1. *The therapist should identify a recent example of an event-related change in eating.*

   - If one is not available, an earlier one should be sought from the patient's monitoring records. If that does not reveal one, then a recent day-to-day difficulty (e.g., a disagreement with a friend; conflict at work) should be identified and used as an example for Step 4 below.

2. *The sequence of events that led to the change in eating should be re-created.*

   - This requires detailed reconstruction in terms of the triggering event and subsequent feelings, thoughts and behavior. Common triggers include pressure at work, an argument, having nothing to do all day, and coming home to an empty apartment.

3. *The therapist should help the patient see that this sequence could have been disrupted.*

   - The aim is to introduce the notion that such changes in eating are not inevitable; for example, the sequence of events could have been interrupted by someone calling the patient to invite him or her out to see a film.

4. *The patient should be taught how to use "proactive problem-solving" to address events of the type that trigger changes in eating.* It should be made clear to the patient that problem-solving is being used here to address the triggers of changes in eating. Some patients tend to view the change in their eating (e.g., binge eating) as "the problem," whereas it is their *response* to the problem.

   - Problem-solving may be taught with reference to the section on problem-solving in *Overcoming Binge Eating* (page 177). The therapist should explain that while many problems may seem overwhelming at first, if they are approached systematically they usually turn out to be manageable or even preventable. Thus by becoming effective problem-solvers most patients can successfully address events of the type that would otherwise disrupt their eating. Effective problem-solving involves the following steps:

     — *Step 1: Identify the problem as early as possible.* Spotting problems early is of great importance. Almost invariably problems are easier to address if they are caught early on. For example, if there is likely to be a problem in the evening (e.g., having nothing to do), it is almost always easier to solve it earlier in the day than at the last minute.

     — *Step 2: Specify the problem accurately.* Working out the true nature of the problem is essential if the best solution is to be found. It may emerge that there are two or more co-existing problems, in which case each problem may need to be addressed individually. Rephrasing the problem can be helpful.

— *Step 3: Consider as many solutions as possible.* All ways of dealing with the problem should be considered. The patient should generate as many potential solutions as possible ("brainstorming"). Some solutions may seem nonsensical or impractical. Nevertheless, they should be included on the list. The more solutions that are generated, the more likely a good one will emerge. Patients who find it difficult to generate solutions may find it helpful to consider what they might suggest to a friend who was in a similar situation.

— *Step 4: Think through the pros and cons of each solution.* The likely effectiveness and feasibility of each solution should be considered.

— *Step 5: Choose the best solution or combination of solutions.* Interestingly, if Step 4 has been conducted thoroughly, choosing the best solution (or combination of solutions) is usually straightforward.

— *Step 6: Act on the solution.*

— *Step 7. Evaluate the process of problem-solving.* Patients should review their problem-solving the next day. When doing so, they should focus on their use of the problem-solving procedure and not on whether the problem was successfully solved. In other words they should focus on honing their problem-solving skills.

5. *The therapist and patient should address the identified problem (using the first six of the problem-solving steps) as if it had been spotted in advance.*
   • This is crucial and it should be collaborative with the therapist encouraging the patient to take the lead whenever possible. If time allows, another recent example should be identified and approached in the same way.

6. *As homework, patients should be asked to practice their problem-solving skills.*
   • Over the following 7 days patients should look out for events of the type that would be liable to trigger changes in their eating and address them using the problem-solving procedure. Specifically, once patients identify a problem, they should write "Problem" in the right-hand column of the day's monitoring record and then turn the record over and address it by writing out the problem-solving steps (see Figure 10.1). Patients should be advised against problem-solving in their head, as this is much less effective.

7. *This homework should be reviewed at the next session and further practice encouraged.*
   • The emphasis should be on helping patients acquire the ability to address or forestall events that would otherwise have triggered changes in eating. As it is especially important that problems are spotted early, patients should be encouraged to screen the remainder of the day for problems each time they have a meal or snack. In this way their problem-solving becomes "proactive."
   • If patients return without having done any problem-solving, the therapist needs to consider why this is the case. Sometimes patients say that they did not have any problems to solve. In these cases the therapist should point out that we all face problems more or less every day. Often examples can be identified by reviewing patients' last 7 days with the help of their records. Then

Big Problem!

Step 1: Going on a date tonight!

Step 2: Worried that he won't like me and will think that I am fat.

Steps 3 and 4: Things I could do and pros and cons:

   a) Cancel on him last minute ...   + I won't have to go and worry
                                             - I really like this guy!

   b) Ask a friend to help me get ready ...   + will make me feel better
                                             - she might not be able to come

   c) Call Mom for reassurance ...   + will make me less nervous
                                           - want to do this on my own

   d) Pick an outfit that I feel comfortable in ... + I will feel at ease
                                           - none

Step 5: Options B and D are the best.

Step 6: Do both of these tonight.

Step 7: It actually worked last night! When I look back at it now, I was able to see a potential problem way in advance, think through some possible ways to handle it and choose two things that worked for me. All in all, I think I did pretty well. And I think he likes me!

FIGURE 10.1. A patient's first attempt at problem-solving (patient A).

patients should be encouraged to practice using problem-solving to address these more minor difficulties so that they are better able to address more major ones when they arise.

As noted above, proactive problem-solving is generally introduced in Stage Three. There is one common exception. This concerns patients whose binge eating is almost exclusively in response to events and adverse moods rather than also being a product of extreme dietary restraint. Many patients with binge eating disorder fall into this category. In common with other patients, the initial focus of these patients' treatment is on establishing a pattern of regular eating (see Chapter 6). Once this is achieved (which often occurs within weeks), it can be appropriate to move directly to the procedures described in this chapter even if nominally still in Stage One.

Addressing Residual Binges

Binge eating is common among patients with eating disorders, and it responds well and rapidly to the "regular eating" intervention of Stage One (see Chapter 6, page 75). With some patients it ceases altogether, but with others binge eating persists into Stage Three albeit at a reduced frequency. Typically these "residual binges" are intermittent and triggered by external events or adverse moods. An elaboration of the problem-solving procedure may be used to address them. We term this "binge analysis."

Binge Analysis

Binge analysis is a strategy for helping patients eliminate their remaining binges (objective or subjective). The first step involves explaining to patients that binges do not come out of the blue: rather, they are the product of one or more of four well-defined processes. These are as follows:

1. *Breaking a dietary rule* and reacting by temporarily abandoning dietary control
2. *Being disinhibited by alcohol or other psychoactive agents* (e.g., marijuana), and thereby being unable to maintain dietary restraint
3. *Undereating* — patients who are persistently or intermittently undereating (i.e., engaging in "dietary restriction" including delayed eating) are under strong physiological pressure to eat.
4. *Being triggered by an external event or adverse mood*

Having explained these processes, the therapist should encourage patients to view each subsequent binge as an "interesting phenomenon" from which they can gain. Specifically, once they have recovered their composure following a binge, patients should consider which of the four mechanisms contributed to it — and often more than one will have operated — and what they can learn as a result. The diagram shown in Figure 10.2 can be helpful in this regard. Analyzing each individual binge in this way has two valuable effects. First, it counters patients' tendency to feel overwhelmed and demoralized by continuing to binge eat, a reaction that may put them at risk of further binge eating. Instead, binges become a behavior to be analyzed objectively and understood (see vignette on page 141). In other words the goal is that patients react to their remaining binges by rolling up their sleeves rather than wringing their hands. The second valuable effect is that

> **The goal is that patients react to their remaining binges by rolling up their sleeves rather than wringing their hands.**

binge analysis highlights and reinforces the use of those specific procedures that are most likely to eliminate the remaining binges. These are listed on the facing page.

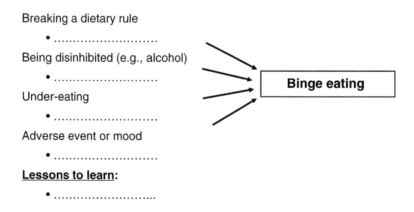

FIGURE 10.2. Binge analysis.

From *Cognitive Behavior Therapy and Eating Disorders* by Christopher G. Fairburn. Copyright 2008 by The Guilford Press. This figure is available online at www.psych.ox.ac.uk/credo/cbt_and_eating_disorders.

1. *Breaking a dietary rule*
   - Addressed by eroding patients' dietary rules and tackling their reaction to rule-breaking (see Chapter 9)
2. *Being disinhibited by alcohol or other psychoactive agents*
   - Addressed by psychoeducation and support
3. *Undereating (dietary restriction)*
   - Addressed by psychoeducation and graded behavior change (see Chapter 11) and focusing on the processes that encourage it (see Chapters 8 and 9)
4. *Being triggered by an external event or adverse mood*
   - Addressed by proactive problem-solving, possibly combined with the development of functional methods of mood modulation (see the next section)

Some patients positively like aspects of binge eating and for this reason are loathe to stop. These patients can be difficult to help. With them, it is best to explore in detail what they gain from binge eating (e.g., immediate enjoyment of eating; relaxation of restraint) and what are the disadvantages (e.g., potential weight gain, expense, secrecy and deceit, self-criticism and perpetuation of the eating disorder in the long-term). The pros and cons approach used with underweight patients (see Chapter 11, page 161) can be helpful in this regard. Once such patients fully appreciate the long-term costs of continuing to binge eat, they are more willing to stop.

Vignette

A patient reported binge eating on a Friday night. Afterward she considered which of the four mechanisms had contributed to this binge. She was not underweight and had eaten enough that day so undereating did not apply, nor had she drunk any alcohol. There was a clear social trigger, however, and once she started to eat she consumed three "trigger" foods, thereby rapidly breaking three dietary rules. So one mechanism was rule-breaking, a problem that she was tackling already. She decided that she needed to learn about the other mechanism, the social one.

Just before starting to binge she wrote on her monitoring record: *"All my friends have gone out. I am on my own. No-one likes me."* The therapist asked her what evidence she had for this thought, and the patient cited the fact that her friends had gone out without her. When asked whether there was any contradictory evidence, she acknowledged that there had been innumerable times when her friends had called round to see her and had included her in events. The patient was asked whether she could think of alternative explanations for what had happened that evening, but she could not.

As homework, it was suggested that she talk to her friends about that evening. The following session she reported that she had discovered that her friends had called her boyfriend, but as they received no answer they assumed that the two of them were already out as they usually spent Friday evening together. They had not thought of contacting her directly as they had not known that her boyfriend was away that weekend.

The patient said that she felt much better once she had heard their explanation and that she would not have binged if she had not jumped to the wrong conclusion. The therapist and patient concluded that the binge had been "useful" in that it had highlighted a general problem of the patient's (social sensitivity and jumping to negative conclusions) that could well have been addressed at the time by problem-solving.

Addressing Mood-Related Changes in Eating

This component of CBT-E is designed for patients whose eating is markedly influenced by their mood. All patients' eating is affected by their mood to an extent, as is entirely normal, and either this area does not need to be addressed or it can be tackled by helping them deal more effectively with the events that trigger the changes in their mood (via proactive problem-solving). However, some patients are either extremely sensitive to certain mood states and have difficulty tolerating them, or they experience unusually intense moods, or both. This may be termed "mood intolerance." Generally the moods in question are adverse moods, but this is not invariably the case. Patients may be sensitive to any intense or strong mood including, for example, excitement. This sensitivity leads them to engage in forms of behavior ("mood modulatory behavior") that help them cope with these moods, either by reducing their awareness of them or by neutralizing them. Binge eating is one example, and vomiting and over-exercising are others. Thus in these patients aspects of the eating disorder help them cope with their moods and are therefore maintained by mechanisms "external" to the core eating disorder. For this reason simply focusing on the usual maintaining mechanisms (as specified in the patient's formulation) is not sufficient to remove these forms of behavior on a permanent basis. Instead, treatment has to directly address the additional maintaining mechanism, namely mood intolerance.

> **In patients with mood intolerance aspects of the eating disorder help them cope with their moods.**

This aspect of treatment is therefore designed for a subgroup of patients. It is especially relevant, but not exclusively so, to patients who are prone to attract the diagnosis of borderline personality disorder (or be referred to as "multi-impulsive"). Originally it was one element of the "broad" form of CBT-E (see Chapter 13), but subsequent experience has shown that it can be readily and appropriately incorporated within the main "focused" version of the treatment. The approach overlaps with elements of dialectical behavior therapy (Linehan, 1993).

Identifying Patients with Mood Intolerance

The patients for whom these strategies and procedures are most relevant are best identified in Stage Two, when reviewing progress (see Chapter 7), or early in Stage Three. By then it is generally clear that some of their eating disorder behavior is being maintained by mood sensitivity. A clue comes from the persistence of certain eating disorder features despite attempts to address them. For example, binge eating may be continuing even though the patient is attempting to comply with "regular eating" (see Chapter 6), or the patient may still be engaging in intermittent non-compensatory vomiting or over-exercising. More direct evidence comes from reviewing in detail recent changes in eating and whether they were preceded by an incipient change in mood that the patient went on to neutralize. The difficulty with this procedure is that patients who are especially mood-sensitive react so quickly to emerging moods that they may not experience an initial mood change. A further clue is a history of other forms of dysfunctional mood modulatory behavior as this is often indicative of some degree of mood intolerance. Two types of behavior are of particular note:

- *Self-injury* (e.g., cutting or burning the skin; hitting oneself). This neutralizes intense mood states almost instantly and is therefore strongly reinforced.
- *Self-medication with psychoactive substances* (e.g., alcohol, marijuana, etc) - This is another way of coping with intense mood states although it is slower to work and less "effective" than self-injury. Intermittent bouts of heavy alcohol consumption (e.g., non-social binge drinking) is particularly suggestive.

Some of these patients engage in a range of forms of mood modulatory behavior. These may be employed interchangeably or patients may go through phases of favoring one over the other. Whatever the pattern, a history of engaging in these forms of behavior should alert the therapist to the possibility that the patient may be mood intolerant.

If it remains unclear whether mood intolerance is contributing to the maintenance of the eating disorder, the best strategy is to address any changes in eating using the problem-solving procedure described above. Doing so will usually reveal any mood sensitivity that is present.

Educating about Mood Intolerance

To educate patients about mood intolerance and the strategy for addressing it, the therapist should identify one or more recent examples with reference to the patient's monitoring records. Then, with each example, the sequence of events that led to the change in eating should be re-created in terms of the presence of any triggering event and the patient's subsequent feelings, thoughts and behavior. Clearly this procedure overlaps with that used to address event-triggered changes in eating. The goal is that patients begin to see that each episode involved a sequence of rapidly unfolding steps:

1. *The occurrence of a triggering event*
   - E.g., an argument on the phone with the boyfriend
2. *Cognitive appraisal of the event*
   - E.g., resentment (*"It is not fair — he is always blaming me"*)
3. *An aversive mood change*
   - E.g., anger
4. *Cognitive appraisal of the mood change, followed by very rapid (within seconds) cognitive amplification of the mood*
   - E.g., *"I can't stand feeling angry like this,"* leading to mood amplification and the thought *"I really can't stand feeling like this,"* leading to yet further mood amplification and the thought *"I REALLY can't stand feeling like this,"* leading to yet further mood amplification and the thought *"I REALLY CAN'T STAND FEELING LIKE THIS."*

5. *The initiation of dysfunctional mood modulatory behavior*
   - E.g., the patient starts to binge or self-injure
6. *The immediate amelioration of the aversive mood*
   - E.g., dissipation of feelings of anger
7. *Later cognitive appraisal*
   - E.g., *"I am such a failure. I have absolutely no control over my eating."*

The therapist should point out that this habitual response is unhelpful in a number of ways: It results in patients not addressing day-to-day difficulties; it leads to unpredictable behavior and often worsens interpersonal problems; it maintains the eating problem; and it makes patients feel bad about themselves.

Slowing Down, Observing and Analyzing

The next step involves patients starting to observe subsequent episodes as they occur in real time. This is extremely difficult and may take quite a few attempts to accomplish, but it is central to overcoming mood intolerance.

As soon as patients detect that there might be a triggering event or mood, they should immediately remove themselves from the situation and write down a brief description of

- What has happened
- Their appraisal of it
- What they are now feeling
- Their appraisal of this feeling

In other words they are recording Steps 1–4 in more or less real time. This has the effect of slowing down the process. It also obliges them to stay in their current state rather than "escaping" by engaging in one of their habitual forms of mood modulatory behavior. Patients need to be forewarned that they will find doing this extremely frustrating, but they should try their utmost to stay "in the moment" for as long as possible. This is important because doing so disrupts the cognitive amplification that lies at the heart of mood intolerance (Step 4 above).

Therapists should be very encouraging and supportive of patients who are attempting this. Even partial successes are true successes.

Intervening

Having begun to slow down, observe and analyze the usual sequence of events and, in the process of doing so, interrupt it by preventing cognitive amplification, the patient is now in a position to intervene at various points in the sequence. The indications for the various strategies and procedures are as follows:

Occurrence of triggering events
   - Prevent when possible using proactive problem-solving

Cognitive appraisal of events
   - Cognitive restructuring and behavioral experiments

Occurrence of aversive moods and their cognitive appraisal
- "Mood acceptance"

Use of mood modulatory behavior
- Practicing the use of functional mood modulatory behavior
- Putting barriers in the way of dysfunctional mood modulatory behavior

Turning to the procedures themselves:

1. *Proactive problem-solving.* This should never be dismissed as a technique. It is generally of great value, even with the most chaotic of patients. It is used to prevent many of the types of problem that would otherwise lead to an episode of mood intolerance.

2. *Cognitive restructuring.* This should be used to help patients assess events and their personal significance. It is especially important to counter dichotomous thinking and negative appraisals (see vignette on page 141).

3. *"Mood acceptance."* This is an umbrella term used to describe the following:

a. *Education about moods*
- Moods are part of normal human experience. It is fine to feel angry or low at times, just as it is to feel happy.
- Moods rarely persist for long (unless one has a mood disorder such as a clinical depression).
- It is helpful to know what mood one is in. Some people misinterpret their mood; for example, by mislabeling excitement as anxiety. Noticing what other features are present can be helpful (e.g., muscle tension may be indicative of anxiety) as can thinking about what others would feel under the circumstances. Note that some patients mislabel their thoughts as feelings (e.g., *"I felt like a failure"*), in which case the therapist should try to help them identify the accompanying emotion.

b. *Acting on moods*
- Moods do not require a reaction. They can just be accepted.
- One can "ride out" a mood and observe it wax and then wane. This is similar to "urge surfing" (see page 79). Doing so will disconfirm the belief that adverse moods just worsen until something has to be done about them.
- If one's current mood is aversive and not one to ride out, there are a variety of ways to modify it that will not do one any harm.

4. *Practicing the use of functional mood modulatory behavior.* Therapists should help patients identify and implement functional methods of changing their mood when the need arises. The methods to use will differ according to the circumstances and the patient's preferences. It is useful to ask patients to prepare a list of methods to have available in advance. The main options include the following:

- Putting on music that is likely to alter one's mood and mindset.
- Communicating with others (especially if it involves talking rather than exchanging texts or e-mails). Face-to-face contact is best.
- Exercising: Brisk walking can be good and is easy to do in most situations.
- Taking a bath is soothing. A candle-lit or bubble bath is even better.

- Taking a cold shower.
- Going out to the cinema. Usually a "light" film is best.

At first, these new forms of behavior may be experienced as "less effective" than the old dysfunctional methods, but with practice they become more effective over time and they have the definite advantage of not having adverse effects. Successfully using functional mood modulatory behavior can help challenge patients' belief that their mood is outside their control. It also can challenge beliefs about dysfunctional mood modulatory behavior (e.g., *"Only binge eating can help me to feel better"*).

5. *Putting barriers in the way of dysfunctional mood modulatory behavior.* This does not apply so much to eating disorder behavior, but it does apply to the use of psychoactive substances and to self-injury (e.g., cutting using razor blades, knives). It is best not to have the requisite substances or equipment at hand. If asked sensitively, many patients will hand over to the therapist their stash of pills, their special knife, etc.

Some Tips and Problems

- Real-time in-the-moment recording is of central importance in helping these patients. It has a major impact in its own right.

  > **One success breeds further successes.**

- As always, employ the principle of parsimony. Avoid overloading patients with a surfeit of techniques. Instead, help them acquire the strategies and procedures that are of most relevance to them.
- Do not forget the value of simple interventions: for example, proactive problem-solving; the use of music to modulate mood; putting barriers in the way of dysfunctional behavior.
- One success breeds further successes.
- Once mood intolerance has begun to be addressed, it should remain a major item on each session's agenda until the pattern has been broken.

Recommended Reading

Recommended reading for Chapters 5–12 can be found at the end of Chapter 12.

CHAPTER 11

Underweight and Undereating

The great majority of patients with an eating disorder undereat at some stage and many become underweight for a time. Generally this phase does not last and they regain the lost weight, often as a result of binge eating, but a minority of patients manage to retain extreme control over their eating and stay underweight. If they have a BMI of 17.5 or below (or are maintaining a body weight that is less than 85% of that expected, as required by DSM-IV), they may meet diagnostic criteria for anorexia nervosa (see Chapter 2). Those who do not have all the necessary diagnostic features (e.g., amenorrhea, the over-evaluation of shape and weight) receive the diagnosis eating disorder NOS instead. Being so underweight is serious because it has major physical and psychosocial consequences, some of which encourage further undereating. Hence this can become a self-perpetuating state.

The focus of this chapter is on how CBT-E needs to be adapted to suit underweight patients (i.e., those with anorexia nervosa or underweight forms of eating disorder NOS) and those who undereat. It is worth noting at the outset that CBT-E does not need major modifications because these patients have the same core psychopathology as the majority of other patients and very similar behavior. As a consequence almost all the strategies and procedures described so far are of relevance to these patients too. Nevertheless they do have certain distinctive features that need to be directly addressed, and these require CBT-E to be modified. The three main features of note are as follows:

1. *Undereating.* Undereating is invariable among underweight patients, although it is also present in many other patients.
2. *Being underweight.*
3. *Having limited motivation to change.* Many underweight patients do not view their undereating or low weight as a problem. This is because it is consonant with their over-evaluation of control over eating, shape and weight. Indeed, they tend to view their undereating and low weight as evidence of their will-power and self-control.

CBT-E has to be adapted to accommodate these three features. The problem with motivation is a particularly difficult one as, unless it is successfully addressed, treatment stands little chance of succeeding. It is therefore a priority from the start. The undereating and low weight are also important. They too need to be tackled early on as maintaining a very low weight is extremely unhealthy; it causes psychosocial impairment; and, as will be explained, it obstructs change.

CBT-E not only needs to be adapted in content; it also needs to be extended in length. This is for two reasons: first, it takes some weeks to engender motivation to change; and second, it takes a long time to achieve, and then maintain, a healthy weight. In patients who have a BMI between 15.0 and 17.5 — the underweight group best suited for outpatient-based CBT-E — treatment generally takes in the region of 40 weeks and involves about 40 sessions (i.e., twice the input of the usual form of CBT-E). With regard to appointment frequency it is our practice to hold sessions twice weekly until the patient is consistently gaining weight. Then the sessions become weekly. In the later stages of weight regain sessions are every 2 weeks, and toward the end of treatment they are every 3 weeks.

How CBT-E is adapted and extended for patients who are underweight is the focus of this chapter. The treatment of underweight adolescents is described in Chapter 14, and an inpatient version of the treatment is described in Chapter 15. *Throughout the chapter it is assumed that the reader is familiar with the 20-session form of CBT-E as described in Chapters 5–10 and 12.*

One other point needs to be stressed. Patients' health and safety are of paramount importance and must never be neglected, and this is especially true of underweight patients because their physical health is invariably compromised. Anyone with clinical responsibility for these patients must be fully aware of the complications that they are prone to develop (see Chapter 4, page 40), and non-medical therapists need to have access to a physician who can advise them on the management of the medical problems of their cases.

Overview of CBT-E for Underweight Patients

The treatment strategy involves the following steps:

1. Starting well by engaging patients and maintaining engagement thereafter. Central to this is showing an intense interest in the patient as a person and not just in his or her eating habits and weight.
2. Educating patients about the psychological, social and physical effects of maintaining a very low weight.
3. Creating a personalized formulation in which the contribution of weight-related effects is highlighted.
4. In the context of the formulation, helping patients to become intrigued by the benefits of change and the possibility of making a "fresh start."

   The goal is that patients themselves decide to regain weight.

   The goal is that patients themselves decide to regain weight. Note that the term "regain" is used: Patients much prefer it to "gain."
5. Ensuring that patients adhere to this decision and helping them regain weight. Typically this takes many months and much perseverance on the part of the patient and therapist.
6. Simultaneously addressing the other features of the eating disorder (e.g., the over-evaluation of shape and weight; body checking; dietary restraint and

dietary rules). Helping patients begin to develop a sustaining and rewarding interpersonal life is especially important.

7. Once a healthy BMI has been achieved, helping patients accept and maintain their new shape and weight.

8. Ending well by maximizing the chances that the changes made are maintained and minimizing the risk of relapse.

The four stages of the 20-session version of CBT-E do not neatly map onto this version of the treatment.

Starting Well

The first two treatment sessions resemble those of the 20-session version, although certain adaptations are needed to accommodate education about the effects of being underweight and the incorporation of this information into the formulation. The subsequent six sessions are also like those of the 20-session version with the important exception that there is a major emphasis on helping patients decide to change. Appointments are twice weekly.

The Initial Session

Engaging the Patient in Treatment and Change

This is especially important, although no special procedures are needed at this point. It is useful to start by asking patients about how they have come to seek treatment. It will emerge that some have come to treatment reluctantly and under pressure from others. With these patients it is important to stress that the therapist will be operating entirely on their behalf and not on behalf of their parents, partner, or anyone else.

Assessing the Nature and Severity of the Psychopathology Present

This assessment is very much like the 20-session one except that the therapist also asks about features likely to be secondary to being underweight. These should not be labeled as such, as otherwise there is a risk that some patients might not disclose them. Rather, inquiry about their presence should be embedded within the usual assessment (see Chapter 5). Table 11.1 lists the main additional features of importance.

Jointly Creating the Formulation

This step is delayed until the next session. This is because underweight patients are less likely to identify immediately with their formulation than are other patients. For this reason, it is especially important that the formulation is created well. Delaying this until the next session gives the therapist time to reflect on the underweight features present, those that are most troubling to the patient, and their likely contribution to the maintenance of the eating problem. It also means that the creation of the formulation can be integrated with education about the effects of being underweight.

TABLE 11.1. Features Commonly Present in Those Who Are Significantly Underweight

Eating disorder features

- Ritualistic eating (e.g., using the same plates or silverware; counting mouthfuls; eating clockwise around the plate; cutting food into specific shapes)
- Eating slowly
- Feeling full even after eating small quantities
- Using large quantities of condiments or spices
- Hoarding food
- Preoccupation with thoughts about food and eating
- Increased salience of food and eating (e.g., reading recipe books; watching TV cookery programs; cooking for others but not eating oneself)

General psychiatric features

- Low mood
- Irritability
- Ritualistic behavior (a strong need for routine; inflexibility)
- Hoarding objects
- Difficulty concentrating
- Loss of previous interests
- Social withdrawal and avoidance
- Loss of sexual appetite

Physical features

- Absent or irregular menstruation
- Decreased sexual responsiveness
- Poor sleep (not refreshing, waking early)
- Sensitivity to the cold
- Dry skin
- Hair loss
- Muscle weakness (on climbing stairs; on standing from sitting or squatting)
- Dizziness

Explaining What Treatment Will Involve

This too is particularly important as these patients tend to have a strong need to feel "in control." The following topics should be covered:

- *Nature and style of the treatment.* This is as described in Chapter 5.
- *Practicalities.* This includes the likely number and frequency of treatment sessions.
- *In-session weighing.* Here there is a departure from the 20-session protocol in that these patients should be weighed every session rather than once weekly. This is because their weight is of medical concern and therefore needs to be closely monitored. Also, weight change is an important aspect of treatment.
- *Instillation of "ownership," enthusiasm and hope.* This too is important. The notion that it is the patient's treatment, not the therapist's, needs to be emphasized, and throughout treatment patients should feel clear about what is happening and why. It is also important to engender hope. Patients with a long history of being underweight may have been told that they will never overcome their eating problem. This undermines any hope of recovery that the patient might have had. We say to patients who are extremely pessimistic about the prospect of change, *"I am sure we can help. It is good that*

you are here" because this is the case. Of course, making false promises must be avoided, but it is rare that we are unable to be of at least some help.

- *Patients' questions and concerns.* Throughout treatment patients should be encouraged to ask questions and air their concerns. Therapists should repeatedly check that patients are "on board."

Introducing In-Session Weighing

In-session weighing follows the same protocol as that used in the 20-session treatment (see page 62) except that it takes place every session (including the initial one), and the educational element about weight checking and avoidance is delayed for a couple of sessions due to constraints on time. In this initial session "collaborative weighing" takes place mid-session rather than at the beginning. This is because it would be inappropriate for the first session to begin with the patient being weighed. Patients are asked to refrain from weighing themselves at home, perhaps by saying:

> *"From now on we will see what your weight is here, twice a week. You will learn a lot about your weight, and you will get good and sufficient information about it from our twice-weekly weighings. Weighing yourself at home in addition to this would just be confusing. Therefore I would like to ask you to do your best to stop weighing yourself at home. We will discuss your weight and how to interpret it in a great deal more detail over the coming weeks."*

Establishing Real-Time Self-Monitoring

This takes place in the initial session, as in the 20-session version, with the same form of monitoring record being used.

Confirming the Homework Assignments

There are two pieces of homework at this stage: starting real-time recording and resisting weighing at home. As in the 20-session version, the therapist should ask the patient to write down on a Next Steps sheet exactly what has been agreed.

Summarizing the Session and Arranging the Next Appointment

The therapist ends the session by summarizing its content, re-stating the homework, and booking the next appointment(s). The patient should be reminded that the next session will begin with weighing.

Session 1

The top priority in the second appointment, as in the first, is engagement. Without the patient being engaged, treatment is likely to get nowhere. There are three other priorities:

- Reviewing the recording
- Providing education about the effects of being underweight
- Jointly creating the formulation

The appointment lasts about 50 minutes, as do all subsequent ones, but, as in the 20-session treatment, the structure of the session is idiosyncratic because of the need to review the records in exceptional detail in order to establish and reinforce high-quality recording. As a result the session has the following format:

1. In-session weighing
2. Reviewing the recording
3. Setting the agenda
4. Working through the agenda, which is likely to comprise:

    • Assessing the patient's attitude toward treatment
    • Providing personalized education about the effects of being underweight
    • Jointly creating the formulation
    • Addressing any other items (i.e., anything else the patient would like to discuss)

5. Summarizing the session, confirming the homework assignments, and arranging the next appointment.

In-Session Weighing

This takes place at the very beginning of the session and opens with "collaborative weighing" (see page 63). The therapist tells the patient his or her current weight in a unit that the patient understands (e.g., pounds) and how it differs (or not) from his or her weight at the initial session.

Patients should be told that it is important that they learn more about body weight and its regulation, weight fluctuations, and weight checking and avoidance, but since these are complex topics the discussion will be postponed for a session or two until there is more time.

Reviewing the Recording, Setting the Agenda, and Assessing the Patient's Attitude toward Treatment

These are as in the 20-session version. The therapist should continue to express interest in the patient as a person. Simple but direct questions, such as those listed below, show that the therapist is truly concerned about the patient's overall well-being and not just his or her eating habits and weight. They also tend to unearth aspects of secondary impairment that might otherwise pass undetected.

> *"I would like to know what is life like for you, at present?"*
> *"Are you happy?"*
> *"Do you have friends?"*
> *"Are you able to do what other people your age do?"*
> *"How is your life compared to theirs?"*

Personalized Education about the Effects of Being Underweight

Education about the effects of being significantly underweight is an essential preliminary to the creation of the formulation. Patients need to know the consequences of what they are doing.

• *Patients should be educated about the significance of their current BMI.* Specifically, they should be told their current BMI and they should be given the BMI thresholds for being significantly underweight, underweight, a low weight, etc. (see page 15). It should be explained that their BMI is well below a healthy level and that they will therefore be subject to a range of adverse physical, psychological and social effects.

• *Patients should be educated about the secondary effects of being underweight.* The main points to stress are summarized in the patient handout shown in Table 11.2. Therapists wanting to learn more about these effects are recommended the chapter by Garner (1997) and the patient–oriented account of Lucas (2004).

• *Patients should be asked to consider which underweight features they are currently experiencing.* This can be done by going though the handout (see Table 11.2). If some features were detected in the initial session yet are not now mentioned by the patient, this omission should be pointed out (indirectly) by saying something along these lines: *"At our first session didn't you tell me that you . . . [e.g., eat very slowly and count mouthfuls; tend to feel cold all the time)?"*

• *The implications of this information should be considered.* There are three points to highlight:

1. Many of the adverse experiences reported by the patient are simply secondary to his or her low body weight. These should be specified.
2. Some of the secondary effects contribute to the maintenance of the eating problem. This is one of the main points to be emphasized when creating the patient's formulation (see the next section).
3. These secondary effects will resolve with weight regain.

Jointly Creating the Formulation

The creation of the patient's formulation follows the principles specified in Chapter 5. It either resembles the "restricting anorexia nervosa" one shown in Figure 11.1 or the composite transdiagnostic formulation if the patient binges and purges (see Figure 11.2).

When personalizing the formulation, it is especially important to highlight the likely contribution of underweight features to the maintenance of the patient's eating problem. The most pertinent are as follows:

• *Preoccupation with thoughts about food and eating.* This is a consequence of dietary restriction. Thinking about food and eating results in patients persisting in their attempts to restrict their eating and being relatively impervious to outside influences. It can be helpful to describe the DVD analogy at this point (see page 119). When underweight, the eating disorder DVD is permanently "in place" and playing at a loud volume. Therapists should note, however, that this is not the time to help patients manipulate their mindset. In our experience, this is a largely fruitless exercise when patients are underweight. Instead, it is better left until they have regained weight and are experiencing times when their DVD is not "in place."

• *Social withdrawal and loss of previous interests.* This prevents patients from being exposed to life experiences that might diminish the importance that they place on con-

TABLE 11.2. Patient Handout on the Effects of Being Underweight

The Effects of Being Underweight

Maintaining an unduly low body weight is unhealthy and harmful. It has numerous adverse effects on one's physical, psychological and social functioning.

Knowledge about the effects of a low body weight has come from a variety of sources, including studies of the effects of famines, and other causes of food shortage, and experimental studies in which volunteers have adhered to a restricted diet for extended periods of time. Consistent findings have emerged. These are summarized below.

If you are underweight you will experience exactly the same adverse effects.

Psychological Effects

Thinking

Thinking is affected by being underweight. This is hardly surprising since the brain requires a lot of energy (i.e., calories) to function properly. Thinking becomes *inflexible* at a low body weight, with the result that it becomes difficult to switch rapidly from topic to topic. It also becomes difficult to make decisions.

Concentration is almost always impaired, although people may not be aware of this because they force themselves to focus on what they are doing. In part the concentration impairment is due to the presence of recurrent thoughts about food and eating (secondary to undereating), which interfere with the ability to focus on other things. Some people find that they even dream about food and eating.

The almost constant thinking about food and eating affects behavior too. It leads some people to become particularly interested in cooking and thus they keep reading recipes and watching TV cookery programs, and they may also do a lot of cooking. At the same time they tend to become *less interested in other things.* They often give up old interests and hobbies.

Feelings

Mood is affected by being underweight. It is generally somewhat low and people are prone to getting *irritated rather easily.*

Behavior

People who are significantly underweight change the way that they behave. If they have been underweight for a long time, they come to think that their current way of thinking, feeling and behaving reflects their "personality" whereas their true personality is being masked by the effects of being underweight.

One of the most prominent changes is *heightened "obsessiveness."* This term refers to the tendency to be inflexible and rigid in one's routines. Some people may also become very particular about cleanliness and tidiness. Often this is accompanied by *difficulty being spontaneous.*

The obsessiveness is often particularly striking when it comes to eating. People may eat in a very particular way. Eating may become like a mini "ceremony" that has to be conducted alone. Some people eat very slowly, chewing each mouthful a certain number of times; others *eat in a ritualized way,* always eating from a certain plate or cutting food into small pieces.

Hoarding objects is yet another feature, although not everyone shows it. The hoarding may be of food or other things. Often people cannot explain why they are doing this.

TABLE 11.2 (*cont.*)

Social Effects

Being underweight has a profound effect on social functioning. There is a tendency to become *inward-looking and self-focused*. This is exaggerated by the heightened need for routine and predictability, and difficulty being spontaneous. As a result people *withdraw socially* and get used to this way of living.

Also there is a *loss of sexual appetite* (due to hormonal changes). This too can contribute to the social withdrawal.

Physical Effects

Being underweight has a marked effect on one's physical health. The exact effects depend upon the extent and nature of the dietary deprivation.

Heart and circulation

There are profound effects on the heart and circulation. Heart muscle is lost and the heart is weaker as a result. Blood pressure drops and the heart rate (pulse) declines. There is heightened risk of heart beat irregularities (arrhythmias).

Sex hormones and fertility

Likewise there are profound effects on hormonal function, with non-essential processes ceasing. As a result sex hormone production declines markedly and people become infertile. There is a loss of interest in sex and sexual responsiveness declines.

Bones

There is a deterioration in bone strength. This is due in part to the hormonal changes, in part due to the decrease in the weight that the bones have to carry, and in part a direct dietary effect. The result is an increased risk of osteoporosis and fractures.

Intestinal function

The gut slows down and as a result food moves slowly along it. Food in the stomach takes much longer than normal to move into the small intestine, which is why people have a heightened sensation of fullness even after eating relatively little. Taste may be impaired and so there may be increased use of condiments and spices to give food flavor. There may be persistent hunger.

Muscles

Muscles waste and weakness can result. This is most obvious when walking up stairs or trying to stand up from a sitting or squatting position.

Skin and hair

The effects vary. A downy hair (called lanugo) may start to grow on the body, especially on the face, abdomen, back and arms. There may also be hair loss from the scalp. Often the skin becomes dry, and it can develop an orange tinge.

Temperature regulation

There is a decrease in body temperature, and people feel profoundly cold.

Sleep

Sleep is impaired when underweight. Sleeps tends to be less refreshing and there is a tendency to wake early.

Postscript: Some of the effects described above are direct effects of sustained undereating, rather than a low weight, and occur in anyone who is markedly undereating whatever his or her actual weight.

(*cont.*)

TABLE 11.2 (*cont.*)

___

The Significance of These Effects

There are five important points to note:

1. **Some of the things that you find difficult or aversive at the moment are likely to be a direct result of having too low a weight.**

2. **Many people who are underweight assume that the way that they are now reflects their personality.** It is most important to stress that your personality is being masked by the effects of being underweight and that your true personality will only be revealed once you cease being underweight.

3. **Some of the effects of having too low a weight are dangerous or do long-term damage to your body** (e.g., the effects on your heart and circulation, and the effects on your bones respectively).

4. **Some of the effects of having too low a weight keep you "locked in" to your eating problem** (e.g., thinking too much about food and eating; being inflexible and having to stick to routines and rituals; having difficulty making decisions; not wanting to socialize; having difficulty concentrating; feeling full so readily).

5. **Almost all these effects will go away if you regain weight to a low, but healthy, level**.

___

trolling their eating, shape and weight. Patients often fail to appreciate how unusual their behavior and lifestyle are.

- *Indecisiveness.* This makes it difficult for patients to decide whether to change. The result is procrastination.

- *Heightened need for routine and predictability.* This also interferes with change.

- *Persistent hunger.* This is not always present, but, if it is, it contributes to the preoccupation with food and eating. Some view it as evidence of their "greediness" and that therefore they need to be especially vigilant about controlling their eating. However, it is not always viewed negatively. Some patients view symptoms of undereating and being underweight (e.g., hunger, dizziness, feeling cold) as evidence of "success" in controlling their eating.

- *Heightened feelings of fullness.* This makes it difficult to increase the amount eaten.

As with other patients the formulation should be drawn out step by step in an unhurried manner, with the therapist taking the lead but with the patient being actively involved. It is best to start with something that the patient wants to change (e.g., binge eating or an aversive feature of being underweight, e.g., feeling cold or sleeping poorly). Whenever possible and appropriate, the patient's own terms should be used. Since the formulation is based on information only just obtained, it should be made clear that it is provisional and will be modified as needed during treatment.

Once the formulation has been created, the therapist should discuss its implications for treatment. These are especially important for underweight patients. There are five points to make. (These points are also made in the patient handout on the effects of being underweight; see Table 11.2).

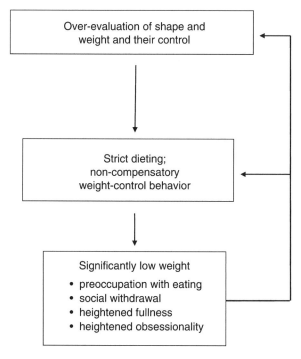

FIGURE 11.1. The "restricting" anorexia nervosa formulation.

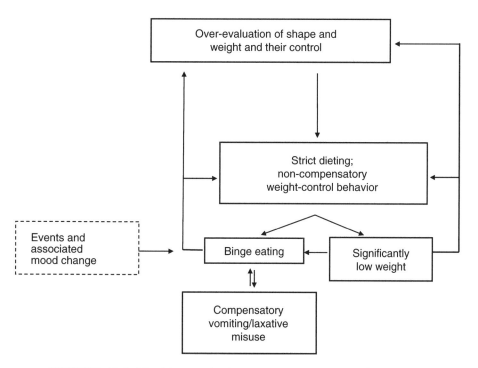

FIGURE 11.2. The binge–eating/purging anorexia nervosa formulation.

1. *Some of the features that the patient is finding aversive or impairing are a direct result of being significantly underweight.* For example:

- Preoccupation with food and eating
- Being inflexible; having to stick to routines; being unable to be spontaneous
- Having difficulty making decisions
- Not wanting to socialize
- Having difficulty concentrating
- Sleeping poorly
- Feeling full so readily
- Feeling very cold
- Feeling physically weak

2. *Often patients assume that their present state (e.g., being socially avoidant, inflexible, insecure) reflects their personality.* It is most important to stress that their personality is being masked by the effects of being underweight and that their true "self" will only become clear if they regain weight. The therapist should try to interest the patient in this phenomenon; for example, by describing how other patients have changed on regaining weight.

3. *Some of the physical consequences of being so underweight are dangerous or risk causing long-term damage to health.* For example:

- Cardiovascular effects
- Effects on the bones

The therapist should identify the physical consequences that are of most relevance and concern to the patient. If aspects of the patient's physical state are particularly serious, the therapist should say so (or ask a physician to do so). There is a tendency for patients (and sometimes their relatives) to turn a blind eye to the seriousness of the patient's physical condition.

4. *Some of the effects of being underweight maintain the eating problem.* For example:

- Preoccupation with food and eating
- Social withdrawal and loss of previous interests
- Indecisiveness
- Heightened need for routine and predictability
- Heightened feelings of fullness

It is important to highlight the vicious circles that exist whereby these secondary effects lock the patient into his or her eating problem.

5. *Almost all the effects of being underweight will resolve if the patient regains weight to a low but healthy level.* Clearly the major implication of the education and formulation is that patients need to stop restricting their eating and start to regain weight. This is obvious. However, in our view it is best not said. Rather, it is preferable to leave patients to think about the information provided and draw their own conclusions. With this point in mind, patients should be given copies of the handout and their formulation, and asked to think about them between this session and the next.

Summarizing the Session, Confirming the Homework, and Arranging the Next Appointment

There are generally three pieces of homework at the end of session 1:

1. Improving upon the recording
2. Reading the handout on being underweight
3. Reviewing the formulation

Reviewing the Formulation and Its Implications

At the next session the therapist and patient should review the formulation, the goal being that the patient understands how being underweight causes the eating problem to persist. The therapeutic implications of this point should then be discussed with the patient being asked to take the lead. The major implication is that weight regain is essential if the patient is to overcome the eating problem.

It is common for patients to object to the prospect of weight regain saying that this is not the answer to their problems and that they will lose all the weight they have regained if they still feel like they do now. It is therefore important to emphasize that treatment will involve much more than weight regain (i.e., it will involve treating the entire eating problem), but that patients cannot overcome their eating problem if they remain underweight.

In-Session Weighing, Weight and Weight Checking

From session 2 onward the therapist and patient plot the available data points onto an individualized weight graph that the therapist has prepared in advance. In later sessions, but still at the outset of them, the therapist and patient jointly interpret the emerging weight data (see page 63), but at this point this is not possible as there are only three data points to review.

Education about weight and weight checking is usually provided in session 2 or 3 depending upon the time available. With one exception, the information is the same as that given to patients receiving the 20-session treatment (see page 70). The exception concerns the BMI. With underweight patients it is important to be absolutely clear about their current weight and BMI, and the BMI (and weight) that they would need to reach to be free from the adverse secondary effects of being underweight. In our experience this is a BMI between 19.0 and 19.9. At this BMI the great majority of patients can eat normally and no longer experience the consequences of being underweight. It is sometimes argued that patients' goal weight (and BMI) should be individualized taking into account their weight history, and that a BMI as high as the mid-20s is appropriate in certain cases. This seems reasonable on theoretical grounds, but there is no direct evidence to support this argument. And there is a more major problem: It is unrealistic. It is difficult enough helping patients achieve and maintain a BMI between 19.0 and 19.9, let alone a higher BMI.

Our position is that the goal of treatment should be to free patients from their eating disorder psychopathology and its adverse effects. In our experience this can be achieved if patients reach a BMI between 19.0 and 19.9 and are successful in address-ing the core maintaining mechanisms (cf., the "house of cards" analogy, page 47). This BMI goal is in fact ambitious, given the disappointing data on the outcome of treatments for anorexia nervosa. Later in treatment we advise some patients (those who have to restrict their eating to maintain their BMI between 19.0 and 19.9) to consider letting their weight rise a little above this level over the year or so following treatment.

Educating the Patient about Eating Problems

Educating patients about eating problems is done in session 3 or 4 using the same guided reading procedure as in the 20-session treatment (see page 74). It might seem odd to recommend that these patients read *Overcoming Binge Eating* but it is highly acceptable to patients and provides the information needed at this stage in treatment. Some patients balk at the title but this is a cue for informing them that while they might not be binge eating at present (many already have subjective binges), most patients with anorexia nervosa will begin to have true objective binges in time, and up to half will develop frank bulimia nervosa. The same is likely to be true of underweight patients with eating disorder NOS. It is our practice to highlight this possibility by adding "Binge eating" to the formulation of patients who are not (yet) binge eating, with it connected to "Dieting" by a dashed line.

Introducing a Pattern of Regular Eating

By session 3 or 4 patients should be ready to adjust their eating habits. It is best to start by helping them establish a pattern of regular eating rather than asking them to eat more. This sequence is used for a number of reasons. First, meals and snacks need to be in place before they can be increased in size. Second, it is a change that most of these patients do not find too hard to accomplish, so long as they do not have to increase the amount that they eat. Since increasing what is eaten is not part of "regular eating," this is not a problem. Patients can simply redistribute their current food intake across the planned meals and snacks. Third, three benefits come from establishing this eating pat-tern:

1. It tackles one form of dieting that is common among underweight patients: the tendency to delay eating.
2. It seems to lessen these patients' propensity to feel full.
3. After a few weeks, there is generally a decrease in the degree of preoccupation with food and eating.

The procedure used for establishing a pattern of regular eating is the same as that described in Chapter 5 (see page 75), although it is important to note that with underweight patients there should be three meals and three snacks (i.e., six episodes of eating rather than the more usual five). Typically the pattern is as follows:

- Breakfast
- Mid-morning snack
- Lunch
- Mid-afternoon snack
- Evening meal
- Evening snack

Helping the Patient Decide to Change

> **The goal in CBT-E is that patients themselves decide to regain weight rather than having this decision imposed upon them.**

The goal in CBT-E is that patients themselves decide to regain weight rather than having this decision imposed upon them. The challenge is how to achieve this goal.

Treatment up to this point (about session 2 or 3) has been designed to prepare the ground for what will be a detailed discussion of the pros and cons of change. Now the therapist directly broaches the topic and puts it at the top of the session agenda for a succession of sessions (often four or more). The therapist starts by validating the patient's experience by acknowledging and empathizing with his or her ambivalence to change (if present). At the same time the therapist conveys belief in the patient's capacity to change. The intention is that the patient becomes intrigued by the benefits of change and the fact that this is an opportunity to make a "fresh start" in life. There are five steps in this process:

1. Creating a "Current pros and cons of change" table (in one session)
2. Creating a "Future pros and cons of change" table (in the next session)
3. Creating a third "Conclusions" table
4. Helping the patient identify and accept the implications of these conclusions
5. "Taking the plunge"

One encounters occasional patients who are already willing to change. With such patients one can omit this part of treatment and move directly to how to change (see page 169). If difficulties with motivation arise later in treatment (as they often do), the pros and cons of change can be discussed at that point.

Step 1: Current Pros and Cons of Change

Patients should be asked to consider their reasons for and against changing. It should be made clear that change would involve overcoming the eating problem and that part of doing this would require regaining weight to a BMI between 19.0 and 19.9 in order to be free from the adverse effects of being underweight. It is best to start by asking patients to list all the reasons why they do not want to change or are afraid of doing so. These can then be put in a table. It is important to acknowledge that patients might view the eating problem as providing something positive that they are worried about losing. Having done this, patients should be asked to innumerate the reasons why they think that they ought to take up this opportunity to change with these reasons also being listed. Patients should be asked to be specific in this regard (e.g., with regard to "better health," the patient should be asked to describe all the positive health changes desired). It is also important to include idiosyncratic reasons to change (e.g., not having to wear two pairs of pantyhose to stay warm). All aspects of life should be considered, including relationships with others, physical and psychological well-being, work performance, and ability to engage in other valued activities. In this context reference may be made to reversing sources of impairment identified on the CIA: Indeed, it can be helpful to ask the patient to complete a new one. As part of the process of considering the pros and cons of change, therapists should normalize the experience of being of two minds about changing (if this indeed appears to be the case).

A typical pros and cons table is shown in Table 11.3. Patients should take a copy of their table home and be asked to reflect upon it before the next session

Step 2: Future Pros and Cons of Change

In the next session the patient's table should be reviewed focusing on any changes that the patient has made. At this stage it is not necessary to question its content.

Then the therapist should ask the patient to adopt a new perspective, one of 5 years hence (less for younger patients) and set the scene by asking the patient questions of the following sort:

TABLE 11.3. Pros and Cons of Change from the Perspective of the Present

Reasons to stay as I am	Reasons to change
It makes me feel in control and special	*I will get rid of the effects of being underweight:*
I get attention from others	*— thinking about food and eating all the time*
I will not get "fat"	*— feeling so cold*
I am good at it	*— not sleeping properly*
It makes me feel strong	*— feeling faint*
It shows I have will-power	*I will feel healthier*
It is familiar and feels safe	*I will be healthier (better bones, stronger heart)*
I have an excuse for things	*I will be able to think more clearly*
I don't have to have periods	*I will have more time*
I am not hassled by men	*I will be able to think about other things*
If I change:	*I will be less obsessive and more flexible and*
— I won't be able to stop eating	*spontaneous*
— my weight will shoot up	*My life will have a broader focus*
— my stomach will stick out	*I will be happier and have more fun*
— my thighs will get fatter	*I will be able to go out with others and get on*
If I change people will think that:	*with people better*
— I am weak and greedy	*I will discover who I really am*
— I have given in	
— I am getting fat	

"What would you like your life to be like in 5 years when you will be . . . years old?"
"What job would you hope to be doing?"
"What responsibilities would you have? Would you be in charge of others? Would you need to travel? Would you have work meetings? Might they involve eating?"
"What sort of relationships would you like to have with other people?"
"What about friends and social life? Would you be active socially?"
"What about relationships with your family?"
"Would you hope to have a partner by then?"
"Would you hope to be married?"
"Would you hope to have had children or to be planning to have them?"
"What sort of person would you like to be? How would you like to be feeling about yourself?"
"What sort of values would you like to have? What would you like to be important to you?"

Once this has been done, patients should be asked whether they have considered how the eating problem would affect their plans and aspirations. Usually they have not thought about this. The therapist should therefore explain what is likely to happen to their eating disorder if they decide not to change, pointing out that much is known about the course of anorexia nervosa. Briefly, in adults with an established underweight eating disorder, the eating problem is very likely to persist. It may remain as it is, but a much more likely outcome is the development of binge eating and accompanying progressive and uncontrolled weight regain. Indeed, as noted earlier, up to 90% start binge eating and up to a half develop frank bulimia nervosa: In other words, they lose control over their eating. This is, of course, these patients' worst fears come true. Once this information has been presented, patients should be reminded of their stated plans and aspirations and asked to consider how they would be affected by having a continuing eating disorder.

Against this background, patients should review the pros and cons of capitalizing on the present opportunity to change, keeping the 5-year perspective in mind. On this basis a second table should be constructed, a typical one being shown in Table 11.4. This table usually differs from the first. Once more, patients should take a copy of their table home and modify it as needed before the next session.

Step 3: Overall Pros and Cons of Change

The third step involves a detailed point-by-point discussion of the patient's second table (illustrated in Table 11.4). During this discussion the therapist should ensure that patients are focusing on the likely impact on their aspirations of not capitalizing on the present opportunity to change. While doing this it is best to reinforce and, if appropriate, amplify their stated reasons to change. These should never be neglected since the benefits of no longer being underweight and overcoming the eating disorder cannot be exaggerated.

The patients' reasons not to change should also be explored in some detail. Below is a list of some of the most common reasons, together with suggested responses. More complex responses are possible, of course, but the ones outlined are generally pertinent and sufficient. Note that, as always in cognitive behavior therapy, particular attention needs to be paid to patients' use of words. Note also that throughout these discussions

TABLE 11.4. Pros and Cons of Change from the Perspective of Five Years' Time

Reasons to stay as I am	Reasons to change
It makes me feel in control and special	*I want to be a success at work*
I will not get "fat"	*I want a long-term relationship*
It is familiar and feels safe	*I want a family*
If I change:	*I want to be a positive role model for my children*
— I won't be able to stop eating	*I want to go on vacations and be spontaneous*
— my weight will shoot up	*I want to be in good health*
— my stomach will stick out	*I don't want to still have the effects of being*
— my thighs will get fatter	*underweight or any other effects of the eating*
If I change people will think that:	*disorder (feeling cold, thinking about eating all*
— I am weak and greedy	*the time, obsessing about my shape)*
— I have given in	*I want to be in "true" control of my eating*
— I am getting fat	*I don't want to waste my life*
	I want to achieve things
	I don't want to be chronically ill

the therapist should adopt an inquisitive questioning approach, rather than the style of questioning that Socrates would have favored (see Table 3.3, page 28).

Reasons to stay as I am:

- *"It makes me feel in control."*
  - — Are these patients truly "in control" or is this spurious? If they were in control, they could elect not to restrict their eating for a few days. They are unable to do this because their need to restrict their eating is out of control. If they make the most of treatment, they will gain true control over their eating.
- *"It makes me feel special."*
  - — What patients mean by being "special" needs to be explored. It often refers to receiving attention from others. If this is the case, then other more positive ways of getting attention should be discussed, ones that might be open to the patient were he or she no longer restricted by the eating disorder.
  - — Is it truly "special" having an eating disorder? Here patients should be reminded how impaired they are, possibly with reference to their CIA.
- *"I don't know who I would be if I did not have an eating disorder."*
  - — Patients should be reminded once again that their personality (i.e., *"Who they would be"*), and therefore their uniqueness as a person, is masked by the effects of being underweight. At the moment they are just like anyone else who is severely underweight: preoccupied with thoughts about food and eating, inflexible and indecisive, socially withdrawn, etc. (see Table 11.2). They have lost their special-ness. Their true personality will only become obvious if they regain weight.
- *"It gives me an excuse for things."*
  - — What is meant by "excuse" needs to be explored. It may have something to do with having an excuse for not meeting their own or others' expectations.

If this is the case, the therapist should question whether the patient would need such an excuse were he or she free from the impairment that is a consequence of the eating disorder. Here the therapist should once more attempt to interest the patient in the benefits of change. We are continually struck by how able and competent these patients are once they have recovered from their eating disorder.

Vignette

A patient was afraid that if she regained weight and recovered from the eating disorder, she would be "normal" and would have no excuse if she failed her impending examinations. She realized that her preoccupation with food and eating was interfering with her ability to concentrate.

She seemed to be in a Catch-22 situation. On the one hand she wanted to remain underweight so that she would have an "excuse" for possibly failing her examinations. On the other hand, it was being underweight that made it more likely that she would fail. It was agreed that if she did not try to change, she would always think that she needed "excuses." Making changes would allow her to find out whether this was truly the case.

- *"It is familiar and feels safe."*
  - Here it is worth agreeing that change is always difficult, but it is especially so if, as a result of being underweight, one has a need for routine and predictability. What a patient means by "safe" also needs to be explored. Usually it simply means not risking change (i.e., sticking to the familiar).
- *"If I change, people will think that I am weak and that I have given in."*
  - Here patients are projecting their own views onto others. The reality is, of course, quite different.
  - Rather than viewing the patient as "weak," people will think that he or she is showing great strength by tackling the eating disorder. It is also worth pointing out that for the patient not eating is easy, whereas eating is difficult.
- *"If I start to eat more, people will think that I am greedy."*
  - Again, patients are projecting their own views onto others.
  - The meaning of greed in the patient's context should be explored. "Greed" refers to an excessive appetite for food. This is quite different from ceasing to undereat, especially in someone who is significantly underweight. People will view the fact that the patient is eating as evidence of his or her willpower and determination, not greed.
- *"If I change, I won't be able to stop eating."*
  - This is a cue to discuss the fact that patients are most at risk of binge eating as matters stand and that with treatment this risk will decline progressively. (See page 140 for a discussion of the mechanisms responsible for binge eating.) As mentioned above, treatment will give the patient control over eating.
- *"If I change, my weight will shoot up."*
  - This concern is addressed by the preceding point as weight cannot "shoot up" if patients are in control of their eating. Also, in reality weight regain is

very difficult. This point can be made now, although it is expanded upon once the patient has decided to embark upon weight regain.

- *"Staying as I am will ensure that I do not get 'fat.'"*
  — This is true, but in reality the patient is emaciated. Is keeping oneself emaciated a good way of avoiding becoming "fat"? The goal of treatment is that patients develop true control over eating, and thereby over their shape and weight as well, at least to the extent that it is possible to control them. Therefore it is most unlikely that the patient would become fat in the normal sense of the word, and the data on the outcome of anorexia nervosa support this. On the other hand continuing to restrict eating and remaining underweight increase the risk of binge eating and consequent uncontrolled weight gain.
  — Patients' use of the term "fat" should always be questioned. These patients are not at risk of obesity or of looking fat. This point can be highlighted with reference to the patient's weight graph.
- *"If I change, my thighs will get fatter."*
  — The patient's thigh muscles will currently be wasted. With weight regain the patient's body will change from being "emaciated" to being "bony," then "scrawny," then "too thin" and eventually the patient will be "slim" or "thin." The notion of becoming "fatter," in the usual meaning of the word, simply does not apply.
  — What also needs emphasizing is that patients may "see" parts of their body as larger than they really are. As explained in Chapter 8 (see page 107), this appears to be due to the way that they look at them and is addressed later in treatment.
- *"If I change, people will think that I am getting fat."*
  — This is another projection of the patient's own views. Others will be relieved to see the patient trying to regain weight and ceasing to be emaciated.
- *"If I change, people will think that I am less attractive."*
  — Again, this is a projection of the patient's views and another untested assumption. It is most unlikely that anyone would have viewed the patient's emaciation as attractive: Rather, most people view a healthy body shape as an attractive one. In this context it can be worth asking patients whether they would be comfortable being seen naked (or wearing a swimsuit). Most underweight patients realize that their bodies do not look good. Once more it is worth pointing out that one goal of treatment is to help the patient regain sufficient weight to become "thin." As matters stand the patient is a long way away from thinness.
  — It can also be helpful to explore the meaning of "attractiveness" by asking the patient to consider the variety of features that contribute to this attribute. These are likely to include other aspects of appearance (e.g., complexion, hair), non-physical attributes (e.g., being entertaining, cheerful, interesting, sociable, chatty, relaxed, caring and so on). The goal is that it becomes clear to patients that in terms of attractiveness body shape is just one element.

This exploration and examination of the patient's reasons not to change should not be hurried and will generally take several sessions. Between these sessions patients should be encouraged to think more about what has been discussed and raise further

> It is important that therapists have a good understanding of the concerns of these patients so that they feel understood, valued and respected.

concerns and questions. Some are defensive about aspects of the eating problem that they value, in part because they are used to other people dismissing them. It is important that therapists have a good understanding of their concerns so that patients feel understood, valued and respected.

Eventually, after all the patients' concerns have been fully discussed, a "Conclusions" table should be drawn up (see Table 11.5).

Step 4: Arriving at the Implications for Change

Next, the full implications of this extended and highly personalized discussion need to be formulated. In practice this happens naturally and gradually for patients begin to make statements such as *"If I regain all this weight . . . "* because by now it is obvious to patients that their present situation is highly problematic and that treatment offers an

TABLE 11.5. Pros and Cons of Change: A Patient's "Conclusions" Table

Conclusions

I want to get better and regain weight because . . .
- *I will be able to have a full life, not one that is just about eating and weight.*
- *I will be healthier: My bones and heart will be stronger; I won't be cold and faint and will be able to sleep properly; I won't be ill!*
- *I will be able to have good relationships with other people and hopefully a partner and children who I can be a good role model to.*
- *I will be able to enjoy my job and be successful at it.*
- *At the moment the eating problem stops me from being able to do things well. When I am better I won't need an excuse.*
- *Regaining weight will mean that I will become slim and healthy. It does not mean that I will become fat.*
- *Getting better won't be giving in. Not getting better would be giving in. Getting better is about choosing to give myself a life.*
- *I want to show how strong I can be by eating as right now not eating is the easy thing.*
- *Eating enough food to be a healthy weight isn't greedy. It is being normal.*
- *Being a healthy weight and eating enough will help to give me true control over my eating. I will be able to make choices about what I eat. At the moment the eating problem has control over me. Becoming well will protect me from out-of-control eating and uncontrolled weight gain.*
- *Being well will enable me to develop my talents as a person and to discover my true self.*
- *Getting better will give me choices in life. The eating problem has been holding me back. Change can only be good.*

opportunity to change. At first, patients tend to make such statements in a tentative manner, but after a while they become more definite, for example, by changing to saying *"<u>When</u> I regain all this weight. . . . ."* At a certain point (but not at the first opportunity) the therapist should acknowledge and confirm what the patient is saying by stating something along these lines: *"It sounds to me as if you have decided to take up this opportunity to tackle your eating problem and make a 'fresh start.' That's great."* Confirmatory statements such as this are important because people who are underweight are indecisive and therefore need help to clinch decisions. Otherwise they are prone to procrastinate almost indefinitely.

It is important to note that patients' motivation to change waxes and wanes and is therefore an ongoing issue in treatment. The therapist always needs to keep motivation in mind and often it has to be addressed beyond the initial pros and cons discussions.

Step 5: "Taking the Plunge"

Having reached this point, and in light of these patients' indecisiveness, the therapist should take the next step on behalf of the patient; for example, by saying:

> *"I suggest that it's time to take the plunge and make a start. The sooner we start, the sooner you will experience the benefits of change, whereas putting it off just prolongs the agony. It's like standing at the edge of a swimming pool and delaying diving in because the water looks cold and uninviting. It's better to just get on with it. Shall we start?"*

Most patients will agree, often with some relief. The occasional patient will want to discuss some outstanding matters or will want to think about it longer. Obviously this position should be respected, but at some point the therapist might have to say: *"We have gone over everything. There is nothing more to say. It really is time to make the decision to get on with it. Shall we just do that?"* Almost always this is successful. If necessary, change may be presented as an experiment and, if patients do not like its effects, they can return to their old way of living after treatment ends. This is not difficult: indeed, it is all too easy. This said, we have not come across any patient who has chosen to do this. Rather, patients tend to say that they wished they had changed sooner because their life now is so much better than it was. The following remarks made by three different patients highlight this point:

> *"It is as if my life has changed from black and white into color."*

> *"My concentration and memory are so much better. It is as if my brain has become twice as large."*

> *"Many of the things that I assumed were my personality aren't. I am not an insecure person. I am quite normal really!"*

Conducting "Stage Two Reviews"

As noted earlier, the treatment stages of the 20-session version of CBT-E do not map neatly onto this extended version of the treatment. Nevertheless it is valuable to conduct a "Stage Two" review after 4 weeks following the guidelines described in Chapter 7. What is different, however, is that equivalent reviews should continue to be conducted at roughly 4-week intervals because it is important to pay particularly close attention to these patients' ongoing compliance and progress. This is because it is often erratic and can stall for weeks at a time. Therapists need to be on the lookout for this stalling and, if it happens, identify and address the cause.

Addressing Undereating and Achieving Weight Regain

Educating the Patient about Weight Regain

Most patients have a large number of concerns about weight regain, many of which are ill-founded. It is most important that they understand what is involved so that they know what to expect. The main points to stress are as follows:

The Weight Regain Process

- There are two phases to weight regain:
    1. *Weight regain* — This involves the patient establishing a daily energy surplus sufficient to regain weight at a reasonable rate, the goal being a BMI "around" 20. It is best to avoid specifying a particular weight.
    2. *Weight maintenance* — This involves the patient learning to maintain a stable BMI "around" 20 (typically between 19.0 and 19.9). This is a most important phase of treatment and ideally at least 6–8 weeks should be devoted to it. Therefore the sooner that patients embark on weight regain, the sooner they will reach a BMI around 20 and be able to practice maintaining their new weight. The fact that there is a weight maintenance phase is popular with patients. Indeed, it helps motivate them to maintain the desired rate of weight regain so that sufficient time is available for it.

- It is remarkably difficult to gain weight if you have an eating disorder and are underweight. This comes as a surprise to most patients who are afraid that their weight will shoot up out of their control. This does not happen.
- To regain weight at an average rate of 0.5 kg per week (roughly 1 lb per week), a rate that is optimal for outpatient treatment, patients need to consume, on average, an extra 500 kcals of energy each day (i.e., an extra 3,500 kcals per week) over and above what they are currently consuming, assuming their weight is stable. The magnitude of this energy surplus comes as a surprise to most patients.
- Over the first week or two of attempting to regain weight the rate of weight regain may be higher than this. This is due to rehydration (i.e., water retention) as people who are undereating are often dehydrated. The initial jump in weight can frighten patients and lead them to cut back on their energy intake which is obviously unhelpful. Therefore they need to be forewarned about this possibility.
- If patients increase their level of activity, they will need to consume proportionately more energy.

The Psychology of Weight Regain

- Patients will need to redirect the drive and determination that they directed at restricting their eating toward regaining weight. Weight regain requires sustained effort over many months.

- Regaining weight is tough and involves taking risks, but the gains are enormous. Being free from the effects of being underweight and the eating disorder mindset (see Chapter 8) is extraordinarily liberating. It really is about *"Getting a life."*

- It takes a long time for the patient to get all the benefits of weight regain. In our experience, the benefits fully develop only once the patient's BMI is 19.0 or more. Until then the benefits are relatively few whereas the effort required is huge. This is an important point that needs to be stressed. Partial weight regain is of limited value because there is *"Pain, but no gain."*

> **Partial weight regain is of limited value because there is "Pain, but no gain."**

Calculating BMI and Weight Goals

Between sessions, the therapist should calculate the patient's weight in kilograms (and in whatever weight unit the patient uses) equivalent to a BMI of 20.0 together with the amount of weight (in both units) that the patient needs to gain to reach this BMI. Then the therapist should draw on the weight graph a diagonal line from the patient's latest weight (projected forward to the next session) up to a BMI of 19.0, the slope representing an average weight gain of 0.5 kg per week. A representative weight graph is shown in Figure 11.3 (of a patient who was already regaining weight).

At the next session these figures should be discussed and the diagonal line representing the expected rate of weight regain explained.

How to Regain Weight

Next the therapist should discuss the various ways of regaining weight. There are three:

1. *Consuming more energy in the form of food and drink.* This may be achieved in the following ways:

- Eating larger quantities (i.e., bigger portions) of the same food. If the patient is eating low-calorie food (e.g., salad), which is often the case, this method is relatively ineffective because it does not result in a significant increase in energy intake.

- Eating more often. This may well have already happened as a result of the regular eating intervention. Like eating larger quantities of the same food, this is relatively ineffective on its own.

- Changing food choice to energy-rich foods and drinks. This usually involves a radical change in food choice, including no longer consuming diet food and drinks. This method is effective so long as enough is eaten. It also has the advantage of not requiring the patient to consume large volumes of food and drink, thereby minimizing feelings of fullness.

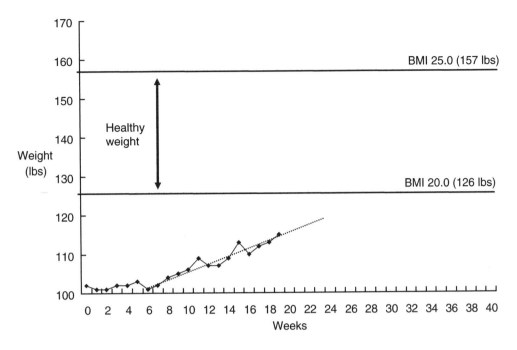

FIGURE 11.3. Weight graph for patient B with weight regain trajectory drawn in.

- Stopping vomiting (if applicable). This helps, but in underweight patients it is almost always not sufficient.
- Making the most of "eating opportunities." This involves the patient "mapping" his or her eating onto that of others and eating more when others do so (e.g., when going out). This is admirable and to be encouraged, but it never produces the energy surplus required.

2. *Decreasing activity level.* This can assist weight regain if the person is exercising very heavily, but it will not be sufficient in its own right.

3. *Consuming energy-rich dietary supplements.* It is an inescapable fact that if weight regain is to be accomplished by changing eating and exercising, patients will have to consume an unusually large amount of energy in the form of food or drink in the later stages of the process. In our view this is contrary to the goal of helping patients establish healthy eating habits. It also necessitates the complex process of patients cutting back on their energy intake once they reach their BMI goal.

Instead, with patients who are willing, we recommend that they take energy-rich drinks in addition to changing their energy intake in the ways described above. At the beginning of the weight regain process we recommend that the therapist simply mention that taking energy-rich drinks might well be very helpful and necessary at some stage, but for the present the patient should focus on increasing his or her energy intake in the form of food and drink.

Next the therapist should ask patients to work out how to increase their energy intake, the goal being that they consume a surplus of 500 kcal daily. They should devise a plan that they think will be both achievable and effective. Ideally it should include most of the elements specified under point 1 above, especially the consumption of energy-rich foods and drinks and the abandonment of diet food. They then should implement the plan. Almost invariably they return having made what they view as substantial changes but in reality they are not nearly sufficient, and so their weight will have changed very little. Discovering this reinforces the therapist's point that gaining weight is surprisingly difficult, and it disconfirms the patients' prediction that their weight will shoot up once they start eating more. (*Note:* Therapists should remind patients, however, of the possibility of an initial rehydration effect.)

Once patients have tried to achieve weight regain their way, the therapist should work out with them a plan that involves consuming foods that are acceptable to them and one that will produce a daily energy surplus of the magnitude required. In general it is best if the plan is highly specific and written down. It is particularly important to pay close attention to portion sizes. Some patients find it helpful to include prepared meals bought from a supermarket as they have a specified calorie content and involve no last-minute decision-making. Patients should then be helped to implement the plan over the following weeks, incorporating whatever modifications seem necessary. In this regard it can be useful to provide them with a list of foods (or food combinations) that have 500 kcals of energy, ideally including items that they liked in the past. Patients can then choose to eat one item from the list each day, in addition to their usual diet.

These procedures will result in weight regain for a variable period of time. With some patients these measures are sufficient to allow them to reach the goal BMI range, but for most there will be a tapering off of their weight regain (i.e., the weight graph will flatten out). This is either due to a decrease in patients' adherence to the agreed plan, an increase in their activity level, or an increase in patients' energy needs as they become less underweight. Whatever the cause, patients will need to increase their energy intake and possibly reduce their activity level. If this works, then the same overall strategy may be continued. On the other hand, if further weight regain seems inordinately difficult, despite the patient's best efforts, then the patient should be strongly encouraged to start consuming energy-rich drinks.

Energy-Rich Drinks and Their Use

Used judiciously these drinks have much to commend them. First, they provide the energy surplus needed without requiring patients to overeat. Second, they can be withdrawn once patients reach the target BMI range without requiring them to cut back on the amount that they are eating. Third, they are relatively simple to use. The main points about their use are as follows:

• Some patients are resistant to the idea of consuming artificial drinks. One reason given is that they are "unhealthy." This is not the case. Many have been explicitly designed to be used with medically ill patients and so have undergone rigorous safety testing. What is undoubtedly unhealthy, however, is being extremely underweight. Another argument is that they are unsuitable for vegetarians. This is also not the case. Yet another is that they are unpalatable. In our view this is simply not true. The great majority of patients find one or more that they come to like. And, even if it were true, patients should balance up the pros and cons of consuming an unpleasant-tasting drink (which can be viewed as "medicine") against the alternative of struggling to eat more or continuing to have an eating disorder.

- It is generally best to use a commercial energy-dense drink designed for medical purposes because they are particularly rich in energy and so are easy to consume in terms of volume. Most manufacturers of these drinks produce a variety of styles and in a range of flavors, and some produce drinks that contain about 250 kcals per carton or bottle. With these drinks patients simply have to consume two each day as well as the amount of food and drink that they need to maintain their weight. This will generally be clear because the patient's weight will already have plateaued.

- We conduct a "taste test" with patients prior to their starting to take the drinks in order to identify one or two flavors that are acceptable. We join the patient in tasting the drinks in order to model their consumption.

- The drinks are highly satiating. They should therefore be consumed after eating rather than before. A good plan is to take one after breakfast and one after the evening snack. Some people find them more palatable if they are chilled.

- If two 250 kcal drinks are being consumed each day, then the patient's weight should rise steadily at an average rate of 0.5 kg per week. If it does not, yet the drinks are being taken, the patient is not consuming enough energy in the form of food and everyday drinks. This can happen if patients cut back their intake in response to introducing the drinks, either because they think that they no longer need to pay attention to their eating or because they are afraid that their weight will suddenly increase. Patients should be forewarned against this possibility, as it is counter to the rationale for taking the drinks. If there continues to be little or no weight regain, the drinks should be withdrawn as the patient must be undereating.

Maintaining Motivation

Motivation should be a running agenda item throughout treatment. At intervals it is worth reviewing the "Conclusions" table (Table 11.5) and therapists should regularly ask patients to restate the reasons why they want to get better, as this can help them stay focused. Some patients find it helpful to have their "Conclusions" table readily accessible or at least the key points highly visible (e.g., in their planner or on notes posted around their bedroom). Concerns about getting better also need to be assessed and addressed repeatedly. As always, both a short-term and a long-term perspective need to be taken. It is important to keep in the forefront of patients' minds the extent to which their life is impaired by the eating disorder. Intermittently filling in a CIA can be helpful in this regard. This awareness can also be heightened by asking patients about things that they have difficulty doing in comparison with their peers. Conversely, once patients are making sustained changes they can be asked whether any of the secondary effects are lessening in severity. Intermittently, and more so as treatment continues, patients should be asked about their future plans and whether or not the eating problem is compatible with them.

It is important to help patients make links between their motivation to change and their behavior. It should be pointed out that in effect they choose whether or not to get better six times each day (i.e., before each of their planned meals and snacks). If patients are struggling to eat as planned, they should be encouraged to review their reasons to change before each meal and snack. In addition, patients should record in real time their concerns about eating (in the right-hand column of the monitoring record) and analyze them there and then (e.g., Concern: *"I feel greedy."* Response: *"I am not eating an excessive amount given my weight. The way I am eating could not possibly be considered greedy."*). In subsequent sessions patients should be helped to fine-tune their responses and act in accordance with them.

Therapists should also explore fluctuations in motivation and their basis. Intermittently patients should be asked how their motivation has changed over the week and what has influenced it. This questioning helps identify factors that facilitate change and should be promoted, and those that are a barrier to change and need to be addressed.

Patients with a BMI between 17.5 and 19.0

As noted in Chapter 6, patients with eating disorders who are somewhat underweight should also be encouraged to regain weight. The same treatment strategies and procedures are used with these patients as with others who are underweight. Generally they can reach a BMI between 19.0 and 19.9 without recourse to energy-rich drinks, but often treatment needs to be somewhat extended in length.

Involving Others

It can be helpful to involve others in the weight regain process and this is the norm when working with adolescent patients (see Chapter 14). The role of others in CBT-E is to facilitate the patient's own efforts.

If the patient lives with a parent or partner, the therapist should raise the possibility that he or she become involved

> **The role of significant others in CBT-E is to facilitate the patient's own efforts.**

in the weight regain process. Generally this involvement is helpful as long as the relationship between the two is a sound one. The nature of the involvement of the third party varies according to the patient's wishes, his or her progress, and the views of the third party. It can involve one or more of the following roles:

- Ensuring that there are adequate supplies of the types of food and drink that the patient is consuming
- Working with the patient in deciding what will be the nature and size of joint meals
- Cooking with the patient
- Eating with the patient and helping him or her eat in a normal fashion
- Helping patients resist urges to binge or purge

Parents of younger patients often take on all these roles whereas such efforts are less appropriate with older patients. It is best that partners do not get too involved as it can affect the balance of the relationship. Of course, the most important role of others is to be encouraging and supportive.

If others are to be involved, they need education and guidance. There should be an initial meeting, much as in the 20-session version of the treatment, in which they are educated about the problem and the CBT-E approach. This should include ample time for them to air their concerns and voice any questions. Then the nature of their involvement should be discussed, having first agreed with the patient upon his or her potential role. Thereafter they should be asked to re-attend at intervals, the natural time being at the regular review sessions. These appointments give the patient, therapist and third party an opportunity to re-examine the other's role, identify successes and problems, and make any adjustments needed.

If others are involved in the weight regain process, they should become less so in the later stages of treatment and should have no involvement with weight maintenance, which patients should master on their own.

Common Difficulties with Weight Regain

Helping adult patients regain weight is rarely easy. It is almost invariably a struggle for the patient and for the therapist. It requires continuous effort for many months and often patients want to abandon the process before it has been completed. As discontinuing treatment is most inadvisable, therapists should do their utmost to help patients reach their goal BMI range. Below is a list of frequent problems and how to address them.

1. *The changes that the patient is making are too small.* This is common. It must be made absolutely clear to patients that they need to have an energy surplus each and every day of 500 kcals on average. Less than this is simply not sufficient. It should be pointed out that making small changes is often just as much effort as making larger ones. One reason patients give for making small changes is that they want to be "safe" (i.e., not overdo it and risk rapid weight gain). In reality, not eating enough is *unsafe* because it risks their not overcoming the eating disorder. Patients are particularly prone to err on the "safe" side (i.e.,

> **Patients need to have an average energy surplus each and every day of 500 kcals.**

undereat) if they are eating unfamiliar food or foods whose calorie content is difficult to estimate. Under these circumstances they tend to overestimate the energy (calorie)

> **Making small changes is often just as much effort as making larger ones.**

content of the food and undereat as a result. It cannot be pointed out often enough that their fear of "overdoing it" or of "eating too much" is not warranted. They are underweight and need to eat *more*. Patients should be encouraged to make the most of situations in which it is normal to eat more than usual (e.g., when eating

> **Playing it "safe" is dangerous!**

out, birthdays, other celebrations) and label them as "eating opportunities." It is also important to explore and question patients' hesitancy regarding weight regain. Why do they want to be so cautious if their true goal is to achieve a healthy weight?

2. *The patient's efforts taper off.* If this is the case the therapist should acknowledge how hard the process is, while bolstering the patient's morale. The canoeing analogy (see below) can be helpful in this regard.

The Canoeing Analogy

Weight regain is like canoeing upstream to a destination that you have been told is wonderful but you are not so sure. Previously you have been canoeing downstream to a place you wanted to go. Now you are being asked to turn the canoe around (i.e., stop undereating) and paddle against the current (i.e., start increasing your energy intake). And you know that you will have to do this every day for a long time if you are to reach the destination (i.e., the amount of weight to be regained is large). And if you stop paddling you will float backward because of the current (i.e., you need to consume an extra 500 kcals every single day, and if you miss one day you will need to consume an extra 1,000 kcals the next day, and so on). And getting only part of the way there is not worth it because you will never have reached the wonderful destination (i.e., the benefits of weight regain only truly develop once your BMI is over 19.0).

———————————

Therapists have to balance having an empathic, encouraging and supportive approach to the difficulties inherent in weight regain with maintaining clear pressure to change. They need to be unambiguous about what needs to be done. This endeavor requires a strong and trusting therapist–patient relationship. "Friendly but firm" is often the best style to adopt.

> Therapists have to balance having an empathic, encouraging and supportive approach with maintaining clear pressure to change.

With patients who are having particular difficulty keeping their mind on the task at hand, it can be helpful for a brief period to have more frequent contact than twice weekly. For example, some patients benefit from sending the therapist a daily e-mail describing their plan for the forthcoming day and what they have achieved since their last e-mail. This is fine in principle. We suggest that it is agreed that the therapist will not respond in any detail and not always immediately.

As mentioned earlier, intermittent review sessions (say, every 4 weeks) are helpful in maintaining momentum. Significant others should be invited if they are actively involved (as is almost invariably the case with younger patients). Whether it is useful to formalize the pressure to change by establishing a weight regain "contract" is a moot point. Doing so has the advantage of operationalizing what is expected and attaching contingencies to the achievement of certain goals, but it has the disadvantage of rigidity and it can sometimes oblige therapists to behave in ways that are counter-therapeutic.

3. *The patient is unable to maintain the increased level of eating due to feelings of fullness.* "Fullness" and how to address it are discussed in detail in Chapter 6 (page 84). The propensity to feel full is heightened in patients who are underweight due to the delay in gastric emptying. This delay is reversed by the restoration of healthy eating habits. It is our impression that regular eating is especially helpful in this regard.

4. *The patient is unable to recall the reasons for regaining weight once he or she has left the therapist's office.* We call this the "parking lot syndrome," referring to the fact that patients can be back in their eating disorder mindset (i.e., playing their eating disorder DVD; see page 119) within minutes of leaving the session. To help counter this, it is important for patients to have ready access to their reasons for wanting to regain weight (see the following vignette).

Vignette

To maintain her motivation, one patient wrote the following:

"I need to concentrate on visualizing myself at a healthy weight with a slim figure that has some shape and that fits clothes well. Not a skeleton with . . .

- *Veins sticking out on my arms*
- *Shoulder bones poking out*
- *Hips poking out*
- *Legs like sticks with no shape*
- *Heart palpitations*
- *No periods*
- *Bones dissolving*
- *Obsessive behavior*
- *No social life . . . no life, really*
- *No confidence*
- *Relationship problems (no interest in sex)*
- *No concentration*
- *Starving much of the time*
- *Obsessed with clothes feeling tight, etc., etc., etc.*

"SO THIS CONSTANT BATTLE IS WORTH IT! I just need to keep fighting and read this when I don't want to carry on."

As noted earlier, we encourage patients to keep their list of reasons to change accessible at all times. Some patients find it useful to read through this list at regular intervals, especially before mealtimes or first thing each morning.

5. *The patient is resistant to change.* A degree of stubbornness and inflexibility is not uncommon among patients who are underweight. Rigidity sometimes reflects a premorbid character trait that has been exaggerated by being underweight. One way of eroding patients' oppositional stance is to identify any unrelated difficulties that they have and help them to overcome them. For example, one patient had significant difficulties with her eyesight. We arranged for her to see a specialist, which not only improved her vision but made her more generally amenable.

6. *The patient wants to stop regaining weight because he or she is becoming "fat."* Patients need to be challenged about their labeling of themselves in this way since, as noted earlier, it does not match reality (their moving from "emaciated" to "slim"). Nevertheless the therapist should acknowledge the difficulty that they face; namely that their experience of themselves is that parts of their body (e.g., their thighs) are too large and that they are getting fat in general (see points 8 and 9 below). It is the therapist's job to help patients understand, reinterpret and override their current experience of their body so that they are more able to accept weight regain. Treatment will also involve addressing the patients' over-evaluation of shape and weight (see Chapter 8).

7. *The patient states that "Eating all this energy-rich food is unhealthy."* There are two points to be made in this regard. The first is that what is truly unhealthy about patients' current state is their low weight, and a period of eating high-energy food is needed to

correct this. "Healthy eating " recommendations are not designed for people who are markedly underweight and have an eating disorder. The second point is that once patients have reached their goal BMI range, they can choose what they eat so long as it is enough and does not involve dietary restraint.

8. *The patient wants to stop regaining weight because his or her stomach (abdomen) is sticking out.* There may be some truth to this, but it is a temporary phenomenon. During weight regain the stomach sometimes does appear to stick out disproportionately. In part this is due to the way in which the body naturally changes when a state of emaciation is being reversed and in part it is a consequence of the marked wasting of the abdominal muscles (so that the stomach is not held in) and back muscles (which no longer broaden out the body and so make any abdominal protrusion more obvious). Thus for a while during weight regain the stomach may appear to stick out, but this does not last. Concern about the phenomenon is exaggerated by patients' tendency to look down at their stomach, especially after having eaten. (This is an excellent example of a situation in which patients make harsh judgments about their own appearance yet have never studied anyone else from the same vantage point; see page 111). The apparent protuberance of the stomach is also exaggerated by certain styles of clothing (e.g., pants that are low-cut at the front) and by the consumption of a bulky high–fiber diet or large quantities of gaseous drinks.

Discussion of the phenomenon should focus on helping patients avoid equating it with having overeaten or with being fat. As noted in Chapter 6, commonsense measures can help reduce it, including choosing energy-dense foods rather than high-fiber ones, limiting the consumption of gaseous drinks, controlling self-scrutiny, and wearing clothes that do not exaggerate it.

9. *The patient wants to stop regaining weight because his or her clothes are becoming tight.* Addressing this concern involves education about the natural temporary change in shape that can follow eating, and the fact that it passes and is not indicative of having overeaten or being "fat"; the effect of paying particular attention to physical sensations that would normally go unnoticed; and the potential value of avoiding tight clothes for the meantime.

The clothing of patients who are regaining weight (and shape), and therefore becoming less emaciated, may well become too small. This can be a major barrier to continuing weight regain. It is therefore best if patients either choose to wear loose-fitting clothes during the weight gain process or, at regular intervals, buy new "less small" clothes. Generally the latter is more realistic. In this regard certain points should be noted:

- It is best if patients keep ahead of the shape change and buy new clothes in advance of the old ones becoming tight
- Patients often need help to accept that they need larger (less small) clothes as one of their measures of success when losing weight (or rather, shape) may have been successive decreases in their clothes size. During weight (or rather shape) regain they have to move in the opposite direction, which many find difficult to do. There are two positive aspects to this: first, they will find that they have a greater range of clothes from which to choose; and second, they will discover that they look better in them. It can be helpful to point out that in order to fit into their current clothes patients will need to stay ill. They should never have fitted into them in the first place.

- Some patients have rather drab and dated clothes. If they can be helped to buy clothes more like those of their peers this can be helpful developmentally.
- Significant others can be of assistance in this regard by providing money to buy new clothes. Buying new clothes can help counter the frugality that characterizes some patients.
- Shopping expeditions with a friend who does not have an eating disorder can be helpful when buying new clothes and it can enhance shape acceptance.
- Certain patients want to keep their old clothes. This should be discouraged. In fact, they should burn their bridges by giving away the old ones.

10. *The patient's attempts to regain weight are adversely affected by comments from others.* Generally others are pleased that patients are eating more normally and looking less ill. However, comments along these lines are likely to be misinterpreted. Comments about eating will be taken to mean that the patient is overeating and being "greedy," and comments about appearance (e.g., *"You look so much better")* will be interpreted as statements to the effect that the patient now looks "fat."

Patients need to be helped to see that their eating disorder mindset or DVD (see page 119) is causing them to misconstrue statements of others. What were positive and encouraging remarks are being converted into criticisms. Patients need help to understand this in the session and then "live" at the time such statements are made.

11. *The patient thinks that he or she has regained enough weight although still being underweight.* It is common to encounter patients whose motivation to reach the target BMI range (19.0–19.9) wanes as they get closer to it. They often think that a weight equivalent to a BMI of 17.0 to 18.0 is high enough, and admittedly it is a lot less unhealthy than the weight at which they started treatment. Although it is important to praise patients for the effort they have put into regaining weight, it is extremely important to point out that if they stop regaining weight at this point, they will have obtained few of the benefits of weight regain. It is like climbing a mountain but stopping just short of the top and so not getting the view. Furthermore,

> **Maintaining a BMI below 19.0 is like walking right at the very edge of a cliff (i.e., it is foolhardy).**

maintaining a BMI at this level is problematic because the eating disorder mindset or DVD will still be "playing," and so they will be prone to relapse. In addition, there will be no buffer zone protecting them from the effects of inadvertent weight loss (e.g., due to illness), which will result in the activation of their eating disorder mindset once their BMI is much below 18.0. Maintaining a BMI below 19.0 is like walking right at the very edge of a cliff (i.e., it is foolhardy).

Moving from Weight Regain to Weight Maintenance

In comparison to the process of regaining weight, maintaining a stable weight is relatively straightforward. This is in marked contrast with in-patient treatment and is one of the major arguments in favor of outpatient treatment. With patients who have been taking high-energy drinks and gaining weight at the appropriate rate, it simply involves removing the drinks one by one. It is our practice to remove the first drink when the patient's BMI is clearly over 19.0 and the second when it reaches 19.5. In the meantime patients should continue to eat as they have been. With patients who have been regaining weight through food and drink alone, the process is more complex as it involves patients reducing the amount that they are eating. This needs to be done cautiously as there is a risk that they will lose weight as a result. It is a matter of trial and error.

Helping patients achieve a reasonably stable weight is also a matter of trial and error. The goal is that patients maintain a weight such that their BMI fluctuates between 19.0 and 19.9. To assist we add a horizontal line to the weight graph at a BMI of 19.0 (as illustrated in Figure 11.4). Patients also need to learn how to balance their activity level and energy intake. Most are surprised at how much they can eat without gaining weight. At the same time therapists should focus on helping patients accept and enjoy their new appearance, and adjust to their new personality as most will discover that they are not the person that they thought they were.

Patients and therapists have opposite concerns at this stage. Patients are afraid that their weight will continue to rise, whereas therapists fear that it will fall. Therapists' fears are the more realistic. The risk of weight loss should be discussed openly with patients together with the dangers that would result from it.

During the weight maintenance phase the therapist will also continue to address the other features of the eating disorder (see the next section). On entering the weight maintenance phase it can be useful to conduct a further assessment of the eating disorder and secondary impairment (using the EDE-Q and CIA respectively) to identify those features still present.

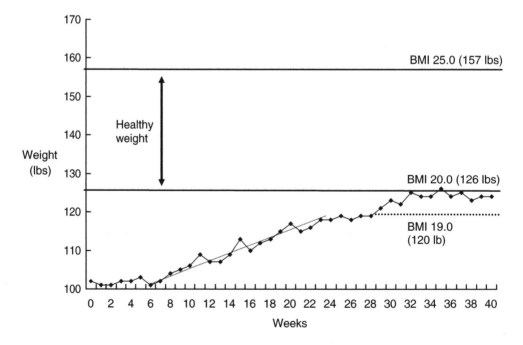

FIGURE 11.4. Weight graph for patient B illustrating weight maintenance.

Addressing Other Aspects of the Eating Disorder

During the weight regain process, other aspects of the eating disorder are addressed in tandem. We suggest that therapists adhere to the guidelines below while noting that during the weight regain process, weight regain is the priority. It should be at the top of the agenda of each session, and the strategies and procedures needed to achieve it should take precedence over others.

- *Dietary restraint.* The addressing of dietary restraint (as described in Chapter 9) is generally delayed until near the end of the weight regain process unless it is proving an obstacle to weight regain. Thus the formal tackling of food avoidance and other dietary rules is postponed. This means that during weight regain therapists may turn a blind eye to idiosyncratic ways of gaining weight so long as they are proving effective. Obviously most patients will have to break many of their dietary rules to achieve weight regain, so although their rules may not have been formally addressed, some will have been tackled to an extent. During the weight maintenance phase it is especially important to help patients eat flexibly and practice eating with others.
- *Binge eating.* There is a subgroup of underweight patients who binge eat and many more have subjective binges. Most purge afterward. These patients have a reputation for being particularly difficult to treat. We do not have enough data to comment on this, but our clinical impression is that they are no harder to treat (with CBT-E) than those who do not binge eat, and in some respects they are easier. This is because they find the binge eating highly aversive and so they are more motivated to change. Furthermore, because they have experienced binge eating, they generally do not need convincing that both their way of eating and their extremely low weight put them at risk of it. Addressing their binge eating proceeds along the usual lines (i.e., starting with the "regular eating" intervention [see page 75] and then moving on to detailed "binge analysis" [see page 140]). With these patients, low weight and binge eating share top place on the session agenda.
- *Purging.* As with other patients, underweight patients may engage in compensatory or non-compensatory purging. As explained in Chapter 6, compensatory purging does not generally need to be tackled, whereas the function of non-compensatory purging needs to be identified and addressed.
- *Excessive exercising.* This is not uncommon among patients who are underweight. As noted in Chapter 6, it is a particular problem in inpatient settings where patients tend to be cooped up and thus are unable to be physically active. Interestingly it appears to be less of a problem in "open-door" inpatient settings (see Chapter 15). Addressing excessive exercising is discussed in Chapter 6 (see page 85). It can be one cause of failure to regain weight and so should be enquired about as a matter of routine. Intense exercising is inadvisable for patients who are very underweight because of their compromised cardiac status, and in patients with osteoporosis the risk of fractures must be kept in mind. This said, we encourage our underweight patients to engage in healthy exercise, as in our experience it helps them accept weight regain.
- *The over-evaluation of shape, weight and controlling eating.* The addressing of the "core psychopathology" and its expressions needs to be integrated with weight regain. With the majority of patients weight and eating are their main concerns in the early stages of

weight regain. Prior to starting treatment they may have judged their self-control in terms of their ability to restrict their food intake and lose weight. As a result eating more and regaining weight are an anathema to them because they have to abandon goals regarding how much to eat and pass through highly significant weight thresholds as they regain weight. Generally these are round numbers and so differ according to the units that the patient uses. In the United States they may be 100 lb, 110 lb, etc., whereas in the United Kingdom they tend to be 7 stone, 8 stone, etc., and in continental Europe they are 40 kg, 50 kg, etc. Thresholds also have to be broken in terms of clothes size. Later on, especially once the patient's BMI exceeds 17.0, shape tends to become the more dominant issue. The addressing of the over-evaluation of shape and weight and their control is described in Chapter 8 and that of controlling eating in Chapter 9.

  • *The marginalization of other domains for self-evaluation.* The importance of enhancing these patients' other domains for self-evaluation (see page 102) cannot be overstated. Most need considerable help to *"Get a life."*

Ending Well

The final stage of this extended version of the treatment follows the same principles as those employed in the 20-session version (see the following chapter). Thus there is focus on maintaining the changes made and on minimizing the risk of relapse. The only significant difference is that detecting early warning signs of a relapse is less easy for patients who do not binge. It is therefore important to identify patients' likely relapse signatures (e.g., delaying or skipping meals or snacks, increasing exercising, reverting to old forms of body checking), especially since patients who have recently regained weight are particularly vulnerable to setbacks. As an additional precaution it is wise to agree on a weight that patients should stay above (their "danger weight"). If their weight drops to this level (generally equivalent to a BMI of 18.5) patients should be advised that alarm bells should ring because their eating disorder mindset will shortly be activated, and they will soon begin to experience the effects of being underweight.

  Patients should be advised to institute their plan for dealing with setbacks either if they spot their early warning signs or if their weight drops to the danger weight. In general, however, they should aim to maintain a weight equivalent to a BMI between 19.0 and 19.9 so that there is a buffer zone between their new weight and the danger weight. In the longer term it may be wise for some patients to allow their weight to increase a little further. This is indicated if they realize that maintaining their weight at a BMI between 19.0 and 19.9 involves dietary restraint and restriction. If this is the case, they should consider increasing their weight to a BMI between 20.0 and 21.0 or even a little higher. This is a topic to discuss in the final treatment sessions and to review at the 20-week post-treatment review appointment.

Recommended Reading

Recommended reading for Chapters 5–12 can be found at the end of Chapter 12.

CHAPTER 12

Ending Well

Stage Four, the final stage in treatment, is concerned with ending treatment well. Just as it is important that treatment starts well (see Chapter 5), so it is important that it ends properly. In routine clinical practice it is not uncommon for treatment simply to fizzle out. This is regrettable as there are important tasks to conduct in the final weeks of treatment, and unless there is a formal ending patients do not benefit from them. The two main tasks are:

> **The end of the treatment is as important as the beginning.**

1. To ensure that the progress made in treatment is maintained after treatment ends
2. To minimize the risk of relapse in the long term

In addition, patients' concerns about ending treatment need to be addressed and certain treatment procedures need to be phased out.

In the main 20-session version of CBT-E, Stage Four consists of three appointments, each 2 weeks apart (sessions 18, 19 and 20). In the extended version of the treatment, Stage Four consists of four or five appointments, 2 or 3 weeks apart. Throughout, the usual session structure is retained, but the sessions become progressively more future-oriented and less concerned with the present.

There are circumstances under which it is appropriate to offer more treatment or to extend treatment (see Chapter 3, pages 33 and 190), but in our experience they are not common. In the vast majority of cases treatment can and should end on time as planned. So long as patients have reached the point where the principal

> **In the vast majority of cases treatment can and should end on time as planned.**

maintaining mechanisms have been disrupted and the "house of cards" is beginning to collapse (i.e., the eating disorder psychopathology is disintegrating), they continue to improve after treatment has ended. Under these circumstances treatment can end, and it is in the patient's interest that it does. Otherwise patients (and their therapists) tend to ascribe continuing improvement to the ongoing therapy rather than the progress that already has been made. In practice this means that it is acceptable to end treatment with patients still dieting to an extent, perhaps binge eating and vomiting on occasions, and having residual concerns about shape and weight.

Addressing Concerns about Ending Treatment

Patients vary in how they view the prospect of ending treatment. If they have been receiving time-limited CBT-E, which we recommend, patients will have known from the outset that treatment will end after a set number of weeks. Despite this foreknowledge, some expect that they will be an exception and that their treatment will continue. To counter this assumption, patients are told at the beginning of each session, the session number and the number of sessions remaining.

The majority of patients are not unduly concerned about treatment ending, especially if they have made good progress. Others fear that they will not cope once on their own. It is important to ask patients how they feel about treatment ending and address their concerns. For example, if patients express sadness and apprehensiveness about treatment ending, these feelings can be normalized. We tell all patients the following:

- *"Although treatment has ended, it is not the end of your progress in overcoming the eating problem."*
- *"It is usual to continue improving after the end of treatment. This is especially true of concerns about shape and weight."*
- *"Although this might seem odd, at the end of treatment it is impossible to gauge the full extent of the progress that you have made."*
- *"A break from treatment is often a good idea."*
- *"This is a good time to practice making use of all the things learned in treatment without outside help."*
- *"The next months are an important time. Even though you will no longer be attending, it is crucial to keep working on making further progress and maintaining the changes that you have made."*

The Driving Analogy

An analogy may be made with learning to drive. You have had lessons on how to do it and have had some practice. Now you need to learn to do it on your own. Unless you do this, you will forget what you have learned.

We also remind patients that there will be a review appointment 20 weeks after treatment finishes, which is an ideal time to take stock. Any problems that might have occurred in the interim can be discussed at this appointment.

Ensuring That Progress Is Maintained

As noted above, the goal of CBT-E is to get patients to the point where the main mechanisms that have been maintaining the eating disorder have been disrupted and the "house of cards" is beginning to collapse. To determine whether this is the case, the therapist needs to assess what progress has been made. This assessment can be done informally by asking the patient what has changed, and what has not, but it is best supplemented with a more systematic evaluation using the EDE-Q to measure eating disorder features and the CIA to

The goal of CBT-E is to get patients to the point where the main mechanisms that have been maintaining the eating disorder have been disrupted and the "house of cards" is beginning to collapse.

measure secondary psychosocial impairment. In this way the nature and extent of any residual eating disorder psychopathology may be detected together with its impact on the patient's life. It is important that this review is done jointly and in a positive way, highlighting what has been achieved and attributing the changes to the patient's own efforts.

Then, usually in the next session, and with reference to the patient's formulation, the therapist and patient need to consider what eating disorder features should continue to be addressed over the 20 weeks until the review appointment. These will be the residue of the maintaining mechanisms that have been the focus of treatment. In this way a personalized short-term maintenance plan can be prepared.

The therapist and patient need to consider what eating disorder features should continue to be addressed over the 20 weeks until the review appointment.

We do this by editing the (purposefully over-inclusive) template plan shown in Table 12.1. Examples of features typically targeted include the following:

- Dietary restraint
  — Food avoidance: Patients may need to address remaining avoided foods.
  — Social eating: Patients may need to continue practicing eating out and eating foods of uncertain composition.

- Over-evaluation of shape and weight
  — Marginalization of other domains of life: Patients may need to persist in trying new activities and persevere with ones that have been started.
  — Body checking: Patients may need to continue using mirrors differently and moderating other forms of checking while remaining aware of the risk of biased comparison-making.
  — Body avoidance: Patients may need to practice further body exposure.
  — Feeling fat: Patients may need to keep questioning what else they are feeling when they "feel fat."

- Event-triggered changes in eating
  — Residual binges: Patients may need to continue proactive problem-solving.
  — Mood intolerance: Patients may need to practice using functional methods of mood modulation.

- Mindsets
  — Patients may need to practice identifying their relapse signature as soon as it occurs and using the two-step method for "ejecting" their eating disorder DVD (see page 122).

The goal is to identify with the patient a limited number of key activities that the patient should engage in over the next 20 weeks. It is important to be realistic and not to overburden patients. The main tasks should be highlighted.

In addition to devising a patient-specific short-term plan, patients should be given the following general injunction, *"Do the right thing."* By this it is meant that patients should

TABLE 12.1. Template for a Short-Term Maintenance Plan (for Editing to Suit the Individual Patient)

Problems to focus on	How to address
Over-concern about shape and weight	• Keep an eye out for unhelpful body shape checking (frequent mirror use, inappropriate clothing checks, pinching/touching, comparing self with others), consider whether information is helpful and accurate, and reduce/stop as discussed. • Be sure not to avoid seeing body shape. If this is happening, try to be more aware of body (e.g., by wearing different clothes, having a massage). • Use mirrors carefully. • Keep an eye out for "feeling fat," and identify the triggers and relabel. • Avoid weighing outside the set weekly time; do not interpret single readings. • Avoid judging self solely on basis of shape and weight. • Maintain and develop other life interests (e.g., _____).
Dietary restraint and restriction	• Try to eat a flexible and varied diet. • Practice eating socially (e.g., with others, in restaurants). • Take care not to avoid certain foods. • Try and eat "enough" and avoid undereating. • Eat regularly (at least every 4 hours). • Avoid strict (rigid and extreme) dietary rules (e.g., concerning amount to eat [calories], when to eat, eating less than others, compensating for food already eaten, "debting" by eating less in advance of eating). • Feeling full is a normal and short-lived sensation. If troubled by recurrent feelings of fullness, identify triggers (e.g., not being used to eating a normal amount, being underweight, not eating regularly, wearing too tight clothing, eating an "avoided" food) and address.
Binge eating	• Conduct "binge analysis," if needed, to identify triggers (undereating, being underweight, going too long without eating, breaking a dietary rule, alcohol relaxing dietary control, responding to a problem in life) and address. • Practice problem-solving the triggers.
Other weight-control behavior	• Avoid vomiting/taking laxatives/over-exercising as they keep the eating problem going (and are relatively ineffective). • Other: _____.
Weight regain and maintenance	• Weekly weighing on a set day is crucial. • Maintain weight within goal weight range (i.e., from _____ to _____). • If weight falls below this weight range — alarm bells! Review pros/cons of weight regain taking a long-term perspective. Remember, one needs to eat 500 extra calories every day to regain on average 0.5 kilogram a week.
Weight loss	• Trying to lose weight is risky if one has had an eating problem. • The goal of weight loss is only appropriate if one is medically overweight. • Remember not to try to lose weight over the next 20 weeks. • Avoid rigid and extreme dietary rules. • If medically overweight, can use "binge-proof" dieting after 20 weeks for a limited time (i.e., modest weight loss goals; flexible guidelines for eating). • Have a realistic goal weight range that is possible to attain without strict dieting. • Remember, it is unrealistic and unhealthy to lose more than 0.5 kilogram a week.

TABLE 12.1 (*cont.*)

Slip-ups and lapses	• Minor slip-ups are to be expected. • Spot slip-ups early and react positively by (1) trying to understand the trigger, and (2) trying to get back on track as soon as possible (see long-term plan). • If struggling to get back on track, contact _____. • Becoming underweight is particularly serious. If body mass index is below 18.5 (_____ pounds) on two readings in a row, contact _____.
Other	• _____

From *Cognitive Behavior Therapy and Eating Disorders* by Christopher G. Fairburn. Copyright 2008 by The Guilford Press. This table is available online at www.psych.ox.ac.uk/credo/cbt_and_eating_disorders.

> **Patients should be strongly advised to "Do the right thing."**

continue to behave in line with the ways identified during treatment (e.g., eating at regular intervals, controlling body checking) because otherwise they will not obtain the full benefits.

Treatment ends with patients being given a copy of their personalized maintenance plan. They are advised to keep this plan readily accessible and refer to it regularly. Note that if clinical perfectionism, core low self-esteem or interpersonal difficulties (see Chapter 13) have been addressed in treatment, the maintenance plan should include tasks relevant to these areas too.

Phasing Out Treatment Procedures

Self-Monitoring

Patients should be asked to stop self-monitoring two sessions before treatment ends (i.e., at session 18 in the 20-session version of the treatment). It is clearly inappropriate and unrealistic to expect them to monitor indefinitely, and it is best if they get used to not monitoring while they are still in treatment.

Patients vary in how they react to being asked to stop recording. Some are relieved, whereas others are concerned that they will no longer be able to observe and analyze what they are doing. It can be helpful to remind them that the records were introduced to help them become aware of their behavior, thoughts and feelings, but now that they have developed this skill, monitoring is no longer needed. Nevertheless, patients should be encouraged to remain alert to how they are eating and to the other matters that have been targeted during treatment (e.g., body checking, food avoidance). At the final session, patients should be asked how they have managed without monitoring. Any problems that have arisen as a result (e.g., the temptation to skip meals or snacks) should be addressed.

In-Session Weighing

Toward the end of treatment in-session weighing needs to stop and patients need to start weighing themselves at home. This transition may be achieved toward the end of Stage Three or, at the latest, at the beginning of Stage Four.

At-home weighing should be done in the same way as in-session weighing; that is, at weekly intervals and on a predetermined day rather than in response to events. Patients should be helped to select a specific day, with a weekday morning generally being best (because if the patient finds weighing unsettling, there are generally more distractions on weekdays). Patients also need to be reminded how to interpret weight data, with emphasis placed on not over-interpreting the latest reading. To help with this, patients should be encouraged to continue to plot their weight on a graph. For a number of weeks at-home weighing should continue alongside in-session weighing, as in this way patients can "calibrate" their scales (i.e., detect and quantify any discrepancy between their scales and the clinic ones). Patients should continue weighing themselves at weekly intervals until the 20-week review session when the need for ongoing weighing can be reviewed.

Minimizing the Risk of Relapse in the Long Term

The other major focus of Stage Four is on minimizing the risk of relapse in the long-term. There are six elements to this:

1. Identifying strategies and procedures to be continued
2. Having realistic expectations
3. Distinguishing a "lapse" from a "relapse"
4. Ensuring that the risk of setbacks is minimized
5. Having a specific plan for dealing with setbacks
6. Drawing up a long-term maintenance plan

> The other major focus of Stage Four is on minimizing the risk of relapse in the long-term.

Crucial preparatory work will already have been undertaken in the latter half of Stage Three with the discussion of mindsets and with patients learning how to influence them (see page 119).

Identifying Strategies and Procedures to Be Continued

Patients should be asked to consider whether there are any elements of treatment that they should continue long-term to minimize the risk of relapse. To this end it can be helpful if patients identify the aspects of treatment that they believe helped them overcome particular aspects of their psychopathology. This can reinforce their importance. Typical examples include regular eating, weekly weighing, problem-solving and binge analysis.

Having Realistic Expectations

There is a tendency for patients who do well in treatment to hope that they will never have eating problems again. Without being unduly negative, the therapist should ensure that patients' expectations are realistic as otherwise they will be prone to react negatively to any setback. Patients should view their eating disorder as an Achilles heel: It is likely to remain their response to times of difficulty and their reaction to certain triggers. Just as some people react to stress by becoming depressed or irritable or by drinking too much, so people who have had an eating disorder are liable to start eating differently. This is because the eating disorder mindset (or DVD) will come back into place under certain circumstances. But, as patients will have learned in Stage Three (see page 119), this mindset is something that they can influence.

Distinguishing a "Lapse" from a "Relapse"

It is also important to stress that the patient's attitude to any setback is crucial in determining what subsequently happens. Viewing any setback as a full-scale "relapse" is likely to create a self-fulfilling prophecy. Adopting such a view encourages a hopeless, passive stance, whereas if the setback is viewed as a "lapse," the patient is more likely to face up to the problem and address it.

Minimizing the Risk of Setbacks

Patients need to minimize the risk of setbacks occurring. They therefore need to be aware of likely triggers. These triggers tend to be of the following nature:

- *Shape or weight-related events*: for example, an increase in weight, an apparent increase in "fatness," critical comments from others, shape and weight change following pregnancy, loss of weight due to illness
- *Adverse eating-related events*: for example, restarting dieting, breaking a major remaining dietary rule, an episode of binge eating
- *Other personally salient adverse events*: for example, negative events in general, especially those that threaten self-esteem
- *Development of a clinical depression;* this may well trigger a setback

Having a Plan for Dealing with Setbacks

Patients need to develop a personalized plan for dealing with any setbacks that occur. Essentially this involves two things:

1. "Ejecting" the eating disorder mindset as soon as possible
2. Addressing the cause of the setback

To eject the eating disorder mindset patients must first recognize it coming back into place. As discussed in Chapter 8, patients need to know what tends to come up on their "screen" when they start to play their eating disorder DVD. In other words, they need to have identified their personal "early warning signs." Next, they need to displace the mindset. This is relatively straightforward if it is done early, but it becomes progressively more difficult the longer that the mindset has been in place as more maintaining mechanisms start to operate and serve to lock in the DVD. In principle, to displace the mindset patients need to ensure that they both "*Do the right thing*" and engage in distracting interpersonal activities (see page 122). The former involves implementing what has been learned in treatment (e.g., regular eating, avoiding unhelpful body checking), whereas the latter requires getting involved in activities that are engaging and likely to displace the newly inserted eating disorder mindset with a healthy one. The best activities are interpersonal in nature, and although engaging in them may be difficult (as it is likely to run counter to what the patient feels like doing), doing so is important if the mindset is to be firmly dislodged.

The second aspect to dealing with setbacks involves identifying and addressing the trigger of the setback. Patients need to take "time out" to consider what might have been its cause and then address it using the problem-solving procedure learned in treatment (see page 137).

Drawing up a Long-Term Maintenance Plan

Lastly, the therapist should draw up a personalized long-term maintenance plan. This may be done by editing the inclusive template plan shown in Table 12.2 to suit the patient. Its purpose is to provide the patient with personalized advice on how to minimize the risk of relapse in the long term.

Post-Treatment Review Session

The post-treatment review session is designed to give patients an opportunity to check in and report on their progress over the previous 20 weeks. We find that 20 weeks is about the right length of time: It is sufficiently long to leave no ambiguity about whether treatment has ended or not, and it ensures that there has been enough time for patients to implement their short-term maintenance plan and address the almost inevitable setbacks. On the other hand it is not too far away: It is close enough for patients to work toward.

The review session has several other purposes:

• *To reassess the patient's state and need for further treatment.* This should be done in the usual way using the EDE-Q and CIA. If there are residual eating disorder features that are significantly interfering with the patient's functioning, then further treatment should be considered. If there has been a setback, a small number of short sessions is often all that is needed for the patient to get back on track. These should include a review of how to handle future setbacks, should they occur. It should be noted that some setbacks follow the development (or return) of a clinical depression. If this is the case, the depression will need to be treated first. Once it has resolved patients are often able to address the setback themselves.

• *To review the patient's implementation of the short-term plan.* The therapist should review each element of the patient's short-term plan, the aim being to see whether the patient needs to continue to address any residual eating disorder features.

• *To discuss the need for ongoing weekly weighing.* Weekly weighing should continue if weight remains an important issue for the patient. If it is not, then a more flexible approach should be adopted, with patients weighing themselves once every few weeks or so.

• *To discuss how any setbacks have been handled.* This is important; the strategy for handling setbacks should be reviewed in some detail.

• *To review, and revise if necessary, the long-term maintenance plan.* This too is important; some new "early warning signs" or triggers may have emerged.

TABLE 12.2. Template for a Long-Term Maintenance Plan (for Editing to Suit the Individual Patient)

How to minimize the risk of setbacks

- Maintain a pattern of regular eating.
- Avoid dieting, especially rigid and extreme diets and ones that exclude lots of foods.
- Maintain weight in goal weight range.
- Beware of engaging in unhelpful body checking or body avoidance.
- Maintain and develop other life interests.
- Use problem-solving to tackle life problems.

Circumstances that might increase the risk of a setback

- Life changes and difficulties; changes to usual routine (e.g., vacations, Thanksgiving).
- Weight loss or weight gain.
- Pregnancy and after pregnancy.
- Low mood and/or the development of a clinical depression.
- Wedding day (being the focus of attention; pressure to look good).

"Early warning signs" of a lapse

Be on the lookout for your "eating disorder DVD" coming back into place. The following early warning signs form part of the first "track" of the DVD:

- Changes in eating, especially eating less, skipping meals or snacks, delaying eating, eating "diet foods"
- Restarting the reading of diet or fashion magazines and/or visiting respective websites
- Restarting or increasing body checking or avoidance
- Restarting or increasing the making of shape comparisons
- Weighing outside set time
- Increasing exercise
- Having urges to vomit or use laxatives
- Having urges to binge eat
- Increased preoccupation with food and eating
- Increased dissatisfaction with shape and weight, and a strong desire to change shape or weight
- Weight dropping below a body mass index of 19.0 (_____ pounds)

If you spot early warning signs, react quickly and positively by taking "time out" to think about what is happening and plan a course of action

Dealing with triggers and set-backs

- Identify trigger.
- Deal with external triggers (life) by problem-solving (see *Overcoming Binge Eating*).
- Beware of labeling a setback as a "relapse" (when one is back to square one).
- Nip setbacks in the bud by following guidelines from treatment (in *Overcoming Binge Eating*); for example, restart monitoring, adopt pattern of regular eating, plan eating ahead and review eating pattern, weigh self each week and interpret carefully, avoid following rigid and extreme dietary rules, question "feeling fat," analyze binges, use distraction activities and problem-solving, reduce problematic body checking or avoidance.
- If pregnant/after pregnancy, then ask health professionals for information on what is usual regarding weight and eating and the typical time taken to lose the weight gained in pregnancy.
- As a general guideline, do the opposite of what the eating disorder mindset (or "DVD") makes you want to do (i.e., *"Do the right thing"*). Get involved in other aspects of your life, such as socializing (thereby putting in other healthier DVDs).
- Other: _____
- Other: _____

If above has not worked within 4 weeks, consider seeking help.
If body mass index falls below 18.5 (_____ pounds) for 2 consecutive weeks, seek help.

From *Cognitive Behavior Therapy and Eating Disorders* by Christopher G. Fairburn. Copyright 2008 by The Guilford Press. This table is available online at www.psych.ox.ac.uk/credo/cbt_and_eating_disorders.

With the great majority of patients the review appointment is a positive one, and it is the last time that the patient and therapist need to meet.

Recommended Reading for Chapters 5–12

Early Change in Treatment Predicting Outcome

See Chapter 3 (page 34).

Education about Eating Disorders

Fairburn, C. G. (1995). *Overcoming binge eating*. New York: Guilford Press.
Garner, D. M. (1997). Psychoeducational principles in treatment. In D. M. Garner & P. E. Garfinkel (Eds.), *Handbook of treatment for eating disorders* (2nd ed., pp. 145–177). New York: Guilford Press.
Lucas, A. R. (2004). *Demystifying anorexia nervosa*. Oxford: Oxford University Press.

Effectiveness of CBT-E

Byrne, S. M., Fursland, A., Allen, K. L., & Watson, H. (2011). The effectiveness of enhanced cognitive behavioural therapy for eating disorders: An open trial. *Behaviour Research and Therapy, 49*, 219–226.
Fairburn, C. G., Cooper, Z., Doll, H. A., O'Connor, M. E., Bohn, K., Hawker, D. M., Wales, J. A., & Palmer, R. L. (2009). Transdiagnostic cognitive behavioral therapy for patients with eating disorders: A two-site trial with 60-week follow-up. *American Journal of Psychiatry, 166*, 311–319.

Engagement and Motivation

Vitousek, K., Watson, S., & Wilson, G. T. (1998). Enhancing motivation for change in treatment-resistant eating disorders. *Clinical Psychology Review, 18*, 391–420.
Wilson, G. T., & Schlam, T. R. (2004). The transtheoretical model and motivational interviewing in the treatment of eating and weight disorders. *Clinical Psychology Review, 24*, 361–378.

Guides to the Practice of CBT

See Chapter 1 (page 6).

Shape Concern and its Modification

Cooper, M. J., Deepak, K., Grocutt, E., & Bailey, E. (2007). The experience of "feeling fat" in women with anorexia nervosa, dieting and non-dieting women: An exploratory study. *European Eating Disorders Review, 15*, 366–372.
Cooper, Z., Fairburn, C. G., & Hawker, D. M. (2003). *Cognitive-behavioral treatment of obesity: A clinician's guide*. New York: Guilford Press.
Delinsky, S. S., & Wilson, G. T. (2006). Mirror exposure for the treatment of body image disturbance. *International Journal of Eating Disorders, 39*, 108–116.
Farrell, C., Shafran, R., & Fairburn, C. G. (2004). Mirror cognitions and behaviours in people concerned about their body shape. *Behavioural and Cognitive Psychotherapy, 32*, 225–229.

Farrell, C., Shafran, R., & Lee, M. (2006). Empirically evaluated treatments for body image disturbance: A review. *European Eating Disorders Review, 14,* 289–300.

Jansen, A., Nederkoorn, C., & Mulkens, S. (2005). Selective visual attention for ugly and beautiful body parts in eating disorders. *Behaviour Research and Therapy, 43,* 183–196.

Jansen, A., Smeets, T., Martijn, C., & Nederkoorn, C. (2006). I see what you see: The lack of a self-serving body-image bias in eating disorders. *British Journal of Clinical Psychology, 45,* 123–135.

Mayer, L., Walsh, B. T., Pierson, R. N., Heymsfield, S. B., Gallagher, D., Wang, J., et al. (2005). Body fat redistribution after weight gain in women with anorexia nervosa. *American Journal of Clinical Nutrition, 81,* 1286–1291.

Reas, D. L., Whisenhunt, B. L., Netemeyer, R., & Williamson, D. A. (2002). Development of the body checking questionnaire: A self-report measure of body checking behaviors. *International Journal of Eating Disorders, 31,* 324–333.

Rosen, J. C. (1997). Cognitive-behavioral body image therapy. In D. M. Garner & P. E. Garfinkel (Eds.), *Handbook of treatment for eating disorders* (2nd ed., pp. 188–201). New York: Guilford Press.

Wilson, G. T. (2004). Acceptance and change in the treatment of eating disorders: The evolution of manual-based cognitive-behavioral therapy. In S. C. Hayes, V. M. Follette, & M. M. Linehan (Eds.), *Mindfulness and acceptance: Expanding the cognitive-behavioral tradition* (pp. 243–266). New York: Guilford Press.

Other Articles of Relevance to Chapters 5–12

Fairburn, C. G., Shafran, R., & Cooper, Z. (1999). A cognitive behavioural theory of anorexia nervosa. *Behaviour Research and Therapy, 37,* 1–13.

Herrin, M. (2003). *Nutritional counseling in the treatment of eating disorders.* New York: Brunner-Routledge.

Linehan, M. M. (1993). *Cognitive-behavioral treatment of borderline personality disorder.* New York: Guilford Press.

Mitchell, J. E., Halmi, K., Wilson, G. T., Agras, W. S., Kraemer, H., & Crow, S. (2002). A randomized secondary treatment study of women with bulimia nervosa who fail to respond to CBT. *International Journal of Eating Disorders, 32,* 271–281.

Ohanian, V. (2002). Imagery rescripting within cognitive behavior therapy for bulimia nervosa: An illustrative case report. *International Journal of Eating Disorders, 31,* 352–357.

Soh, N., Surgenor, L. J., Touyz, S., & Walter, G. (2007). Eating disorders across two cultures: Does the expression of psychological control vary? *Australian and New Zealand Journal of Psychiatry, 41,* 351–358.

Steffen, K. J., Mitchell, J. E., Roerig, J. L., & Lancaster, K. L. (2007). The eating disorders medicine cabinet revisited: A clinician's guide to Ipecac and laxatives. *International Journal of Eating Disorders, 40,* 360–368.

Tareen, A., Hodes, M., & Rangel, L. (2005). Non-fat-phobic anorexia nervosa in British South Asian adolescents. *International Journal of Eating Disorders, 37,* 161–165.

Teasdale, J. D. (1997). The relationship between cognition and emotion: The mind-in-place in mood disorders. In D. M. Clark & C. G. Fairburn (Eds.), *Science and practice of cognitive behaviour therapy* (pp. 67–93). Oxford: Oxford University Press.

Teasdale, J. D. (1999). Metacognition, mindfulness and the modification of mood disorders. *Clinical Psychology and Psychotherapy, 6,* 146–155.

ADAPTATIONS OF CBT-E

CHAPTER 13

Clinical Perfectionism, Core Low Self-Esteem and Interpersonal Problems

Christopher G. Fairburn, Zafra Cooper, Roz Shafran,
Kristin Bohn and Deborah M. Hawker

It will be recalled that there are two main forms of CBT-E. There is the "focused" form, which is suitable for the majority of patients and is the default version. It focuses directly and exclusively on the eating disorder psychopathology and was described in the previous eight chapters. This chapter is devoted to the other form of CBT-E, the "broad" form. It is designed for patients in whom certain mechanisms external to the eating disorder psychopathology maintain this psychopathology and thereby obstruct change. The broad version of the treatment has additional "modules" that are designed to address these external mechanisms, the intention being that in appropriate patients they are used to facilitate change. Returning to the house of cards analogy (see page 47), the strategy is to pull out one or more peripheral cards (usually one) that appear to be propping up the eating disorder, in addition to pulling out key eating disorder cards. Originally the broad form of CBT-E consisted of four treatment modules directed at the modification of mood intolerance, clinical perfectionism, low self-esteem and interpersonal difficulties respectively. Recently, the first of these modules, that focused on mood intolerance, has been incorporated into the focused version of the treatment (see Chapter 10, page 142).

> The focused form of CBT-E should be viewed as the default version.

> In the broad form of CBT-E the strategy is to pull out one or more peripheral cards that appear to be propping up the eating disorder.

Deciding Whether to Use the Broad Form of CBT-E

The broad form of CBT-E is designed for patients in whom clinical perfectionism, core low self-esteem or marked interpersonal problems are pronounced and appear to be maintaining the eating disorder. Clinically, the decision whether or not to use the broad form of the treatment is a major one because it governs the form and content of the treatment from Stage Two onward. Also the decision can have

> **The broad form of CBT-E is designed for patients in whom clinical perfectionism, core low self-esteem or marked interpersonal problems are pronounced and appear to be maintaining the eating disorder.**

an impact on the patient's outcome, either for the better or for the worse. Fortunately, research evidence is available to guide the decision as the relative effects of the focused and broad forms of CBT-E have been tested in a large two-center treatment trial (see Fairburn et al., 2009). In brief, it was found that the two forms of the treatment were equally effective overall, but this equivalence disguised two important findings. First, for patients in whom at least two of the original four external mechanisms were judged by their therapist (at the beginning of Stage Two) to be a "moderate" or "major" clinical problem (about 40% of the patients), the broad form of the treatment was superior to the focused form. In contrast, for the remaining patients (about 60%) the opposite was the case; that is, the focused form of the treatment was superior to the broad form (and this was also true of those with intermediate levels of "complexity"). Although these findings require replication, they are consistent with the theory underpinning CBT-E and our own clinical experience. We therefore recommend that the findings be used to govern clinical practice. Thus the broad form of the treatment should be used only with patients who have severe additional problems of the type described in this chapter, with the remaining patients receiving the focused form of CBT-E.

The decision whether or not to use the broad form of CBT-E is made in Stage Two after eight sessions of treatment. Stage Two is a good time to make this decision because by then the therapist knows the patient reasonably well and barriers to change are becoming increasingly clear. We recommend that therapists base the decision on the following two guidelines:

1. The default form of CBT-E is the focused version. With most patients it is more effective than the broad version and it is easier to implement. Also, it now incorporates the mood-intolerance module.
2. The broad form of CBT-E is used only if it is concluded in Stage Two that clinical perfectionism, core low self-esteem or marked interpersonal problems are pronounced and appear to be maintaining the eating disorder.

Implementing the Broad Form of CBT-E

There are three phases in the implementation of the broad form of CBT-E. In the first (in Stage Two), it is decided which of the three additional maintaining mechanisms to address. Guidance for doing so is provided below, module by module. In practice it is not uncommon for several modules to seem relevant, and it can be difficult to decide which one to select. Below is some guidance:

- If just one module seems relevant, this module should be used. An exception is core low self-esteem, which can be addressed either using the core low self-esteem module or the interpersonal one.
- If two modules seem relevant:
  - — In general, and if using the 20-week version of the treatment, follow the principle of parsimony and select one module based on the extent to which the target mechanism appears to be obstructing change.
  - — If the extended version of the treatment is being used (see Chapter 11), there may be sufficient time to address two of the external mechanisms. This is usually done sequentially (e.g., by addressing clinical perfectionism first and then interpersonal problems).

The second phase of broad CBT-E involves tackling the identified external mechanism(s) using the relevant module(s) while also addressing the core eating disorder maintaining mechanisms (as described in Chapters 8–11). This takes place throughout Stage Three. With regard to the organization of the sessions, it has been our practice to allocate half of the core part of the session (i.e., the time allocated to the addressing of items on the session agenda; see page 73) to the broad CBT-E module(s). As we have adhered to the standard 50-minute-session format, this means that approximately 15 minutes per session have been allocated to the addressing of the external maintaining mechanism(s). To accommodate this, less time has been devoted to the core eating disorder mechanisms than is usually the case.

It is worth noting that the broad version of CBT-E could be implemented differently. For example, CBT-E could be increased in length (e.g., to 30 sessions) to allow more time for the external mechanisms to be tackled. Alternatively, the treatment sessions could be extended in duration to, say, 80 minutes. We favor this latter option as our clinical experience suggests that doing so allows therapeutic momentum to be maintained and a variety of mechanisms to be addressed while providing a treatment that is acceptable in overall length. If this approach is adopted, it is best to have a short mid-session break to let the therapist and patient stretch their legs and collect their thoughts.

The third phase of broad CBT-E takes place in Stage Four (see Chapter 12). It involves drawing up a "maintenance plan," as usual, but one that incorporates elements from the additional module(s) that have employed in Stage Three.

The three broad CBT-E modules will now be described. They are described only in outline as an entire book could be written about each of them and, indeed, in each case this has been done already.

Clinical Perfectionism

Background

Clinical experience and research evidence indicate that the trait of perfectionism is common among people with eating disorders and often is evident before the onset of the eating disorder. What has not been established is whether it influences treatment outcome. At the extreme end of the trait is what may be termed "clinical perfectionism" (Shafran, Cooper & Fairburn, 2002), a state in which this trait is so pronounced that the person's life is significantly impaired. It is our strong impression that clinical perfectionism interferes with treatment response.

The psychopathology of clinical perfectionism is similar in form to that of an eating disorder. At its heart is the over-evaluation of achieving and achievement. People

> **The psychopathology of clinical perfectionism is similar in form to that of an eating disorder.**

with clinical perfectionism judge themselves largely, or even exclusively, in terms of working hard toward, and meeting, personally demanding standards in areas of life that are important to them. If they have a co-existing eating disorder, they also apply their extreme standards to their eating, weight and shape, and their control, and so they diet especially intensely and are similarly rigorous in their exercising, body checking, etc. Thus the psychopathology of clinical perfectionism intensifies aspects of the eating disorder and makes it harder to treat.

The main features of clinical perfectionism are listed below. They are not all invariably present:

- Over-evaluation of achieving and achievement in valued domains of life (expressed in areas such as work, performance at sports or music, etc., and in the eating disorder)
- Marginalization of other aspects of life
- Rigorous pursuit of personally demanding standards despite this having adverse effects on actual performance and causing impairment in other aspects of life
- Discounting successes and resetting standards if goals are met (e.g., if a work goal is met, it is immediately replaced by a new, even more demanding one)
- Repeated performance-checking (i.e., checking that one's performance meets one's personal standards and comparing it with that of others)
- Fear of failing to meet personal standards
- Avoiding crucial tests of performance (e.g., not submitting work) for fear that one's performance will not be good enough
- Preoccupation with thoughts about performance

With Whom to Use this Module

Clinical perfectionism is usually evident from early on in treatment. It may be seen in patients' recording, which tends to be over-detailed, and in their dietary restraint, which is often especially extreme and rigid. Thus the "Regular eating" intervention may be resisted because it clashes with the patient's standards. Clinical perfectionism may also be expressed in patients' behavior in sessions with some patients slowing down treatment with innumerable questions about its finer details.

In the presence of such features therapists should enquire directly about clinical perfectionism. This is done in Stage Two (see Chapter 7). Useful questions include the following:

- *"Some people with eating disorders could be described as 'perfectionists'; that is, they set themselves very high standards and are always striving to meet them. Might this apply to you? Would others say this of you?"*
- *"Would you say you have high standards compared to those of others? Would others agree? In what areas of your life does this occur (e.g., work, tidiness, sports, music)?"*

- *"How important to you is it to work hard and do well? Is it very, or even extremely, important?"*
- *"Do you think a lot about achieving and achievement? Is this on your mind much of the time?"*
- *"If you meet one of your goals, do you immediately set yourself a new, higher goal?"*
- *"Do you repeatedly check your performance (at how you are doing at meeting your goals) and compare it to that of others?"*
- *"Do you ever fear that you might not meet your goals?"*
- *"Do you ever avoid doing things for fear that your (work, etc.) will not be good enough?"*
- *"Do you tend to judge yourself on the basis of achieving and achievement?"*

If some or all of these questions are answered affirmatively *and* clinical perfectionism appears to be an obstacle to change, then clinical perfectionism should be an additional target of treatment and should be added to the patient's formulation (see Figure 13.1).

Treatment Strategies and Procedures

The strategy for addressing clinical perfectionism mirrors that used to address the over-evaluation of shape and weight (see Chapter 8), and the two are tackled more or less in tandem, as explained below.[1]

> **The strategy for addressing clinical perfectionism mirrors that used to address the over-evaluation of shape and weight.**

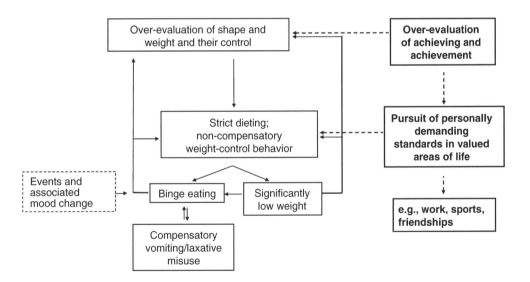

FIGURE 13.1. The transdiagnostic formulation with clinical perfectionism added.

From *Cognitive Behavior Therapy and Eating Disorders* by Christopher G. Fairburn. Copyright 2008 by The Guilford Press. This figure is available online at www.psych.ox.ac.uk/credo/cbt_and_eating_disorders.

---

[1]Therapists wanting ideas about additional procedures of relevance to clinical perfectionism are recommended the book by Antony and Swinson (1998). It is written as a self-help book for people with perfectionist tendencies, but we think that with patients with clinical perfectionism it is best used as a therapist's guide.

Identifying the Over-Evaluation of Achieving and Its Consequences

This is best done in the session after the same topic has been addressed with respect to shape and weight. It will emerge that the patient's system for self-evaluation (as represented by his or her pie chart; see page 98) has a dominant slice representing the over-evaluation of achieving and achievement, and that this slice covers the area occupied by the shape and weight slice as well as other areas (i.e., those subject to the perfectionism, typically work but also other areas that the patient values, e.g., sports, housekeeping, music).

Vignette

One patient created a pie chart with over 20 slices, each meticulously labeled. She reported that these were the areas of life on which she based her self-evaluation. On (lengthy) discussion with the therapist it emerged that almost all of them were the focus of her extreme striving and that they could be amalgamated into a single large "achieving and achievement" slice.

In discussing the pie chart it should be made clear that having such a dominant slice is "risky," self-perpetuating, and tends to narrow one's interests, just as with the over-evaluation of shape and weight (see page 99). The therapist should help the patient see that judging oneself primarily in terms of achieving and achievement results in a relentlessly driven life in which there is little room for spontaneity or for pleasures that are not performance-related.

The "expressions" of the clinical perfectionism should then be identified and, on this basis, an extended formulation constructed. An example is shown in Figure 13.2. If this extended formulation is drawn using the same format as the equivalent one for the over-evaluation of shape and weight (see Figure 8.3) this should help make it clear to the patient that the perfectionism is being similarly expressed in the eating disorder as well as in other personally important areas of the patient's life.

Enhancing the Importance of Other Domains for Self-Evaluation

The over-evaluation of achieving and achievement results in the marginalization of other areas of life, just as happens with the over-evaluation of shape and weight, but in patients with clinical perfectionism this may be even more marked. The strategy for addressing such marginalization is described in Chapter 8 (see page 102). With these particular patients it is important to encourage them to take part in activities simply for the sake of enjoyment, although in our experience it is hard for them to do so (see vignette below). Involving significant others can be of help. It is also worth identifying with the patient activities that cannot be measured with regard to performance yet are generally valued although are viewed by the patient as being a "waste of time." Such activities might include reading books or newspapers, listening to music, staying in touch with friends, etc. Spontaneity is also something to encourage for these patients find unpredictability difficult to tolerate, and this interferes with their ability to socialize. One of our patients tried to counter this difficulty by planning "spontaneous" social

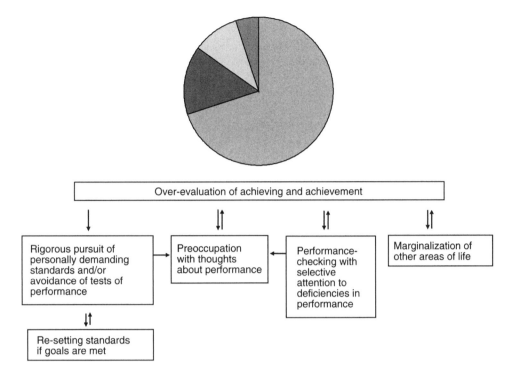

FIGURE 13.2. The over-evaluation of achieving and achievement: An "extended formulation."

From *Cognitive Behavior Therapy and Eating Disorders* by Christopher G. Fairburn. Copyright 2008 by The Guilford Press. This figure is available online at www.psych.ox.ac.uk/credo/cbt_and_eating_disorders.

events. Therapists can introduce increasing degrees of flexibility by adapting the dice procedure described in Chapter 11 (page 134).

Vignette

In the context of enhancing other domains for self-evaluation, a patient chose to spend weekends exploring the local countryside with his girlfriend. As part of this process they would have lunch or tea in cafes or restaurants. It emerged that he started to systematically rate these places along various dimensions with the goal of possibly producing a written guide to them. Thus what had been intended to be a non-measurable form of relaxation became yet another focus of his perfectionism.

Addressing Goals and Striving

People with clinical perfectionism tend to work exceptionally hard and be dismissive of "wasting time." Despite this, their performance is usually suboptimal because they are working excessively and are therefore less effective due to fatigue, and because they tend to be indecisive as getting things right is so important to them. To address this therapists need to help patients establish more appropriate work habits, thereby allowing time for the development of marginalized domains for self-evaluation. To achieve this, therapists should discuss with patients how they could become "more effective." Education about work habits is of particular value as patients commonly believe that the harder they work, the better they will do. This is often not the case. Indeed, their performance may improve with less striving (see vignette on page 206).

Discussing what patients really want to achieve in their life (i.e., their long-term aspirations and true goals) can also be of value. Accepting a slightly lower level of performance may be necessary to "Get a life" and, paradoxically, it may result in enhanced performance. Ideally, patients should decide to do this, but suggesting that they lower their standards goes down extremely badly. Rather, it is

> Suggesting that these patients lower their standards goes down extremely badly. Rather it is better to talk about how they might become "more effective"!

better to talk about how they might become "more effective." To this end it can be helpful to ask patients to specify in detail their goals in the various domains of life to which they apply their perfectionism and what would need to be done to achieve them. What usually emerges is an obviously impossible list of goals that they are simultaneously trying to meet (see Table 13.1)

TABLE 13.1. A Patient's Goals in Three Areas of Life

Work (as a teacher)

- To be seen to be working harder than my colleagues
- To be first into school in the morning and last to leave
- To do more than is expected of me
- To complete work well ahead of deadlines
- To ensure that my classroom is neat and tidy at all times
- To be viewed as the best teacher in my school year
- To initiate new ideas and policies at meetings
- To volunteer for extra work

Exercise

- To engage in daily exercise, however inconvenient and however I am feeling
- To set myself new short-term and long-term challenges and targets (e.g., faster lap times, longer races, tougher competitions)
- To be one of the best runners in my club
- To never perform less well than the last time
- To exercise to an extent that is viewed as a massive achievement by others

Eating, shape and weight

- To stick to my rules about what and when I eat
- To never eat "bad" foods
- To always eat less than others around me
- To always choose the lowest-fat option when there is a choice
- To ensure that my stomach is flat
- To never let my weight go up
- To be the thinnest among my friends and colleagues

Addressing Performance Checking

At the same time as enhancing the importance of other domains for self-evaluation, the therapist should directly target the patient's over-evaluation of achieving and achievement. Often it is best to begin with its expression in the form of performance checking as this tends to be particularly potent in maintaining the over-evaluation. This is because it highlights what patients are not achieving thereby encouraging yet further striving. This vicious circle should be discussed to establish whether patients identify with it. The performance checking will be evident in all areas of life that are the focus of the clinical perfectionism including, of course, shape and weight and controlling eating. Thus performance checking should be addressed in general as well as in relation to weight (weighing or weight checking) and shape (shape checking). In practice this means identifying its expressions across the various domains of life affected.

As with body checking, the first step is to identify the forms of performance checking present. Two periods of 24-hour recording are usually sufficient, one being a work day (if applicable) and the other being a day off work. Having done this, the therapist should discuss with the patient the consequences of his or her particular forms of checking, the main point being that the checking is generally driven by a fear of failure with there being a focus on what the person is not achieving rather than on what is being accomplished. In addition, it is helpful to explore any adverse effects; for example, repeated checking can reduce productivity. The therapist and patient should then proceed to categorize the various forms of checking into two groups: forms of checking that are probably best stopped (e.g., furtively looking at other people's work), and behavior that needs to be moderated (e.g., repeatedly testing one's work performance). In the context of the formulation and education, and with the therapist's help, patients can usually make changes along these lines while exploring the consequences of doing so. They should be forewarned that in the short term making such changes will result in them becoming more preoccupied with their performance (just as happens with the in-session weighing intervention in Stage One; see page 62), but within weeks this declines.

One particular form of performance checking involves making repeated comparisons with the performance of others. Patients' appraisal of their own performance is often meticulous and characterized by selective attention to things that they are not succeeding in doing. In contrast, patients' assessment of others is generally superficial and uncritical. The therapist should highlight this unfavorable bias and devise homework tasks that highlight and counter it (in line with the principles described with regard to shape; see page 110).

Patients with clinical perfectionism also tend to select top performers as the subject of their comparisons. Often this occurs across all the domains affected by the perfectionism, such that the amalgamated comparison is even more unrealistic (e.g., simultaneously comparing oneself to a top executive, a professional athlete, a super-mom and a top chef). For example, one of our patients was trying to be a "superwoman" in 10 different areas of her life and had extreme standards for her performance in each one. Highlighting this and pointing out the impossibility of meeting these standards can be helpful in its own right. In this context it can be also helpful to have a general discussion about the need to achieve a balance between acceptance and change (see page 214).

Addressing Avoidance

Avoidance may take two forms. First, patients may avoid making their own assessments of how they are performing. This will result in them having little or no information about their true progress or ability: Instead, they "fear the worst." An example with respect to eating disorder psychopathology is avoidance of weighing (see page 63). Second, there may be avoidance of crucial external tests of performance; for example, not attending a job interview, not handing in course work, or not competing at an athletics competition. This is driven by the fear that they will fail or be judged not good enough. Both types of avoidance need to be addressed, the former by helping patients introduce normative ongoing performance checking, and the latter by helping them balance the immediate and longer-term pros and cons of completing tests of performance.

Vignette

Although this patient described herself as a "weak perfectionist," this was far from the case. She had extreme clinical perfectionism which was expressed in her work. She had to be first in the office in the morning and the last to leave at the end of the day, and she spent much of her evenings working. It was also expressed in her exercising — a 6-mile run before breakfast whatever the weather — and in her dieting and body checking.

Treatment was complicated by the clinical perfectionism. She came to treatment sessions with long lists of questions for the therapist and was unduly detailed in her recording. Every element of treatment had to be described to her in meticulous detail, and she found it very difficult to modify her behavior in any way.

In Stage Two it was agreed that her "standards" should be an additional focus of treatment. It gradually became clear to the patient that she had extreme standards for virtually everything that she did and that these were counterproductive because they were impairing her performance in a range of areas. Common processes were identified across the various domains of life affected (e.g., repeated performance checking, avoidance of tests of performance, extreme striving, resetting goals if standards were met) and, with difficulty, she began to address them. At the same time the therapist tried to help her develop marginalized domains of life and engage in new performance-free activities (e.g., listening to music).

By the end of treatment she had improved, but she still tended to restrict her eating. The clinical perfectionism was also still evident, but it was causing less impairment: Indeed, she could see that by adjusting her standards she achieved more.

The Effects of These and Other Cognitive Behavioral Interventions

As with the addressing of the over-evaluation of shape and weight, these strategies and procedures result in the progressive erosion of the main expressions of the over-evaluation and, by removing their reinforcing effect, this has a gradual but profound impact on the over-evaluation itself, an effect that continues even after treatment has ended. This effect is augmented by an increase in the importance of other domains of life (i.e., an increase in the number and size of these slices in the patient's pie chart). As with all aspects of CBT-E, this work is combined with other cognitive behavioral interventions.

Perfectionist behavior with respect to treatment itself also needs to be addressed. Recording only needs to be "good enough"; over-detailed recording tends to distract the patient and the therapist from the main issues at hand. Similarly, lengthy in-session questioning can bog down sessions and interfere with progress. Both may be used as examples of the impairing effect of extreme striving.

Two additional strategies complement this work, both of which are best used toward the end of treatment. These are exploring the origins of over-evaluation and learning to manipulate the perfectionist mindset (as with the over-evaluation of shape and weight; see Chapter 8).

Exploring the Origins of Over-Evaluation

It is often helpful to ask patients to consider the origins of their concerns about performance. This can help make sense of how the perfectionism developed and has evolved, and most importantly it can highlight how it might have served a useful function before it became so extreme. As it is often difficult to time the onset of clinical perfectionism, it is only possible to look for events or circumstances that might have sensitized the patient to performance rather than examine their contribution at various stages in the development of the problem (as is done with concerns about shape, weight and eating; see page 117). The sensitizing events and circumstances may include a family history of clinical perfectionism, family values concerning achievement, pressures to succeed, early "successes" and "failures," the reactions of significant others, and the influence of the patient's education.

Learning to Manipulate the Perfectionist Mindset

Like the core psychopathology of eating disorders, that of clinical perfectionism may be viewed as a "mindset" or a frame of mind (see page 119) and, just as the cognitive behavioral procedures of CBT-E erode the mechanisms that have been holding the eating disorder mindset in place, so the procedures directed at clinical perfectionism have an equivalent effect. As a result, more appropriate mindsets are able to move into place. At first this happens only transiently, but it happens more and more as the maintaining mechanisms are further eroded.

Just as it is important that patients learn about manipulating their mindset with respect to their eating disorder (see page 122), so they should learn to do so with respect to clinical perfectionism. To achieve this, therapists should employ equivalent strategies and procedures, the goal being that patients learn three things: first, to identify stimuli that are prone to put the perfectionist mindset (or DVD) back in place; second, to recognize the first signs that it is "playing"; and third, to displace it.

Maintaining the Changes Made and Minimizing the Risk of Relapse

The strategies and procedures used to maintain progress and minimize the risk of relapse are the same as those used more generally with respect to the eating disorder (see Chapter 12). The therapist should identify what problems remain and devise a specific perfectionism-oriented "maintenance plan" for the patient to implement over the following months. The same applies to relapse prevention in the longer term, with particular attention being paid to the identification of patients' likely relapse signature and what action they should take if they experience a setback.

Vignette

A patient wrote at the end of treatment:

> "Being able to relax is a big change. I have a much better work–life balance than before. I am still competitive, but I can see that how trying to achieve perfection was counterproductive. More hours worked, more miles run, and less food eaten doesn't mean you are succeeding. The hard way isn't always the right way. Life is so much better now."

Core Low Self-Esteem

Background

Clinical experience and research evidence indicate that low self-esteem is common among people with eating disorders and, like clinical perfectionism, may predate the onset. There is also some evidence from the research on bulimia nervosa that low self-esteem is associated with a poor response to treatment. Despite this, low self-esteem does not generally need to be addressed in treatment because it does not necessarily obstruct change. Furthermore, self-esteem commonly improves with the successful treatment of the eating disorder, even if it has not been explicitly targeted. Nevertheless, there is a subgroup of patients who have extreme, or "core," low self-esteem in whom change in the eating disorder is particularly difficult to achieve as a result of two main processes:

> **Low self-esteem does not generally need to be addressed as it does not necessarily obstruct change.**

1. The intensity of these patients' low self-esteem leads them to strive especially hard to control their eating, shape and weight to gain some sense of self-worth. This makes it very difficult for them to moderate their dieting, exercising, body checking, etc. Thus in these cases there is an additional mechanism driving the eating disorder.
2. The unconditional and pervasive nature of these patients' negative view of themselves results in their seeing little or no prospect of recovery. Essentially, these patients write themselves off from the beginning and therefore do not fully engage in treatment.

In this specific subgroup of patients with low self-esteem, treatment stands little chance of succeeding unless their self-esteem is also addressed. It is for these patients that this module is designed.

The main features of core low self-esteem are as follows:

- An unconditional and pervasive negative view of self-worth that is longstanding and not explained by the presence of a clinical depression. (See page 246 for a description of the features of clinical depression among patients with eating disorders.) These patients believe that they have little or no value as people, and they describe themselves using terms such as "worthless," "useless," "stupid," "unlovable" or a "failure."
- A negative view of the future and the possibility of change
- Pronounced negative cognitive processing biases

With Whom to Use This Module

Core low self-esteem is usually evident from the outset of treatment and can be ascertained from the history. The key point is that it is a longstanding and pervasive negative view of the self that is unconditional. It is not based on patients' current appraisal of their ability to achieve things; rather, it is a persistent and profoundly negative view of the self that is largely independent of current circumstances and performance. It is difficult to identify core low self-esteem in the presence of a clinical depression because it too results in patients having a profoundly negative view of themselves. Therefore, if there is a co-existing clinical depression, this should be treated first (see page 248) and the patient's self-esteem reassessed after this has been done.

During Stage One core low self-esteem may be evident in these patients' excessively self-critical responses to anything that does not go well. While it may not prove to be an overt barrier to change, few of these patients do well in Stage One.

In the presence of features suggestive of core low self-esteem, therapists should conduct a thorough assessment in Stage Two. Useful questions include the following:

- *"How do you view yourself?"*
- *"Would you say you are someone who is self-critical? . . . extremely so?"*
- *"Would others agree?"*
- *"How do you think you compare as a person with other people?"*
- *"Do you think that you have any positive qualities?"*
- *"Do you see yourself as always having been like this?"*

If these and other questions suggest that the patient has core low self-esteem, and progress in Stage One suggests that it might be an obstacle to change, then it should become an additional focus of treatment. It can be addressed in two ways. It may be directly tackled using cognitive behavioral procedures, in which case it should be added to the formulation (see Figure 13.3). Alternatively, it is possible to tackle core low self-esteem indirectly by enhancing the patient's interpersonal function-

> **Core low self-esteem can be addressed in two ways: directly using CBT strategies and techniques, or indirectly by enhancing interpersonal functioning.**

ing (see later in this chapter). Occasionally, if time allows (generally only in the extended version of the treatment; see Chapter 11), both strategies may be used as they can be complementary, but if the patient is receiving the 20-week version it is not often realistic to consider both options. The direct method is generally better with those patients who have obvious cognitive biases and who accept that they would benefit from working on them (see vignette on page 214). The indirect method is better if there appears to be the potential to create a self-maintaining positive interpersonal environment.

Treatment Strategies and Procedures

In outline, the work on core low self-esteem starts with personalized education about the processes that maintain it. Subsequently there is sustained focus on helping these patients recognize and correct in real time those cognitive processes that are maintaining their negative self-evaluation. This is combined with efforts to help patients identify, and start to engage in, new and rewarding aspects of life. Toward the end of treatment there is a "historical review" designed to explore how patients acquired their negative view of themselves. Finally, and on the basis of all the preceding work, patients are helped to formulate, accept, and live consistently with, a more balanced appraisal of their self-worth.[2]

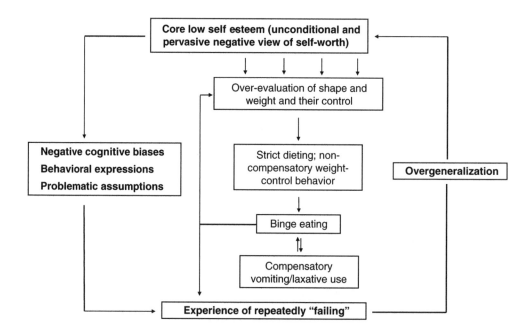

FIGURE 13.3. The bulimia nervosa formulation with core low self-esteem added.

From *Cognitive Behavior Therapy and Eating Disorders* by Christopher G. Fairburn. Copyright 2008 by The Guilford Press. This figure is available online at www.psych.ox.ac.uk/credo/cbt_and_eating_disorders.

---

[2]For further guidance on addressing core low self-esteem, see the articles by Fennell in the Recommended Reading section at the end of this chapter. Fennell's (2006) book on low self-esteem is a particularly rich source of information. While it is a self-help book, we think it is best used as a therapist's guide with patients who have core low self-esteem.

Personalized Education

To start, the therapist should provide personalized education about core low self-esteem and its contribution to the maintenance of the eating problem. The main overall point to stress is that powerful vicious circles operate that serve to maintain both the low self-esteem and the eating disorder. The specific points are as follows:

- People with core low self-esteem see themselves and the world from an extremely self-critical perspective while other views are either not noticed or are discounted.
- Core low self-esteem, when it co-occurs with a dysfunctional scheme for self-evaluation (i.e., an unbalanced pie chart, see page 98), as in patients with an eating disorder, leads people to strive particularly hard to perform well in the areas of life that they (over-)value.
- It also makes it likely (through the operation of negative cognitive biases) that they perceive themselves as repeatedly failing in this regard.
- In addition, it makes it likely that they will generalize from these perceived failures to seeing themselves as being a "failure" in general, thereby confirming their negative view of themselves.

Addressing Cognitive Processes that Maintain Core Low Self-Esteem

Patients need help to appreciate that the way that they "see" themselves and the world is likely to be biased (i.e., they have been filtering information negatively) and that things may not actually be as they seem. The therapist may use the following analogy:

Sunglasses Analogy

Imagine that overnight someone puts sunglasses on you without your knowing. You wake up in the morning and it seems dark outside. This is your reality: It is how you are seeing and appraising the world. You conclude that since the weather is so gloomy, you will need to wear warm clothes.

You then go to the bathroom and see in the mirror that you are wearing sunglasses, and you take them off. Now everything looks quite different. Outside it is light. You realize that you were seeing things incorrectly. There will be no need for those warm clothes.

So it is with people who have low self-esteem. They see the world from an unduly negative perspective. They look on the black side of everything . . . things are half empty rather than half full . . . and they are pessimistic. But their way of looking at things is biased: It is as if they were wearing dark sunglasses and were not aware of it. Life is not how they see it.

People with low self-esteem need help to recognize this bias in the way that they filter information about themselves and the world, and then they need help to overcome this bias so that they can see things how they really are.

The main cognitive processes that create this negative bias are listed below, and each is addressed using conventional cognitive behavioral procedures.

• *Discounting positive qualities.* This is best addressed from the outset. Most patients with core low self-esteem notice and recall their negative qualities while overlooking their positive ones. Identifying positive qualities, however apparently trivial, can help patients achieve a more balanced view of themselves. To do this, patients should make a list of their positive attributes, noting their skills and strengths. They may find this a difficult task, and it is therefore best to start the list in the session. Useful questions to ask are as follows:

— *"What have you achieved in your life so far?"*
— *"What skills have you acquired?"*
— *"What challenges have you faced?"*
— *"What do other people like or value in you?"*
— *"What qualities and actions that you value in others do you share?"*
— *"What aspects of yourself would you value in others?"*
— *"What bad qualities do you not have?"*

The next step is for the patient to note down instances of these positive qualities as they occur in everyday life and, indeed, to actively look out for them. For example, patients should note examples of their behavior (e.g., phoned an ill relative) that show the operation of their positive attributes (i.e., being kind and caring). Therapists should encourage patients to note on their monitoring record at least one (and preferably more) such event each day. Once this procedure has been introduced, it should continue throughout the rest of treatment.

In addition, at the end of each week patients should ask themselves, *"What things have gone reasonably well this week?"* and *"Why have they gone well?"* At first this is best done in the session with the therapist's help, but later on patients should do this themselves, noting down the main points on the back of the day's monitoring record.

• *Selective attention.* Patients with core low self-esteem have selective attention to information that is consistent with their negative view of themselves. They look for failure and, just as *"If you look for fatness, you will find it,"* so too *"If you look for failure, you will find it."*

> Just as "If you look for fatness, you will find it," so too "If you look for failure, you will find it."

To address selective attention, the first step is education. In general, we all pay particular attention to stimuli that are salient to us. For example, if one buys a new car one starts to notice many more cars like it. This is not because their number has increased; rather, it is due to paying particular attention to these specific cars. The equivalent happens in patients with low self-esteem: They look out for failure experiences and find them, and as a result their negative view of themselves is repeatedly confirmed. Having explained this, the therapist should ask patients for possible examples from their life.

Next, the therapist should help the patient become progressively more aware in real time of situations in which they engage in selective attention. The goal is that they learn to broaden their focus of attention at these times instead of paying particular attention to "failures."

• *Double standards.* Typically patients with core low self-esteem have one set of (harsh) standards for judging themselves and another (more lenient) set for others. Addressing double standards primarily involves helping patients recognize that they operate in this way and then reviewing in detail any justification for such double standards. With the majority of patients just highlighting the phenomenon in-session, and then identifying it in real time, is sufficient to undermine it.

- *Over-generalization*. Patients with core low self-esteem tend to view any instance of not succeeding as a failure, and then generalize from such failure experiences to being "a failure" in general. This cognitive process is addressed in much the same way as double standards. The therapist first helps patients identify when they do this and then, in-session, asks them to question the basis for their thinking, the aim being to erode the phenomenon. Subsequently patients should be helped to practice doing this in real time.

- *Dichotomous appraisals of self-worth*. This cognitive process is also common among patients with core low self-esteem (e.g., *"If I am not strong, I must be weak"*). It is an example of black-and-white thinking and is addressed in the usual way.

- *Dysfunctional beliefs*. Dysfunctional beliefs are almost ubiquitous among patients with core low self-esteem. These include views such as *"I need to be really good at . . . to be worthwhile."* Beliefs of this kind may be addressed using standard cognitive behavioral procedures (e.g., surveys, formal cognitive restructuring, orthogonal continua).

Exploring the Origins of the Core Low Self-Esteem

It is of value with patients with core low self-esteem to conduct a thorough "historical review," similar to that done in the course of addressing clinical perfectionism. The question to be addressed is how they acquired their negative view of themselves. This review is best done collaboratively in-session, as some of these patients find the process distressing and confirmatory, and may become preoccupied with particular adverse experiences.

Circumstances and events of note typically include a family history of low self-esteem, a negative family environment (e.g., lack of affection or warmth, frequent criticism, undue control, extreme discipline, rejection, unpredictability), and adverse childhood experiences (e.g., abuse, teasing, bullying, lack of stability, lack of friends, other negative life events). An essential part of this review is re-evaluating patients' views of past events and experiences from the vantage point of the present. To do this, therapists need to help patients examine and question their old appraisals of the past and develop new ones.

Arriving at a Balanced View of Self-Worth

The strategies and procedures described above are concerned with modifying patients' negative views of their worth, or value, as people. This work is complemented by the erosion of the over-concern about shape and weight (see Chapters 8 and 9) and the establishment of new domains for self-evaluation (see page 102), as it is important to help these patients engage in new and rewarding aspects of life.

The final step in addressing core low self-esteem involves helping patients formulate and accept a more balanced (and therefore less negative) view of themselves. Patients should be helped to review their judgments about themselves, the goal being to arrive at a more realistic appraisal of their qualities. For example, the judgment *"I am weak"* may be questioned by reviewing times when patients have been strong, and times when it would be acceptable or understandable not to be strong, appreciating that no one is strong all the time. Although such a reappraisal may result in the identification of matters that patients might choose to work on, therapists should help patients see that this does not warrant the conclusion that they are "weak."

This type of reappraisal should include the notion of "acceptance" because a balance needs to be struck between "acceptance" and "change." There are aspects of life one can change (e.g., how one eats [within certain limits], whether one induces vomiting, the standards one sets oneself, how one judges oneself) and, if they are problematic, then one should seriously think about changing them. However, there are other aspects of life that one cannot change (e.g., one's physique and height; one's early experiences) or that can change only to a limited extent (e.g., one's weight in the long term, one's family, other people) or with great difficulty. One has to learn to accept those things that cannot be changed, and, as Wilson (2004) has pointed out, doing so is a sign of strength and self-affirmation. The goal is that patients start to behave consistently with this new balanced appraisal of themselves, and observe the results. Examples might include talking to others about things they have achieved, however minor; asking for help, when previously help seeking was viewed as a sign of weakness; challenging criticism, if it is not deserved; experimenting with Internet dating; and applying for a new job.

Vignette

This patient made limited progress in Stage One largely because of his negative thinking and, in particular, his extreme self-criticism. It emerged in the Stage Two review that he doubted his value as a person and did not think that he could ever change. He was aware that he had a generally negative perspective as others had pointed this out in the past. As his view on himself was clearly a problem, and it was affecting his progress at overcoming the eating disorder, the therapist suggested that his self-esteem become an additional focus of treatment. He agreed.

Stage Three of treatment included all the usual elements, together with a focus on self-esteem. He was provided with information about possible cognitive biases that might be contributing to his view of himself and was encouraged to look out for these in real time. Most prominent in his case were selective attention to minor interpersonal difficulties (labeled as "failures") combined with overgeneralization ("*I am a failure*"). It was also clear that he made biased comparisons with other people, and either neglected or discounted positive experiences. The therapist helped him identify and correct these cognitive biases in real time and also taught him to recognize and accept his positive attributes. Gradually he began to question his prior assumptions about himself as he could see that they did not match reality.

At the end of treatment he admitted to being "perplexed" about his true personality. With the eating disorder largely resolved, his view that he was ugly, unattractive and unlovable did not seem correct. He decided that he needed to get on with his life and stop assessing himself. This he did with great success.

Interpersonal Problems

Background

Most patients with eating disorders have difficulties in their relationships. In general these lessen as the eating disorder improves. Indeed, patients' interpersonal lives often improve markedly once they are free from the effects of the eating disorder. However, there are patients for whom this does not happen — where, instead, there is a noxious interaction between the eating problem and the patient's interpersonal life such that both need to be addressed in treatment if the patient is to overcome the eating disorder (Fairburn, Cooper, & Shafran, 2003). It is for these patients that this module is designed.

With Whom to Use This Module

It will become clear in Stage One if interpersonal problems are contributing significantly to the maintenance of the eating disorder. This interaction may take several forms: Interpersonal events and circumstances may lead to an intensification of dietary restraint, even to the extent that patients may cease eating for a while; they may trigger an episode, or succession of episodes, of binge eating; or they may trigger vomiting, laxative-taking or over-exercising.

Isolated interpersonal events may be addressed using proactive problem-solving (see page 137), supplemented if needed with work on mood intolerance (see page 142), but if there are recurrent interpersonal difficulties, and these are impeding progress, they should become an additional focus of treatment in their own right. Clearly this decision needs to be made in collaboration with the patient, but under these circumstances patients are generally eager for this to happen.

The Nature of the Module

> The interpersonal module has two goals: The first is to resolve the identified interpersonal problem(s); and the second is to generally improve patients' interpersonal functioning.

The interpersonal module has two interrelated goals: The first is to resolve the identified interpersonal problem or problems; and the second is to generally improve patients' interpersonal functioning. In CBT-E these goals are achieved using a somewhat controversial strategy: this is to use a psychological treatment other than CBT. The treatment is interpersonal psychotherapy or "IPT."

IPT is a well-known, empirically supported, psychological treatment that is designed to improve current interpersonal functioning. It was originally devised as a short-term treatment for clinical depression (Klerman, Weissman, Rounsaville, & Chevron, 1984), but it has since been shown to have a specific beneficial effect in bulimia nervosa. Indeed, it is the leading empirically supported treatment for bulimia nervosa after CBT. There are four reasons why we use IPT rather than CBT to effect interpersonal change:

1. IPT was explicitly designed to achieve the type of interpersonal change needed, and within the appropriate time frame.
2. There is no form of CBT that has similar goals and an equivalent evidence base.
3. The research on bulimia nervosa has shown that IPT is highly acceptable to patients with eating disorders.
4. IPT has one other compelling property. This is that most patients leave treatment feeling convinced that they were fully responsible for the changes made, and that they could now successfully address other interpersonal problems, should they arise. In other words, IPT produces a strong sense of interpersonal competence and empowerment. This is a most attractive characteristic as it results in patients believing that they have control over their interpersonal lives (at least to the extent that anyone has), something that many of these patients have never had in the past.

The difficulty with this strategy is that it involves delivering two very different psychological treatments at one time. This is difficult to accomplish and potentially unwise. As Wilson (2004) has argued, receiving conceptually and procedurally different treatments is likely to confuse patients and risks diluting their individual effects. Furthermore, there is a practical problem as these two particular treatments are "immiscible" (Fairburn, 1997), like oil and vinegar. But just as oil and vinegar may be combined to dress a salad, so CBT and IPT may be combined in one single treatment. They cannot be integrated because of their procedural differences, particularly in terms of therapist style, but they can co-exist so long as this is done carefully. This is what is done in CBT-E, and in our experience it works well. (Therapists not trained in IPT could, in principle, use CBT strategies and procedures to achieve the same ends, but this approach has not been tested.)

> **Just as oil and vinegar may be combined to dress a salad, so CBT and IPT may be combined in one single treatment. They cannot be integrated because of their procedural differences, but they can co-exist.**

Interpersonal Psychotherapy (IPT)

IPT, as usually conducted, involves 12–16 weekly outpatient sessions, each lasting about 50 minutes. It has three phases. Below is a very brief outline. For details about the practice of IPT, the IPT manual should be consulted (Weissman, Markowitz, & Klerman, 2000). For details about how IPT has been adapted for patients with bulimia nervosa, see Fairburn (1997).

- *Phase One* generally occupies up to three weekly sessions. The goals are threefold:
  1. *To describe the rationale and nature of IPT.* In the CBT-E context the rationale is that interpersonal difficulties appear to be contributing to the maintenance of the eating problem, and the outcome of treatment is likely to be better if these difficulties are addressed.
  2. *To identify one or more current interpersonal problems.* This is done in several dif-

ferent ways, the most important involving examining interpersonal precipitants of changes in eating.

3. *To agree jointly which of the identified interpersonal problems should become the focus of the rest of treatment.*

- *Phase Two* is the main part of treatment and occupies up to 10 weekly sessions. The goal is that the patient first characterizes the identified interpersonal problems and then addresses them. IPT categorizes interpersonal problems into one of four overarching "problem areas": grief, interpersonal role disputes, role transitions and interpersonal deficits, and both problem area-specific and generic IPT strategies and procedures are used to address them.

- *Phase Three* generally occupies the final three sessions. There are two goals; the first being to ensure that the changes made in treatment are maintained, and the second being to minimize the risk of relapse in the longer term. Thus at this stage the goals are the same as those of the focused form of CBT-E (see Chapter 12), albeit with the emphasis being on the maintenance of interpersonal change.

The therapeutic style in IPT is active but not directive. Patients are helped to explore the identified problem or problems, and then consider ways of addressing them. Subsequently, patients' actual attempts to change and their implications become the subject of the sessions. The therapist's role is to keep patients focused on these interpersonal tasks, to encourage patients to think, and to provide clarification when needed, but it does not extend to suggesting solutions or particular courses of action. The therapist points out themes and inconsistencies; helps patients analyze how they communicate with others; assists patients in thinking through decisions; and highlights points that patients might miss — but this does not extend to making "interpretations." Rarely is reference made to the patient–therapist relationship and throughout treatment the focus is primarily on the present and future.

Implementing the Interpersonal Module

Implementing the interpersonal module poses a number of challenges:

1. The therapist needs to be competent at delivering IPT. This includes being clear about its strategies and techniques, and how they differ from those used in CBT.

2. The therapist needs to be comfortable having IPT sessions that are unusually brief. In reality the abbreviation is not as extreme as it might seem in that all the in-session time available for the interpersonal module is "pure" IPT. This is because many non-specific preliminaries will have taken place during the preceding CBT part of the session. In this context it should be noted that the number of sessions available (11 or 12; i.e., Stages Two, Three and Four of CBT-E) and their time frame are not atypical for IPT and so treatment is able to progress through the three phases at the usual rate.

3. Patients need to understand that they are receiving two different psychological treatments delivered in one treatment session, and they need to be clear about their different rationales and styles. This needs to be explained at the outset (i.e., at the end of Stage Two).

4. The IPT and CBT parts of the sessions need to be clearly demarcated from each other. This is done both verbally and behaviorally. When it is time for the IPT segment of the session agenda to start (generally after the CBT segment), the therapist states that it is now time for the "Life" part of the session and sits back pushing aside the patient's monitoring records, etc. Then the IPT session begins, usually initiated by the therapist beginning with the standard IPT prompt, *"How have things been since we last met?"* When the time available for the IPT part of the session is over, the therapist states that it is time to wrap up and provides a succinct summary of what has been covered. The therapist then sits forward, gathers together the CBT paperwork, and rounds off the session in the usual way (see page 62). Thus the CBT session has an IPT segment "floating" within it, but the two do not mix — just as with oil and vinegar.

Combining CBT and IPT might seem impossibly difficult, but in practice it is perfectly feasible, and patients are generally very positive about the "life" part of their sessions and make good use of it.[3]

Vignette

This patient was in her 40s. She had a history of having had an eating disorder in her adolescence, but she had subsequently been well until the breakup of her marriage 18 months earlier. Since then she had severely restricted her eating and had restarted self-induced vomiting and laxative misuse. Her weight had dropped considerably, although she was not underweight.

In Stage One it became abundantly clear that the patient's interpersonal circumstances had a substantial influence on her day-to-day eating. On days when she was stressed she would abandon "regular eating" and eat almost nothing. She was also prone to vomit on these days. In Stage Two it was therefore agreed that the patient's interpersonal life would become an additional focus of treatment.

In Stage Three each session had an IPT section within it. The identified IPT problem area was "role transition" as she was having to adjust to no longer being married and to living alone and supporting herself financially. The therapist helped her focus on identifying the tasks that the transition involved, and she began to make the necessary changes of her own accord. These included identifying and establishing a lifestyle that suited her; forming new friendships (as most of her old friends had been lost as a result of the marital breakup); and starting a new business. At each session she would think over what had happened over the previous week and what could be learned from it. At times she got "stuck," and little would happen for a few weeks. At other times she made major changes. Overall she made excellent progress and at the same time she gradually relaxed her extreme control over eating. By the end of treatment she

---

[3]Often, to supplement the IPT work, and with the goal of generally improving interpersonal functioning, we recommend that patients read and implement relevant sections from the self-help book on assertiveness by Alberti and Emmons (1970). Many patients with eating disorders have difficulty being appropriately assertive, and this book provides much commonsense guidance.

was beginning to forge a new life for herself. There were some residual eating disorder features, but these largely resolved during follow-up.

Recommended Reading

Broad CBT-E

Fairburn, C. G., Cooper, Z., Doll, H. A., O'Connor, M. E., Bohn, K., Hawker, D. M., Wales, J. A., & Palmer, R. L. (2009). Transdiagnostic cognitive behavior therapy for patients with eating disorders: A two-site trial with 60-week follow-up. *American Journal of Psychiatry, 166*, 311–319.

Fairburn, C. G., Cooper, Z., & Shafran, R. (2003). Cognitive behaviour therapy for eating disorders: A "transdiagnostic" theory and treatment. *Behaviour Research and Therapy, 41*, 509–528.

Clinical Perfectionism

Antony, M. M., & Swinson, R. P. (1998). *When perfect isn't good enough*. Oakland, CA: New Harbinger.

Bardone-Cone, A. M., Wonderlich, S. A., Frost, R. O., Bulik, C. M., Mitchell, J. E., Uppala, S., et al. (2007). Perfectionism and eating disorders: Current status and future directions. *Clinical Psychology Review, 27*, 384–405.

Glover, D. S., Brown, G. P., Fairburn, C. G., & Shafran, R. (2007). A preliminary evaluation of cognitive-behaviour therapy for clinical perfectionism: A case series. *British Journal of Clinical Psychology, 46*, 85–94.

Shafran, R., Cooper, Z., & Fairburn, C. G. (2002). Clinical perfectionism: A cognitive-behavioural analysis. *Behaviour Research and Therapy, 40*, 773–791.

Core Low Self-Esteem

Fennell, M. J. V. (1997). Low self-esteem: A cognitive perspective. *Behavioural and Cognitive Psychotherapy, 25*, 1–25.

Fennell, M. J. V. (1998). Low self-esteem. In N. Tarrier, A. Wells, & G. Haddock (Eds.), *Treating complex cases: The cognitive behavioural therapy approach* (pp. 217–240). Chichester: Wiley.

Fennell, M. J. V. (2006). *Overcoming low self-esteem self-help course*. London: Robinson.

Interpersonal Psychotherapy (IPT)

Agras, W. S., Walsh, B. T., Fairburn, C. G., Wilson, G. T., & Kraemer, H. C. (2000). A multicenter comparison of cognitive-behavioral therapy and interpersonal psychotherapy for bulimia nervosa. *Archives of General Psychiatry, 57*, 459–466.

Alberti, R., & Emmons, M. (1970). *Your perfect right*. Atascadero, CA: Impact.

Fairburn, C. G. (1997). Interpersonal psychotherapy for bulimia nervosa. In D. M. Garner & P. E. Garfinkel (Eds.), *Handbook of treatment for eating disorders* (2nd ed., pp. 278–294). New York: Guilford Press.

Fairburn, C. G., Jones, R., Peveler, R. C., Hope, R. A., & O'Connor, M. E. (1993). Psychotherapy and bulimia nervosa: Longer-term effects of interpersonal psychotherapy, behavior therapy, and cognitive-behavior therapy. *Archives of General Psychiatry, 50*, 419–428.

Klerman, G. L., Weissman, M. M., Rounsaville, B. J., & Chevron, E. S. (1984). *Interpersonal psychotherapy of depression*. New York: Basic Books.

Weissman, M. M., Markowitz, J. C., & Klerman, G. L. (2000). *Comprehensive guide to interpersonal psychotherapy*. New York: Basic Books.

Wilfley, D. E., Welch, R. R., Stein, R. I., Spurrell, E. B., Cohen, L. R., Saelens, B. E., et al. (2002). A randomized comparison of group cognitive-behavioral therapy and group interpersonal psychotherapy for the treatment of overweight individuals with binge eating disorder. *Archives of General Psychiatry, 59,* 713–721.

Another Article of Relevance to Chapter 13

Wilson, G. T. (2004). Acceptance and change in the treatment of eating disorders: The evolution of manual-based cognitive-behavioral therapy. In S. C. Hayes, V. M. Follette, & M. Linehan (Eds.), *Mindfulness and acceptance: Expanding the cognitive-behavioral tradition* (pp. 243–266). New York: Guilford Press.

CHAPTER 14

CBT-E and the Younger Patient

Zafra Cooper and Anne Stewart

Eating disorders typically develop in adolescence, and they contribute substantially to the psychiatric problems seen in this age group. As there is evidence that younger patients respond better to treatment than adults, the detection and prompt treatment of these patients are of great importance. The need for prompt intervention is magnified by the medical complications that may accompany eating disorders, which are particularly serious in young people.

> **The prompt treatment of younger patients is of great importance.**

The eating disorders seen in younger patients are classified in the same way as those seen in adults (see Chapter 2). Thus there are the two specified eating disorders, anorexia nervosa and bulimia nervosa, and the residual diagnosis of eating disorder NOS. The proportion of cases with anorexia nervosa is higher than in adults, but, as with adults, eating disorder NOS is the most common eating disorder diagnosis. The clinical features seen in this age group are much the same as those seen in adults, although as noted previously there is a subgroup who show no evidence of over-concern with shape and weight; rather, their undereating stems from an over-evaluation of control over eating per se (see Chapter 9, page 134).

There are a number of reasons for thinking that CBT-E might be particularly suitable for younger patients. First, the clinical features seen are very similar to those found in adults and this, together with clinical experience, supports its use. Second, there is evidence that younger patients respond well to CBT for other disorders suggesting that treatment of this type and style is suitable for this age group. Third, "control" is a topic of concern for younger patients, and they therefore respond well to a treatment such as CBT-E that is designed to enhance their sense of control. Thus the treatment fits well with their need to develop autonomy and independence. Fourth, CBT-E has well-specified ways of enhancing the motivation of patients, a property that is particularly relevant to the treatment of adolescents. Fifth, the transdiagnostic nature of CBT-E is also a major advantage, as it is a treatment for all forms of eating disorder, whereas to date the limited research on the treatment of adolescent patients has focused largely on those with anorexia nervosa. Nevertheless, CBT-E does need to be modi-

> **CBT-E needs to be modified to suit younger patients.**

fied to suit younger patients. In particular, it needs to take account of the fact that most are still living with their family and are dependent upon them, and it needs to be adjusted to suit their stage of emotional and cognitive development and their social environment.

In this chapter the general principles underlying the modification of CBT-E for younger patients are discussed first. Then a description of CBT-E for younger patients is provided, focusing in detail only on the ways it differs from the form of CBT-E described in Chapters 5–13. These differences are based on the need to modify the treatment along the lines described above and on clinical experience in Oxford and elsewhere. The adaptations vary to some extent according to the age of the patient and their developmental stage. As yet, CBT-E has not been evaluated in this age group.

Principles Underpinning the Modification of CBT-E

Developmental Stage

When working with young people it is important to consider the normal developmental tasks of adolescence. Crucial issues include developing a sense of identity, learning to become independent, developing new and changing interpersonal relationships, and adjusting to the changes of puberty. Young people with an eating disorder tend to regress developmentally and become dependent on their parents. In addition, they may withdraw socially and lose their identity and interests. Even in the early stages of treatment it is important to keep in mind the aim of promoting a return of normal adolescent development. The style of treatment should therefore enable the young person to develop autonomy and personal responsibility. As far as is possible the young person should be helped to make choices and take appropriate control, not only over their eating, but also over other aspects of his or her life.

It is also important to consider the cognitive development of the young person and adapt the language, content and style of the treatment accordingly. The use of metaphors, images, cartoons and pictures can be helpful but needs to be age appropriate.

Motivation

Ambivalence toward treatment is particularly common in younger patients and hence the request for treatment is often initiated by their parents. The young person may not be committed to treatment and may even be resistant to it. Refusal to engage in treatment may be a way of asserting identity and independence. Thus, it is crucial to address motivation and, as with adults, not just at the start of treatment but throughout as it may change over time. CBT-E incorporates a range of strategies and procedures designed to engage patients and enhance and maintain their motivation for change (see Chapters 5 and 11).

Interpersonal Functioning

Peer relationships are very important in adolescence, particularly for girls who make up the majority of younger patients. Adolescent girls tend to seek approval from peers for their developing identity, and therefore their relationships play a vital role in this process. Girls who have poor peer relationships, often accompanied by low self-esteem or an insecure sense of identity, may turn to controlling their eating, shape and weight as a way of boosting their self-esteem and enhancing peer approval. Therefore the treatment of younger patients needs to address a number of aspects of peer relationships. These may include improving social communication, developing assertiveness, and enhancing the ability to resolve conflicts.

Schools are a particularly crucial component of the younger person's social environment and may need to be involved in treatment. For example, even with patients who do not need to take time off from school, it may still be useful to establish a link with their teachers so that they can facilitate treatment, perhaps by providing support at mealtimes or planning activities to replace physical activity when this is not advisable.

Medical Complications in Adolescents

Many adolescent patients are underweight and being underweight is a particular concern in young people. They are still growing and their body organs are not yet mature. Even modest weight loss can cause significant medical complications as well as impairment of growth. The growth impairment is particularly likely in boys due to their relatively prolonged period of growth. While catch-up growth can occur with weight regain, these adolescents are at risk of never reaching their full height potential. Similarly, puberty may be delayed and, in girls, there may be prolonged amenorrhea. The osteopenia and osteoporosis that accompany being significantly underweight are especially relevant to this age group as adolescence is a critical time for laying down new bone. While there may be recovery of bone mass in those who overcome their eating disorder (with an accompanying resumption of normal hormonal functioning), in those who remain underweight there is an increased likelihood of permanent low bone density with heightened risk of fractures.

To minimize the short- and long-term medical complications of undereating and being underweight, the threshold for intervening with younger people is lower than with adults, and it is important that treatment starts without undue delay. A detailed physical assessment is important too, and there is a need for regular and comprehensive physical reviews.

The Need to Involve Others

The Family

With adults CBT-E is primarily a one-to-one treatment, although significant others are commonly involved but only in a facilitative way (see page 87). With younger patients, parents and other family members are invariably involved in treatment and they may play a central role. This is for a number of reasons. First, with younger patients there is the matter of parental responsibility and consent. Second, parents and other family members are a major influence, which can be, at best, helpful in overcoming the eating problem and, at worst, unhelpful and an obstacle to change. It is therefore important that they are informed and involved in a way that establishes them as a useful resource for the young person, but it is equally important that their involvement is not perceived as a threat to the patient's autonomy and independence. Third, as younger patients generally live and eat at home, and are dependent on their parents for food, parents can be of direct assistance in helping patients change how they eat.

The Multidisciplinary Team

In Chapter 3 it was argued that complications arise from the involvement of multiple therapists at one time (e.g., a psychologist, dietician and physician) as this practice encourages patients to partition their problems and talk about particular topics with particular people. As a result there is the risk that no one sees and appraises the full clinical picture. Nevertheless this practice is not unusual. To an extent it is inevitable in inpatient units, but it also occurs in some outpatient settings particularly those involving younger patients.

   With younger patients a case may be made for the involvement of multiple therapists and therapies, the strongest argument being that there is a need to combine individual treatment (in this case, CBT-E) with some form of family intervention. If multiple forms of treatment are used, it is essential that they are conceptually and procedurally compatible and, hopefully, synergistic; and, if multiple therapists are involved, steps need to be taken to ensure that the therapists communicate with each other on a regular basis. (See Chapter 15 for a description of how this is achieved with inpatient CBT-E.) It is also important that the young person is aware that his or her care is shared and discussed within the treatment team.

Assessing Patients and Preparing Them for Treatment

The aim of the initial interview is to begin to engage the patient and forge a positive therapeutic relationship, in addition to establishing the nature of the eating problem. There are three further goals: to begin to engage the parents, to assess the patient's physical state, and to decide what form treatment should take.

   Like adults with an eating disorder, young patients should be seen on their own. This is to gain an understanding of their perspective on the referral and the nature of their problems and to begin to develop a relationship with them. As young patients are often brought unwillingly to the initial session, considerable time and effort need to be devoted to engaging them. They often feel that they are not listened to, so taking time to hear and understand their perspective is crucial.

   A joint interview with the parents or other relevant family members is needed to obtain a developmental history and to understand their view on the eating problems. A separate parental interview may be indicated if the young person is agreeable to this, in order to give the parents a chance to raise any issues relating to personal or marital difficulties that may be having an impact on the eating disorder. However, the decision to do this should be balanced against the risk of alienating the patient.

   The routine use of certain assessment questionnaires is recommended because they provide standardized information about eating disorder features and other psychopathology. The adult version of the EDE-Q (see Appendix B) is suitable for patients age

16 or over, and there is a modified version for use with younger patients (Carter, Stewart, & Fairburn, 2001).

As with adult patients, young patients need to be weighed and have their height measured. In addition, they should undergo a detailed physical assessment to identify any physical consequences of the eating disorder that might pose immediate medical risk. With atypical presentations, clinicians should have a higher index of suspicion than with adult cases of the possibility of there being a general medical disorder. Centile charts should be used to establish the presence and degree of any weight loss. BMI centile charts are available (e.g., www.cdc.gov/growthcharts); a cutoff of less than the 2.4 centile indicates being underweight. It is important to note that in adolescence failure to gain weight may be indicative of serious relative weight loss.

By the end of the initial evaluation, it should be possible to decide whether or not to use CBT-E. In our view and context, there are four options:

1. *Observe.* If the eating disorder is mild or remitting, then CBT-E is not indicated. Instead, it is appropriate simply to give advice and encouragement to the patient and family. In such cases a number of review meetings should be held to ensure that progress is being maintained. Self-help literature may be recommended.

2. *Initiate immediate CBT-E.* This is appropriate for patients whose weight is within the healthy range or those who are only moderately underweight (no more than 20% weight deficit) and are willing to engage in a one-to-one treatment.

3. *Initiate CBT-E following a preliminary intervention.* With some patients it is not appropriate or possible to embark directly on CBT-E. This is for a number of reasons:

- Degree of weight loss is too great (e.g., more than 20%)
- Physical risk (e.g., rapid weight loss, frequent vomiting or laxative misuse)
- Severe co-existing psychiatric problems
- Suicide risk
- Refusal to engage in individual treatment

With these patients a preliminary intervention is required. In our view this may take one of two main forms:

- *The "Maudsley method" of family-based treatment* (Lock, le Grange, Agras, & Dare, 2001). This is an empirically supported outpatient-based method for helping young patients regain weight. It is best used with younger adolescent patients.
- *Day patient or inpatient treatment or intensive outpatient treatment.* Note that intensive treatments of this type can take the form of CBT-E (see Chapter 15). These treatments are likely to involve the patient's family.

Either of these interventions can be followed by CBT-E if required, although they may result in the resolution of the eating problem. This is especially likely in young patients with an eating disorder of recent onset.

4. *Provide some other form of treatment.* There are some patients for whom CBT-E is not appropriate. Because of their level of cognitive development, CBT-E may not be suitable for some patients below the age of 15 years, and it is rarely appropriate for patients under 14 years. These patients often benefit from a family-focused approach.

There are a number of additional contraindications to embarking on CBT-E immediately (see page 38). Two need to be highlighted in relation to young people. The first is the presence of a co-existing clinical depression. This needs to be treated first for the reasons given in Chapter 4 (see page 40), but as there are concerns about the use of antidepressant medication in younger patients, it is important that clinicians adhere to up-to-date national guidelines in this regard. The second relates to the presence of obstacles to regular attendance. As noted in Chapters 5 and 6, a central feature of CBT-E is establishing and maintaining therapeutic momentum. This requires that appointments be frequent (especially in the early stages) and regular. If this is impossible, for example, because of a prebooked family vacation, then it is best to defer treatment rather than risk a "false start."

Adaptations to CBT-E

CBT-E for younger patients is largely the same as that for adults, but certain adaptations are routinely needed and others may be necessary as a result of the preliminary treatment. The routine adaptations are described below.

> **CBT-E for younger patients is largely the same as that for adults.**

The treatment has the same format, stages and content as CBT-E for adults. Treatment length, as with adults, depends on whether patients are significantly underweight or not. Those who have a BMI of 17.5 or less (or a weight deficit equal to, or greater than, 15%) need an extended period of weight restoration and so the 40-week form of treatment is appropriate (see Chapter 11), although the full 40 weeks are often not required with patients who have had a preliminary treatment. The 20-week version is suitable for most of the remainder, other than those who are moderately underweight and who would benefit from having treatment extended somewhat to accommodate a degree of weight regain.

Clinical experience suggests that, as for adults, it is helpful to work within a specified time frame, with treatment having a definite predefined end point. Lack of a clear time frame can enable the younger patient to put off making the decision to change and thereby protract the eating disorder. It may also deprive the patient of the valuable final stage of treatment (see Chapter 12). It is important to keep in mind the need for full physical recovery with younger patients (i.e., restoration of menstruation and normal physical functioning) because of its long-term significance. This does not preclude ending treatment when the patient is still somewhat symptomatic so long as the main maintaining mechanisms have been disrupted and the disorder is on the wane (see page 183). What is important is to follow up patients to ensure that they are continuing to make good progress.

Involving Parents

CBT-E with younger patients invariably involves the parents, and they play a major role (especially with younger adolescent patients). The parents are involved from the outset. They need to know about the nature of the eating problem and what treatment involves. They need to understand the importance of establishing therapeutic momentum and the fact that the young person will be recording (and that the monitoring records are private). It is useful if patients are willing to show their parents their formulation so that they understand more about the eating problem. Regular joint meetings with the patient, therapist and the parents are important so that the parents are kept abreast of how they can facilitate the young person's efforts to change. For example, parents may help them eat

> **CBT-E with younger patients invariably involves the parents.**

at regular intervals, introduce avoided foods, and address aspects of body checking (e.g., by removing bathroom scales and surplus mirrors). Later in treatment parents need to step back and let the young person take progressively more responsibility for his or her behavior. Some parents need help to do this. Psychoeducational groups can be of value in educating and supporting parents during the young person's treatment.

Engaging the Patient in Treatment and Change

Engagement is particularly important with adolescent patients, especially those who have come to treatment reluctantly and those who have had a preliminary treatment when others have largely been responsible for their eating. For the latter group it is essential to stress that CBT-E is a different form of treatment to the one that they have received so far, and that the therapist will be operating entirely on their behalf and not on behalf of their parents. To maintain this distinction, any ongoing family-focused work should be conducted by a separate therapist, although the CBT-E therapist may attend. The fact that the CBT-E therapist is working exclusively on the young person's behalf is highlighted by the provision of a clear explanation of what treatment will involve (see pages 38 and 54) and how it will differ from what has happened so far.

Jointly Creating the Formulation

The formulation should be created in the same way as with adults (see pages 51 and 153). It is important that the terms and concepts used are familiar to patients and make sense to them. It should be a new formulation, created afresh, even if a different formulation was used in the preparatory treatment. Jointly creating the formulation provides a further opportunity to engage the young person and it once more emphasizes the notion that it is the young person, with the therapist's help, who will be in control of making the changes needed. As with adults, the formulation should be kept simple and focus only on the main maintaining mechanisms with other elements being added later if needed.

Establishing Real-Time Self-Monitoring

This takes place in the initial session, as in the adult version of CBT-E. Younger patients are often reluctant to record so its purpose needs to be carefully explained (see page 57). Any difficulties should be sensitively explored and the therapist should explain that recording is an essential part of treatment. Patients who are following a prescribed eating plan (initiated during the preparatory treatment) may find it particularly irksome to record. In such instances creative ways of recording may need to be devised, for example, by making copies of the eating plan for patients to tick off what they are eating but with space on the right for comments about eating and other matters (e.g., shape, weight and exercising). Patients will also need to record any episodes of unplanned eating. In general, however, it is best if the patient uses the usual monitoring record. Whatever method is used, it is important to ensure that the recording is done in real time and that the patient understands its purpose.

In-Session Weighing

The in-session weighing protocol is the same as that used with adults (see page 62). It is not uncommon for young people to be reluctant to be weighed or only agree on condition that they are not told their weight, sometimes claiming that it will be easier for them to regain if they do not know the number. It is important to explain carefully why it is best that they know their weight and that this is an integral part of treatment. It is essential that this is agreed early on in treatment and implemented consistently throughout without it becoming a focus for negotiation over several sessions.

Education about Weight, Weight Checking and Eating Problems

While education needs to be provided in an age-appropriate way, its content does not need to differ much from that for adults. Three points deserve special mention. First, as with adult patients, young people are anxious about weight change, tend to misinterpret single readings on the scale and are likely to be particularly anxious if a goal weight range is proposed. It is best to be clear that the aim of treatment is to free the young person from his or her eating problem and its effects and, if underweight, this usually requires regaining weight to achieve a BMI of about 20 (or 100% weight for height in the case of younger adolescents). Second, when discussing the adverse effects of the eating disorder, and also the pros and cons of change, it is important to note that young people tend to have a different time perspective from adults. Hence discussion focused on long-term adverse consequences or problems 5 years ahead may not seem relevant or important to them. While longer-term adverse effects of the disorder should not be omitted from the discussion, the therapist needs to focus particularly on the more immediate future (6 months to a year) and emphasize those adverse effects that are likely to motivate the young person (e.g., missing school for a protracted period; not being able to complete important examinations; not being able to go on a trip abroad; not being able to go to college). Third, whereas we recommend *Overcoming Binge Eating* for the education of older adolescents, with younger patients it is best to recommend books specifically written for their age group.

Introducing a Pattern of Regular Eating

Younger patients may need more guidance about what they should eat than adult patients. This information can be provided by a dietician or equally well by the therapist. Parents may need to be involved too, as it is likely that they are the ones who buy, prepare and serve food. Parents can also play a helpful role in encouraging the young person to adhere to a pattern of regular eating.

Regaining Weight

The strategies used to help young patients regain weight are the same as those used with adults (see Chapter 11). It is essential that the decision to embark upon weight regain is made by the young person and not imposed upon him or her. Parents have a greater role in the treatment of younger adolescents than is usually the case with adults. It is important to provide nutritional education and advice because young patients are more likely to be ill-informed in this regard. As with adults, regular review meetings (see page 168) are needed to ensure that progress is maintained and to identify emerging obstacles to change. These reviews should be attended by all those involved in helping the young person.

Toward the end of treatment time should be allocated for practicing maintaining a stable healthy weight (see page 179). Usually about 8 weeks is sufficient.

Addressing Other Aspects of the Eating Disorder Psychopathology

The other aspects of younger patients' eating disorder psychopathology are addressed using the strategies and procedures employed with adults (see Chapters 5–12). As was noted earlier, a subgroup of younger patients has a variant of the "core psychopathology" in which there is over-evaluation of control over eating per se rather than control over eating in order to influence shape or weight. The addressing of this psychopathology is described in Chapter 9.

Addressing Clinical Perfectionism, Core Low Self-Esteem and Interpersonal Problems

The "broad" form of CBT-E (see Chapter 13) may be used with younger patients, if clearly indicated, but, as with adults, the focused version is the default version. Given the need in younger patients to promote a return to normal development, it could be argued that there should be a lower threshold for using the broad form of CBT-E than in adults and especially with those patients who have low self-esteem or major interpersonal difficulties. On the other hand the data on adults suggest that only in patients with extreme problems of this type is the broad version superior to the focused version. In the remainder (the majority), the opposite is the case. Clearly what is needed is research on the relative effects of the two forms of CBT-E in younger patients.

Ending Treatment

Ending treatment well is essential. How to do this is described in Chapter 12. As noted earlier, some degree of residual eating disorder psychopathology is the norm on finishing treatment, and this is acceptable so long as the main maintaining mechanisms have been disrupted and the disorder is on the decline. What is important is to follow up patients to ensure that they are continuing to make good progress. In exceptional circumstances CBT-E may be extended for some months, particularly if the young person is improving but has significant residual features. It is important in such cases to review progress at regular intervals to ensure that continuing treatment is justified. If patients' response to CBT-E has been limited and further full-scale treatment is indicated, it is our view that, as with adults, they should be offered more intensive treatment rather than an alternative form of outpatient treatment. Intensive outpatient CBT-E, day patient CBT-E and inpatient CBT-E are three good options, as they are conceptually and procedurally compatible with outpatient-based CBT-E. These forms of CBT-E are described in the following chapter.

Recommended Reading

Carter, J. C., Stewart, D. A., & Fairburn, C. G. (2001). Eating Disorder Examination Questionnaire: Norms for adolescent girls. *Behaviour Research and Therapy, 39*, 625–632.

Commission on Adolescent Eating Disorders. (2005). Eating disorders. In D. L. Evans, E. B. Foa, R. E. Gur, H. Hendin, C. P. O'Brien, M. E. P. Seligman, et al. (Eds.), *Treating and preventing adolescent mental health disorders* (pp. 257–332). New York: Oxford University Press.

Fairburn, C. G. (1995). *Overcoming binge eating.* New York: Guilford Press.

Fairburn, C. G., & Gowers, S. G. (2008). Eating disorders. In M. Rutter, D. Bishop, D. Pine, S. Scott, J. Stevenson, E. Taylor, et al. (Eds.), *Rutter's child and adolescent psychiatry* (5th ed.). Oxford: Blackwell.

Katzman, D. K. (2005). Medical complications in adolescents with anorexia nervosa: A review of the literature. *International Journal of Eating Disorders, 37,* S52–S59.

le Grange, D., & Lock, J. (2007). *Treating bulimia in adolescents: A family-based approach.* New York: Guilford Press.

Lock, J., & le Grange, D. (2007). *Help your teenager beat an eating disorder.* New York: Guilford Press.

Lock, J., le Grange, D., Agras, W. S., & Dare, C. (2001). *Treatment manual for anorexia nervosa: A family-based approach.* New York: Guilford Press.

National Institute for Clinical Excellence. (2004). *Eating disorders: Core interventions in the treatment and management of anorexia nervosa, bulimia nervosa and related eating disorders.* London: National Institute for Clinical Excellence.

Nicholls, D., Chater, R., & Lask, B. (2000). Children into DSM don't go: A comparison of classification systems for eating disorders in childhood and early adolescence. *International Journal of Eating Disorders, 28*, 317–324.

Schapman-Williams, A. M., Lock, J., & Couturier, J. (2006). Cognitive-behavioral therapy for adolescents with binge eating syndromes: A case series. *International Journal of Eating Disorders, 39*, 252–255.

Wilson, G. T., & Sysko, R. (2006). Cognitive-behavioural therapy for adolescents with bulimia nervosa. *European Eating Disorders Review, 14*, 8–16.

CHAPTER 15

Inpatient, Day Patient and Two Forms of Outpatient CBT-E

Riccardo Dalle Grave, Kristin Bohn, Deborah M. Hawker and Christopher G. Fairburn

> **The mainstay of the treatment of eating disorders is outpatient treatment.**

The mainstay of the treatment of eating disorders is outpatient treatment. It is less disruptive to the patient's life than inpatient or day patient treatment, and the changes made are more likely to last because patients make them while living in their usual environment. Nevertheless, there are patients who need more intensive treatment. Two forms of intensive CBT-E are described in this chapter, one being inpatient-based (although it includes a day patient component) and the other being a form of outpatient treatment. Both were developed by the first author and his colleagues in Italy. A group version of CBT-E is also described.

Inpatient CBT-E

Goals and Indications

The inpatient treatment outlined below was derived from the form of CBT-E described in this book and it has been in use since 2004 (in the Department of Eating and Weight Disorders of Villa Garda Hospital outside Verona). It is currently being evaluated in a randomized controlled trial. Its main indications are as follows:

- Poor response to well-delivered, outpatient-based treatment.
- Presence of features that make outpatient treatment inappropriate. These include very low weight, rapid weight loss and marked medical complications (e.g., pronounced edema, severe electrolyte disturbance, hypoglycemia).

Significant suicide risk and severe interpersonal problems are also indications for hospitalization. Contraindications are daily substance misuse (intermittent substance misuse is not a contraindication) and acute psychotic states.

Inpatient CBT-E retains three of the core characteristics of CBT-E: First, the treatment is designed to be suitable for all forms of eating disorder; second, the form of the treatment is dictated by the particular psychopathological features present and the processes that are maintaining them; and third, the treatment addresses these mechanisms using CBT-E strategies and procedures. However, the treatment also has some properties that distinguish it from the outpatient-based CBT-E for adults:

- It is designed to be suitable for both adult and adolescent patients.
- The patients are inpatients initially, and then day patients.
- It is delivered by multiple therapists from different professional backgrounds.
- There is assistance with eating.
- Some elements of the treatment are delivered in a group format.
- There is a family therapy module for younger patients.

The goal of the treatment is to help patients reach a state such that they can benefit from outpatient-based CBT-E.

Preparation for Admission

Patients need to be prepared for admission. There are six main tasks that generally occupy two sessions:

> **The goal is to help patients reach a state such that they can benefit from outpatient CBT-E.**

1. *To assess the patient's eating disorder and general psychiatric status.* See Chapter 4 (page 35).

2. *To assess the patient's physical health.* This is important because the physical health of many of these patients is significantly compromised.

3. *To engage the patient in treatment.* See Chapters 5 and 11 (pages 48 and 161).

4. *To educate the patient about his or her eating disorder and create a provisional personal formulation.* See Chapters 5 and 11 (pages 51 and 153). Like outpatient CBT-E, the goal is that patients start to become interested in, and intrigued by, their eating problem.

5. *To explain what inpatient CBT-E involves.* This involves the therapist describing the aims, duration, organization, procedures and effects of inpatient CBT-E. It is emphasized that the hospital admission is an opportunity to change and make a "fresh start." Patients are also taken on a tour of the unit.

6. *To involve significant others.* With adult patients who are willing to have significant others involved, the therapist provides them with basic information on eating disorders, the processes involved in their maintenance, and on the nature of the treatment. The significant others are asked if they would agree to participate in up to three 30-minute sessions during the course of treatment (described later in the chapter). With adolescent patients the therapist provides more detailed information on eating disorders, the role of significant others (usually parents) in treatment, and the organization of the CBT-E family module (described later in the chapter). The therapist maintains a neutral stance regarding the origins of the eating problem and underlines the fact that the ultimate decision to be admitted must be made by the patient but that it might be useful for everyone present to discuss the pros and cons of hospitalization.

The first preparatory session ends with the therapist asking the patient to do the following three homework tasks:

1. Consider the pros and cons of being admitted to the unit.
2. Read the informative pamphlet on inpatient CBT-E.
3. Create a list of questions to discuss with the therapist.

The second session is generally held 1 week after the first. The therapist reviews with the patient the pro and cons of admission while reinforcing interest in change. Then patients' questions are addressed and, if they agree to be admitted, they are placed on the waiting list (up to 6 weeks).

The Unit

Inpatient CBT-E is best provided in a specialized unit for the treatment of eating disorders. The unit should be "open," and patients in a stable medical condition should be free to go outside. Similarly, significant others should be free to visit the patient at any time other than mealtimes and when treatment sessions are occurring. The unit atmosphere should be psychological rather than medical, and not institutional. As it will be the patients' "home" for some months, they should be allowed to decorate their rooms with posters, etc., and there should be appropriate recreational and study facilities.

The unit atmosphere should be psychological rather than medical.

The Clinical Team

Inpatient CBT-E is implemented by a multidisciplinary team comprising physicians, psychologists, dietitians and nurses. In our opinion it is best if CBT-E is the sole psychotherapeutic treatment employed as this guarantees that patients are provided with a single consistent approach to the understanding and treatment of their eating problem. If this is the model adopted, all the team needs to be fully trained in CBT-E and all should use the same concepts and terms. To maintain fidelity to the treatment and ensure cross-therapist consistency in its implementation, a review meeting is held each week in which the therapists for each patient (i.e., a physician, psychologist, dietitian and nurse) meet the patient to discuss the various elements of the treatment and their relationship to one another.

The Stages of Inpatient CBT-E

The treatment lasts 20 weeks, 13 weeks of which are spent as an inpatient followed by 7 weeks as a day patient during which the patient lives close to the hospital and spends weekends at home. There are four stages, which mirror those of outpatient-based CBT-E:

- *Stage One (weeks 1–4).* The focus of this first stage is on engaging and educating patients, reinforcing and modifying, as needed, their personalized formulation, obtaining maximal early behavior change, including the initiation of weight regain in underweight patients.

- *Stage Two (weeks 5 and 6).* This stage involves a detailed review of progress and the identification of any barriers to change. In addition, there is a formal assessment of the possible contribution of the four additional "external" maintaining mechanisms (i.e., mood intolerance, clinical perfectionism, core low self-esteem and interpersonal difficulties; see Chapters 10 and 13).
- *Stage Three (weeks 7–17).* The precise content of this stage is dictated by the patient's psychopathology. In almost all patients it includes addressing the over-evaluation of control over eating, shape and weight (see Chapters 8 and 9) together with food avoidance and other dietary rules (see Chapter 8). In subgroups of patients one or more of the external maintaining mechanisms may also be tackled using the "broad" CBT-E modules (see Chapters 7, 10 and 13). During this stage most underweight patients reach their target BMI range and start to practice weight maintenance.
- *Stage Four (week 18–20).* The focus of this final stage in treatment is on preparing a revised formulation that identifies the maintaining mechanisms still operating and, on this basis, preparing for subsequent outpatient-based CBT-E.

Distinctive Treatment Procedures

Most of the treatment procedures are the same as those used in outpatient CBT-E, but some need to be modified to suit the inpatient setting, and certain others are specific to inpatient CBT-E.

Use of More Than One Therapist

Patients are assigned to four therapists: a dietitian, psychologist, physician and nurse, each of whom has a specific role in treatment. The dietitian is primarily concerned with overseeing the modification of eating habits and weight. The psychologist focuses on the more cognitive aspects of CBT-E, especially the modification of the over-evaluation of control over eating, shape and weight. In addition, the psychologist is responsible for implementing the "broad" CBT-E modules. The physician is responsible for the physical health of the patients and the use of any medication. The nurse has the usual tasks of overseeing the running of the unit, generally supporting the patients, as well as conducting the weighing.

Monitoring of Weight and Eating Habits

Body weight is measured by the nurse for the first 8 weeks of treatment, and thereafter by the patients themselves. The weighing scales provide information accurate only to the nearest 0.5 kg to help patients counter their concern with trivial changes in weight. Patients complete a weekly checklist on which is recorded the frequency of key eating disorder behavior (e.g., binge eating, self-induced vomiting, laxative and diuretic misuse) and the intensity of body checking and avoidance, feeling fat, and preoccupation with thoughts about eating, shape and weight. These data and those on body weight are discussed at the weekly review meeting.

CBT-E Sessions with the Psychologist

The CBT-E sessions conducted by the psychologist are on a one-to-one basis. They are held twice weekly for the first 4 weeks and thereafter weekly. They focus on the following topics:

1. Helping underweight patients adjust to and accept the rapid changes in shape and weight (see Chapter 11).
2. Once patients are day patients, helping them deal with events and moods that affect their eating (see Chapter 10).
3. If indicated (see Chapter 7), addressing clinical perfectionism, core low self-esteem or interpersonal difficulties, as in outpatient-based CBT-E (see Chapter 13).
4. Preparing a discharge treatment plan in order to achieve a smooth transition from inpatient to outpatient CBT-E.

Assisted Eating

The main reason some patients need more intensive treatment than outpatient CBT-E is that they are unable to make the necessary changes to their eating. This is for various reasons including the intensity of their over-concern about controlling eating, shape and weight, and their resulting ambivalence about change, the presence of marked rituals affecting eating, and preoccupation with thoughts about food and eating. Such features prevent outpatient-based weight regain or, sometimes, the addressing of binge eating. The major strength of inpatient treatment is that it can provide the intensity of support and psychotherapeutic input needed to overcome these problems.

The dietitian oversees what may be termed "assisted eating." This typically takes place over the first 6 weeks. Exactly what assisted eating addresses depends upon the nature of the patient's problems, but it usually tackles not eating enough (to regain weight), not eating often enough, and not eating a reasonable range of foods. An eating plan is devised for each patient that is designed to address his or her particular difficulties. This is done collaboratively and is combined with suitable education about eating, nutrition and energy balance.

Weight regain is a goal for about two-thirds of patients. To achieve this, patients eat three meals and a snack each day (breakfast, lunch, mid-afternoon snack and dinner) in the dining room with the assistance of the CBT-E–trained dietitian who uses cognitive behavioral procedures to help the patient eat. Patients are encouraged to view food like "medication," and to eat mechanically for the meantime. This type of eating continues until patients can eat autonomously and appropriately. The main therapeutic techniques used are education and support, distraction, and in those who are not too preoccupied, de-centering from problematic thoughts and urges. In some patients ritualistic ways of eating are also addressed. During the phase of assisted eating patients stay in a dedicated room for 1 hour after eating and do not have access to a bathroom.

It is important that patients feel in control of the changes in their eating. They are therefore active participants in deciding their goal BMI range (which is generally between a BMI of 19.0 and 19.9; see Chapter 11) and the nature of their diet. For the first week of treatment their energy intake is set at 1,500 kcal per day, and it is then increased to 2,000 kcal per day in the second week, and to 2,500 kcal per day in the third week. Subsequently, patients' energy intake is adjusted collaboratively on the basis of their rate of weight regain, the goal being a gain of 1.0–1.5 kg per week (i.e., much greater than the 0.5 kg per week goal of outpatient CBT-E; see page 169). If patients need to have an intake of over 2,500 kcal per day to achieve this, they are given the option of doing so using food alone or with the addition of high-energy supplementary drinks. Once patients' weight reaches a BMI of 18.5, their energy intake is gradually decreased to enable them to reach and maintain their body weight within the goal BMI range.

About a third of patients are admitted because of binge eating and purging that have proved impossible to control on an outpatient basis. They too engage in assisted eating designed to show them that they can eat a healthy diet comprising three meals and a snack without gaining weight and that they can eat these meals without binge eating or purging. Both are tasks that they were not able to accomplish on an outpatient basis. It is also stressed that the interruption of binge eating in an inpatient setting is evidence that there were circumstances operating in their day-to-day life (e.g., family tension, ready availability of food) that encouraged binge eating and purging and that these will need to be addressed later during their hospital stay to avoid relapse.

Addressing Dietary Restraint and Dietary Rules

Once the 8-week period of assisted eating is over, patients are encouraged to eat autonomously and to start eating outside the unit. Patients plan their eating in advance and record it much as is done in outpatient CBT-E. They are no longer supervised after eating. There are individual weekly meetings with the dietitian to discuss their eating habits and address any remaining problems. Dietary restraint and dietary rules are addressed using the strategies and procedures described in Chapter 9. From week 14 patients live outside the hospital and can cook for themselves. During the final weeks of treatment weekends are spent at home and gradually all meals are consumed outside the unit.

Group Treatment Sessions

Group treatment sessions are used to supplement the individual ones. This has the advantage of efficiency, and it encourages self-disclosure, mutual support and learning from patients who are doing well, while helping patients address secrecy and shame.

Two types of group are held: psychoeducational and CBT-E focused. The psychoeducational groups are held twice a week and address facts about eating disorders and CBT-E strategies. The CBT-E groups are weekly and focus on eating disorder behavior (e.g., binge eating, non-compensatory purging, driven exercising) and the over-evaluation of shape and weight.

Involvement of Significant Others

With adult patients significant others are seen if the patient is willing and doing so is likely to facilitate treatment. The significant others are people who have a major influence on the patient's eating. Typically they attend three times during the course of treatment, and the aims and content of these sessions are much like those in individual CBT-E (see Chapter 6).

There is much greater involvement of significant others with patients under the age of 18 years and they take part in a "CBT-oriented family module." This consists of six family sessions with the psychologist, two family meals in the unit, and two sessions with the dietitian to plan meals at home. The module has three components:

1. *Education.* This occupies two sessions and covers the following topics: the cognitive behavioral theory of the maintenance of eating disorders; the patient's personal formulation; the strategies used to assist the patient's eating; the expression of emotion within the family; and the developmental challenges of adolescence.

2. *Eating as a family.* The family consumes two meals in the unit with the assistance of the dietitian. These take place after the first 6 weeks of treatment. The first meal is provided by the hospital whereas the second is prepared by the parents. In both the emphasis is on the patient applying what has been learned in the context of assisted eating and with the parents trying to help the patient do this. After each meal there is a debriefing meeting with the patient and parents to discuss what happened and what can be learned from it. In the day hospital phase the dietitian meets the patient and parents to plan and review the family meals that will take place during the weekends at home.

3. *Creating the optimal family environment.* In these four sessions the parents are helped to create a positive home environment that is likely to support the patient's efforts to change. In addition, they are taught how to use problem-solving (see Chapter 10) to address everyday difficulties and more significant family crises.

Maintenance of Change after Discharge

One of the major limitations of inpatient treatment is the high relapse rate. This is likely to be due in part to the fact that the changes take place while the patient is in the protected environment of the hospital and in part because of the major disruption that typically occurs on discharge.

To maximize the chances that the changes made with inpatient CBT-E are maintained on discharge, the following elements are employed:

- The unit is open so that patients are not in a sheltered environment as in many inpatient units.
- There is a day treatment phase near the end of the admission during which patients face some of the difficulties that they will encounter after discharge (e.g., socializing with others, cooking) while still having the support of treatment.
- During the final few weeks of treatment patients spend weekends at home, again while still having the support of the hospital.
- Significant others are involved in treatment and helped to create a positive home environment for the patient to return to.

In addition, toward the end of treatment considerable effort is put into arranging suitable outpatient treatment, preferably in the form of CBT-E, so

> **The ideal arrangement is for outpatient-based CBT-E to start prior to discharge so that the transfer is seamless.**

that the subsequent treatment is consistent with the inpatient approach. The ideal arrangement is for outpatient-based CBT-E to start prior to discharge so that the transfer is seamless.

Problems Implementing Inpatient CBT-E

Inpatient treatment is rarely straightforward. In part this is because of the severity of the problems being treated and in part because the inpatient setting has certain negative effects. Three problems are of particular note: medical complications, over-exercising and the negative influence of other patients.

Medical Complications

One of the reasons why patients with eating disorders receive inpatient treatment is because of acute medical complications, and many of those without acute complications are nevertheless medically compromised as a result of their undereating and very low weight. Inpatient units must therefore pay careful attention to their patients' medical status and have suitably experienced physicians available. Non-medical staff also need to be aware of their patients' compromised physical state and of physical symptoms and signs of particular concern (see Chapter 4; see page 41).

Over-Exercising

Over-exercising in general, and driven exercising in particular, are common in underweight patients and are a particular problem in closed inpatient units where patients are cooped up.

The management of over-exercising was discussed in Chapter 6 (see page 85). The same principles apply with inpatient CBT-E. One important aspect of managing such exercising is to encourage patients to engage in light healthy exercise instead. This helps discharge their urge to exercise and as a result patients are better able to accept weight gain with its attendant changes in shape. If the exercising is used in part as a means of mood modulation, then the strategies described in Chapter 10 need to be employed. If all else fails the CBT-E team needs to discuss with the patient whether it would be helpful to have his or her exercising restricted for a period of a few weeks until the urge to exercise dies down. This is rarely necessary and should only be done with the consent of the patient.

The Negative Influence of Other Patients

In inpatient units patients influence each other and this can be for the better or for the worse. It is the staff's job to try to engender a positive atmosphere in which patients help each other overcome their eating disorder. Even in the best inpatient units, however, some patients have a negative effect on others. This is a difficult problem to overcome. The "saboteurs" need help to stop harming others. Their motives need to be explored and understood, and if possible addressed. If this proves impossible, they need to be asked to leave. This is a very unusual occurrence. At the same time the "victims" need to be protected and the saboteurs' behavior reframed as symptomatic of their psychiatric problems.

Intensive Outpatient CBT-E

Goals and Indications

This is a form of outpatient-based CBT-E that has yet to be formally evaluated. It is primarily designed to help patients who are having difficulty modifying their eating habits in response to conventional outpatient-based CBT-E. Its goal is to help such patients get to a state whereby they can benefit from conventional CBT-E.

The majority of patients for whom intensive outpatient CBT-E is indicated are underweight and not succeeding in eating more and regaining weight. An important question is how to identify them as it is common and clinically appropriate with CBT-E for there to be a 6- to 8-week delay before underweight patients start to regain weight (see Chapter 11). There can be no firm answer to this question, but the absence of weight regain by week 12 would be one reasonable guideline, as would incomplete weight regain such that the patient's BMI remained below 17.5. The treatment may also be used with patients who have severely disturbed eating habits (e.g., frequent binge eating and vomiting) but who are not underweight. If they are unable to modify their eating habits by week 8 (of their 20-week treatment), this more intensive form of treatment can be of value.

Preparation for Intensive Outpatient CBT-E

As most patients who receive intensive outpatient CBT-E are already in treatment, the aim of the preparation phase is not to help patients decide to start treatment but rather to get their agreement to the intensification of CBT-E. The rationale provided is that the intensity of conventional CBT-E is not proving sufficient, and this more intensive intervention might help them make the necessary changes that would obviate the need for the much more disruptive options of inpatient or day patient treatment.

The Unit

Intensive outpatient CBT-E is ideally provided in a specialized outpatient center for the treatment of patients with an eating disorder. It requires standard treatment offices as well as a kitchen and a dining room where assisted eating can take place. In addition, there needs to be a recreational room and facilities for patients to work or study.

The Clinical Team

Like inpatient CBT-E, intensive outpatient CBT-E is implemented by a multidisciplinary team that has been trained in CBT-E, and this is the sole psychotherapeutic treatment provided. The team comprises physicians, psychologists and dietitians. Ideally the psychologist is the same person who was providing the conventional outpatient-based treatment. Again, like inpatient CBT-E, there is a review meeting each week in which the therapists for each patient meet with the patient to discuss the various elements of the treatment.

The Form of Intensive Outpatient CBT-E

With underweight patients intensive outpatient CBT-E has a fixed duration of 12 weeks. With patients who are not underweight, but who have highly disturbed eating habits, treatment can be much shorter (2–4 weeks).

Treatment involves attending from lunchtime through to dinnertime (12:45 P.M. to 7:45 P.M.) every weekday (see Table 15.1). It includes the following procedures:

- The consumption of two meals and a snack each day supervised by a dietitian (lunch, snack and dinner)
- Two CBT-E sessions a week with a psychologist
- Two CBT-E sessions a week with a dietitian
- Periodic medical examinations
- A weekly review session with the therapists and patient

TABLE 15.1. Timetable for Intensive Outpatient CBT-E

	Monday	**Tuesday**	**Wednesday**	**Thursday**	**Friday**
12:45–1:00 p.m.	Body weight measurement				Body weight measurement
1:00–2:00 p.m.	Assisted lunch	Assisted lunch	Assisted lunch	Assisted lunch	Assisted lunch
2:00–3:00 p.m.	Review meeting	Free time for studying or doing other activities	Free time for studying or doing other activities	Free time for studying or doing other activities	Free time for studying or doing other activities
3:00–4:00 p.m.	Individual session with dietitian (weekend review and meal planning)	Individual session with psychologist	Medical examination[a]	Individual session with psychologist	Individual session with dietitian (weekend preparation)
4:30–5:00 p.m.	Assisted snack	Assisted snack	Assisted snack	Assisted snack	Assisted snack
5:00–6:30 p.m.	Free time for studying or doing other activities	Free time for studying or doing other activities	Free time for studying or doing other activities	Free time for studying or doing other activities	Free time for studying or doing other activities
6:30–7:30 p.m.	Assisted dinner	Assisted dinner	Assisted dinner	Assisted dinner	Assisted dinner
7:30–7:45 p.m.	Food provision for breakfast	Food provision for breakfast	Food provision for breakfast	Food provision for breakfast	Food provision for weekend

[a]Weekly in severely underweight patients (BMI < 16.0) and those with medical complications.

During the last 4 weeks underweight patients consume progressively more meals outside the outpatient unit, and the treatment gradually evolves into conventional outpatient CBT-E.

Distinctive Treatment Procedures

Most of the treatment procedures are the same as those used in outpatient CBT-E, but some are specific to this treatment.

Monitoring of Weight and Eating Habits

With underweight patients weight is measured by the dietitian for the first 8 weeks of treatment, and thereafter at home by the patients themselves. Patients complete the same weekly checklist as is used with inpatients. These data and those on body weight are discussed at the weekly review meetings.

CBT-E Sessions with the Psychologist and Dietitian

The sessions with psychologist are similar to those of conventional outpatient-based CBT-E, the main difference being the major focus on accepting the rapid changes in eating, weight and shape. The sessions with the dietitian are concerned with the patient's eating habits and nutritional needs, and with ensuring that the changes in eating are maintained over the weekends.

Assisted Eating

Patients consume lunch, a snack and dinner on the unit. The food is frozen or pre-packaged so that it requires minimal preparation, and it is designed to meet the dietary needs of the individual patient. With underweight patients the dietitian takes the lead in determining the energy content of the meals for the first 4 weeks, but from the 5th week onward the patient gradually takes over. Breakfasts and weekend meals are preprepared too and provided by the unit. In the last 4 weeks there is a gradual phasing out of the consumption of the prepared meals, and patients begin to eat outside the unit.

Most other aspects of the assisted eating procedure are the same as those used in inpatient CBT-E, and with underweight patients there is the same goal rate of weight regain.

Involvement of Significant Others

This follows the protocol used in inpatient CBT-E.

Maintenance of Change after Discharge

To maximize the chances that the changes made during intensive CBT-E are maintained on discharge, patients are helped to become progressively more responsible for

their eating as treatment progresses and the CBT-E sessions either continue uninterrupted or resume without a break.

Problems Implementing Intensive Outpatient CBT-E

The problems attendant upon inpatient treatment are less of a problem with intensive
outpatient CBT-E. Medical complications occur and are managed in the same way.
Over-exercising is rarely a difficulty, nor is negative interaction between patients. This is
probably because patients are not together 24 hours a day and so are less prone to get
over-involved with each other.

Group CBT-E

Although CBT-E is designed to be delivered on a one-to-one individualized basis,
group versions of the treatment are being tried. In Oxford we created a version in
which there were 17 group sessions and three individual ones over a 21-week period.
One individual session took place at the beginning of treatment in order to help engage
the patient and create a personalized formulation; the next occurred after 4 weeks (i.e.,
at the beginning of Stage Two; see Chapter 7) to review progress and assess treatment
priorities; and the third took place at the end of treatment to plan for the future (see
Chapter 12). Meetings were held on a weekly basis until the last two, which were every
2 weeks. In order to maintain therapeutic momentum at the start of treatment patients
also received one planned telephone call lasting approximately 15 minutes in each of the
first 4 weeks, halfway between the group meetings. Its purpose was to review patients'
progress and their homework, and to address any difficulties they were experiencing in
implementing what had been agreed in the previous group meeting.

The treatment followed the CBT-E protocol as described in this book and the
treatment was designed to mirror the 20-week treatment. There were two therapists,
both of whom were intimately familiar with CBT-E, and six patients. Each patient was
assigned to one of the two therapists. (Originally there were eight patients. Two were
removed from the group because they were not benefiting, and they were offered individual treatment instead. One had a BMI below 18.0 and the other had developed a
marked clinical depression.)

The group meetings followed a similar format to that used in the individual treatment, and covered the same material. They lasted 90 minutes. In advance of each meeting the patients met their designated therapist for 10 minutes to be weighed, have their
weight graph plotted (see page 63), and for a brief joint review of their monitoring
records. Patients were not required to disclose their weight to other group members or
reveal their monitoring records.

The group meetings began with the setting of an agenda that was then worked
through. Its content was much the same as it would have been with one-to-one treatment but without the individualization. Homework assignments were given just as in
individual treatment. In addition, the therapists used the group format to encourage
patients to share common experiences, provide support for each other, and collectively
problem-solve difficulties that they were encountering. This support occurred only dur-

ing the group sessions as patients were asked not to contact each other outside the group (because this could lead to group splitting and to unhelpful conversations). Patients were also asked to maintain confidentiality.

It is not possible to say whether this version of CBT-E was as effective as CBT-E delivered in the usual way. What was clear was that arranging group treatment was far more difficult than organizing treatment on an individual basis (in terms of patient availability and avoiding breaks in treatment) but, perhaps even more importantly, the treatment could not be individualized to nearly the same extent as one-to-one CBT-E. For example, it was not possible to focus on individual setbacks and difficulties as much as would have been desirable. Part of the problem lay in the

> Group CBT-E could not be individualized to nearly the same extent as the one-to-one version.

heterogeneity of patients' eating disorder features (e.g., some people only restricted their eating and did not binge eat, whereas others had frequent episodes of binge eating). On a more positive note, the psychoeducational aspects of treatment, and the shape and weight interventions, seemed ideal for delivery in a group setting and were very well received.

Concluding Remarks

The form of inpatient CBT-E described in this chapter represents the first attempt to apply in a "real world" inpatient setting the strategies and procedures of CBT-E. Experience to date indicates that the treatment is well accepted by patients and staff alike. The emerging data on treatment outcome are very positive, and the changes appear to be well maintained.

Intensive outpatient CBT-E is a new approach that has yet to be evaluated formally. It is designed to be an alternative to inpatient or day patient treatment for patients who are not benefiting from conventional CBT-E. It seems to fulfill this role. Whether it has other indications requires further examination.

Group CBT-E is more problematic as it is difficult to organize and a critical element of the treatment is lost or watered down, namely its individualization. In our view these disadvantages probably outweigh its potential strengths.

Recommended Reading

Andersen, A. E., Bowers, W., & Evans, K. (1997). Inpatient treatment of anorexia nervosa. In D. M. Garner & P. E. Garfinkel (Eds.), *Handbook of treatment for eating disorders* (2nd ed., pp. 327–353). New York: Guilford Press.

Dalle Grave, R. (2005). A multi-step cognitive behaviour therapy for eating disorders. *European Eating Disorders Review, 13*, 373–382.

Dalle Grave, R. (2005). *Terapia cognitivo comportamentale dei disturbi dell'alimentazione durate il ricovero* [Cognitive behavior therapy for inpatients with an eating disorder] (Seconda edizione ed.). Verona: Positive Press.

Dalle Grave, R., Bartocci, C., Todisco, P., Pantano, M., & Bosello, O. (1993). Inpatient treatment for anorexia nervosa: A lenient approach. *European Eating Disorders Review, 1*, 166–176.

Dalle Grave, R. (2011). Intensive cognitive behavioural therapy for eating disorders. *European Psychiatric Review, 4*, 59-64.

Dalle Grave, R., Ricca, V., & Todesco, T. (2001). The stepped-care approach in anorexia nervosa and bulimia nervosa: Progress and problems. *Eating and Weight Disorder, 6*, 81–89.

Garner, D., Vitousek, K., & Pike, K. (1997). Cognitive-behavioral therapy for anorexia nervosa. In D. M. Garner & P. E. Garfinkel (Eds.), *Handbook of treatment for eating disorders* (2nd ed., pp. 94–144). New York: Guilford Press.

Lock, J., le Grange, D., Agras, W. S., & Dare, C. (2001). *Treatment manual for anorexia nervosa: A family-based approach*. New York: Guilford Press.

Pike, K. M. (1998). Long-term course of anorexia nervosa: Response, relapse, remission, and recovery. *Clinical Psychology Review, 18*, 447–475.

Vandereycken, W. (2003). The place of inpatient care in the treatment of anorexia nervosa: Questions to be answered. *International Journal of Eating Disorders, 34*, 409–422.

CHAPTER 16

"Complex Cases" and Comorbidity

Christopher G. Fairburn, Zafra Cooper and Deborah Waller

> **Complexity is the norm rather than the exception with patients who have an eating disorder.**

The notion of there being a subset of "complex cases" does not really apply to the eating disorders, or at least to adults with an eating disorder. Almost all these cases are complex as the great majority have other significant problems. Most meet diagnostic criteria for one or more additional Axis I disorders and many attract personality disorder diagnoses. Physical complications are not rare and a significant subgroup has a co-existing, and interacting, general medical disorder. Interpersonal difficulties are common too and, finally, the chronic nature of these disorders often has a major impact on these patients' psychosocial development. Complexity is the norm rather than the exception with patients who have an eating disorder.

This chapter discusses how to evaluate and manage such co-existing problems while providing CBT-E. There are three main sections: the first concerns co-existing psychiatric disorders; the second, general medical disorders; and the third discusses what to do when the patient experiences a life event or crisis before or during treatment. Interpersonal and developmental difficulties are discussed in Chapter 13.

Co-Existing Psychiatric Disorders

As noted above, most patients with an eating disorder meet diagnostic criteria for at least one other psychiatric disorder. The most common co-existing Axis I disorders are mood disorders, especially clinical depression, anxiety disorders and substance misuse. When evaluating features suggestive of these disorders, the following questions should be kept in mind:

1. *Are the features of the co-existing disorder directly attributable to the eating disorder or its consequences?*
   - If so, the apparent comorbidity may be spurious since the co-occurring disorder may simply be a feature of the eating disorder.

2. *Are the features of the co-existing disorder likely to interfere with the successful treatment of the eating disorder?*

   • If so, they will need to be addressed, either in advance of treatment or at the same time.

3. *Are the features of the co-existing disorder likely to dissipate if the eating disorder is successfully treated?*

   • If so, and they are unlikely to interfere with treatment, they probably do not need to be addressed.

Clinical Depression

A substantial proportion of patients with an eating disorder have a co-existing clinical depression that requires treatment in its own right. Often these patients' depressive features are viewed by clinicians as simply being typical of patients with an eating disorder and are dismissed as such. We view this as a mistake — one that we used to make ourselves.

> A substantial proportion of patients with an eating disorder have a co-existing clinical depression that requires treatment in its own right.

We have come to the conclusion that embedded among patients with eating disorders, and across the three major diagnostic groups, is a sizeable subgroup who have a semi-independent clinical depression, and that when this is the case it interferes significantly with the treatment of the eating disorder. This is for a number of reasons: first, depressive thinking results in patients being hopeless about the possibility of change, which undermines their ability to engage in treatment; second, the reduction in drive seen in depression also has this effect; and third, the impairment in concentration can result in information not being retained. The importance of detecting and treating these clinical depressions cannot be overstated and, whenever possible, this should be done before starting CBT-E.

Identifying these patients is not straightforward. Some features of depression are to be expected in patients with an eating disorder for the following reasons. First, low self-esteem is frequent among those with an eating disorder (see Chapter 13) and so self-critical thinking is commonly present. Second, low mood and certain other features usually suggestive of a clinical depression are also characteristic of being very underweight (e.g., impaired concentration, decreased energy and drive, poor sleep, loss of interest in sex, heightened obsessionality — see Chapter 11) and so are to be expected among those with a low BMI. Third, binge eating typically arouses shame, guilt, low mood and self-criticism, all otherwise suggestive of a clinical depression. Fourth, sustained dietary restraint and restriction can result in irritability and impaired concentration, both features of clinical depression. Lastly, the impaired interpersonal functioning that is a common product of an eating disorder can result in patients feeling worthless and unlikable, also suggestive of depression.

It is now our practice to look extremely carefully for clinical depressions in our patients because these depressions are eminently treatable and doing so makes the eating disorder easier to overcome. Detecting these depressions requires particular attention to be paid to discriminatory depressive features that are not otherwise typical of patients with an eating disorder. Table 16.1 lists these features and others that we view as suggestive of a depression. The more of these features that are present, the more confident are we that a diagnosis of a clinical depression is warranted. It is worth noting that patients who are reluctant to take antidepressant medication may minimize or deny their symptoms. If this appears to be the case, it is best to discuss the matter with the patient and stress the need to be open and frank. Often it is worth assessing such patients on a number of occasions as their minimization tends to break down over time. It is important to add that suicide risk must be assessed when evaluating these patients. This means that all eating disorder therapists should be competent at assessing suicide risk. The risk is largely, but not exclusively, restricted to patients who have a co-existing clinical depression.

If a clinical depression appears to be present, we explain this to patients saying that it is important to treat it first as recovering from the depression will result not only in

TABLE 16.1. Discriminatory Clinical Features Suggestive of a Co-Existing Clinical Depression

Recent intensification of depressive features (in the absence of any change in the eating disorder or the patient's circumstances)

Heightened extreme and pervasive negative thinking (i.e., broader in content than concerns about eating, shape and weight)
- Global negative thinking
- Hopelessness in general (i.e., seeing the future as totally bleak; seeing no future; resignation)
- Recurrent thoughts about death and dying
- Suicidal thoughts and plans (e.g., thoughts that one would be better off dead; having a specific plan for ending one's life)
- Undue guilt about events and circumstances unrelated to eating disorder psychopathology

Decrease in interests and involvement with others (over and above any impairment that already accompanied the eating disorder)
- Decreased socializing (e.g., no longer seeing friends)
- Ceasing to engage in activities that had been pursued (e.g., ceasing to read newspapers or follow the news; ceasing to listen to music)

Decrease in drive and impaired decision-making
- Decline in ability to motivate oneself to do things (e.g., to work; to play sports)[a]
- Procrastination (i.e., due to impaired decision-making)

Other suggestive features
- Tearfulness (when previously would not have cried)
- Neglect of personal appearance and hygiene (compared to usual standards)
- Neglect of day-to-day activities (e.g., not opening mail; not paying bills)
- Late onset of the eating disorder (i.e., after the age of 30 years)
- Atypical manner in treatment sessions (e.g., a persistently low mood)
- Poor response to the first stage of CBT-E
- Through lack of drive and negative thinking, inability to undertake agreed homework tasks

Clinical tip: With patients who are distressed about their eating habits, ask about their mood on a "good day" (in their terms) as this helps disentangle their mood from their eating problem.

[a]A relative of one of our patients memorably reported that his daughter's "'Get up and go' had got up and gone!"

their feeling better, but it will also mean that they will be more capable of overcoming their eating problem.

Our preferred mode of treatment is antidepressant medication. This surprises (and even shocks) some colleagues as we are well known for our particular interest in psychological methods of treatment. The important point to note is that we favor the use of antidepressant medication in this context. This is because it works well and is rapid, thereby allowing us to move quickly onto the psychological treatment of the eating disorder.

Briefly, and with exceptions, our use of antidepressant medication is as follows:

1. We positively recommend that the patient take antidepressant medication. We do not think it appropriate to be tentative about this. We discuss in detail the pros and cons of taking the medication (see page 249) with the aim of helping the patient make a well-informed decision.

2. We generally treat the depression with fluoxetine. This is not to imply that other antidepressants would not be as effective. It is just that in our experience fluoxetine works well in most cases and presents few complications. We usually start at a dose of 40 mg (once daily, first thing in the morning) as we have yet to encounter a patient with an eating disorder who has responded to 20 mg. (Some patients induce vomiting in the mornings, although this is unusual. In these cases there is the risk that they will not retain the medication. This possibility needs to be discussed with the patient and means of delaying the vomiting identified.) The patient is then reassessed after 2 weeks. If 40 mg is sufficient, signs of response will begin to be evident after about 10–12 days. It is worth noting that the extent of the initial response is sometimes less than it appears because patients are so pleased with the change in their state that the response seems greater than it actually is.

3. If there are no signs of a response, we increase the dose to 60 mg and wait for another two-to-three weeks to see if there is an effect. If this dose is insufficient, we increase the dose still further because in our experience there is a significant group of patients who make an excellent response to fluoxetine but only at higher doses than this. (This is an interesting observation. It may be a physiological effect of these patients' chronic dietary restriction.)

4. Once the patient has made a full response (generally after 4–6 weeks on the active dose), the drug is continued at this level for the next 9 months to minimize the risk of return of the depression. During this time the eating disorder is treated using CBT-E. After 9 months of continuation medication, and assuming the patient is not facing particular stresses at the time, the drug is discontinued.

5. The adverse effects of fluoxetine in these patients are generally minimal. They fall into two main groups. There are those that develop upon starting the drug or on increasing the dose. These last for about 5 days and usually consist of varying degrees of nausea (from minor to marked). The second group is not common but they tend to persist as long as the patient continues to take the drug. One is a fine tremor of the hands (visible if patients stretch out their arms and fingers) especially at higher doses and in those who are underweight. If the tremor is mild, some patients prefer to continue with the drug rather than switch to another antidepressant and possibly jeopardize their response. If the tremor is marked, however, another antidepressant will need to be cho-

sen. Another feature occasionally encountered is slight difficulty swallowing, although this is rarely troublesome. A third feature is a reduction in (or loss of) sexual appetite and responsiveness. This is usually surmountable. Very few patients choose to discontinue the drug for this reason.

One other point needs to be emphasized. In our experience antidepressant drugs work equally well (as antidepressant agents) whatever the weight of the patient. It is not uncommon to hear it said that antidepressants do not work in patients with anorexia nervosa. This is simply not true in our view. Antidepressants do not work as a treatment for anorexia nervosa, but they do work as a treatment for clinical depression, even in patients who are very underweight.

It is not uncommon for patients to have reservations about taking antidepressant medication. Some of these reservations stem from the depression itself and reflect patients' self-criticism, indecisiveness and procrastination. It is important to explore these reservations in some detail to correct any misconceptions while at the same time highlighting the potential benefits of the medication. The main points to stress (as needed) are as follows:

- Taking antidepressant medication is not a sign of weakness. Antidepressants do not interfere with one's ability to deal with life difficulties; indeed, one is in a much better position to do so once the clinical depression has resolved.
- Overcoming a clinical depression by taking antidepressant medication will mean that one is more capable of making full use of the psychological treatment for the eating problem.
- Antidepressant drugs are not addictive. They are easy to stop and in the case of fluoxetine there is no discernible withdrawal syndrome.
- Antidepressants are not mood enhancers. They are drugs for the treatment of clinical depressions.
- There are very few side effects; indeed, most patients say that they are unaware that they are taking fluoxetine once the initial side effects have worn off.
- Fluoxetine does not increase appetite or weight. Indeed, at higher doses (60 mg) it can reduce the propensity to binge eat.
- Another important point to emphasize is that the patient will be more sensitive to the inebriating effects of alcohol and so should drink with caution.

Treating clinical depressions in this way sometimes has an effect on the eating disorder. Either this is a direct pharmacological effect of the antidepressant drug or it is as a result of the improvement in the patient's psychological state. For example, as noted, in those who binge eat there may be a reduction in the frequency of binge eating and, as a consequence, a lessening of certain secondary features (e.g., fears of losing control over eating, level of secondary depressed mood). This is probably a direct pharmacological effect as research indicates that it even occurs in patients who are not depressed initially. Rarely, in our experience, does the improvement extend to the core psychopathology of the eating disorder or its direct expressions and, possibly for this reason, it is often not sustained. Recovery from the depression may affect the eating disorder in other ways. Patients who are underweight may either start to undereat even more strictly as a result of an increase in their drive and determination, or they may eat more as a result of a return of their appetite and willingness to socialize.

Thus, to summarize with reference to the three questions listed earlier:

1. *Are the features of the co-existing disorder directly attributable to the eating disorder or its consequences?*

   - Many features suggestive of a clinical depression can be secondary to an eating disorder giving rise to the spurious impression that there are two psychiatric disorders present. However, in patients with a co-existing clinical depression there are discriminatory depressive features that are not typical of patients with an eating disorder (see Table 16.1).

2. *Are the features of the co-existing disorder likely to interfere with the successful treatment of the eating disorder?*

   - Depressive features, if prominent, do interfere with the patient's ability to benefit from CBT-E. Therefore patients who have a co-existing clinical depression should have this treated first. Antidepressant drugs work well in these patients whatever their body weight and eating disorder diagnosis.

3. *Are the features of the co-existing disorder likely to dissipate if the eating disorder is successfully treated?*

   - Secondary depressive features typically dissipate if the eating disorder is successfully treated. This is not true of cases in which there is a clinical depression.

Other Mood Disorders

Occasionally we are referred patients with bipolar I or II disorder and an eating disorder. So long as the patient is euthymic, CBT-E can proceed as usual with these patients, and often they do well. Setbacks, if they occur, are often triggered by incipient mood change. More common and difficult to manage is the co-existence of an eating disorder and some forms of bipolar disorder not otherwise specified (e.g., when there is rapid and frequent alternation [over a matter of days] between subthreshold, but nevertheless significant, manic and depressive states). These patients are quite different from those with borderline personality disorder with whom they can be confused. They are difficult to help with CBT-E while their mood is unstable so mood stabilization has to be the first priority. Unfortunately some mood stabilizing drugs undermine control over eating and result in weight gain, side effects that are unacceptable to patients with eating disorders.

Anxiety Disorders

Anxiety disorders commonly co-exist with eating disorders but do not pose nearly as great a management problem as clinical depression because they do not generally interfere with treatment. (Note that if anxiety features or substance misuse co-exist with a clinical depression, they may be secondary to it. In these cases we recommend that the clinical depression be treated first along the lines specified above.)

Starting with the three key questions listed earlier:

1. *Are the features of the co-existing disorder directly attributable to the eating disorder or its consequences?*

   - Features suggestive of an anxiety disorder are often present in patients with an eating disorder. For example, avoidance of socializing due to difficulty eating in front of others is not uncommon, especially among underweight patients. It is not indicative of a social phobia, however, as the fear is attributable to the eating disorder. The same is true of the ritualized eating and hoarding that is a non-specific effect of being significantly underweight (see Chapter 11) and that might otherwise be viewed as evidence of an obsessive–compulsive disorder.

2. *Are the features of the co-existing disorder likely to interfere with the successful treatment of the eating disorder?*

   - In the case of anxiety disorders, this is not common. Occasionally we have been referred patients with such extreme agoraphobia that they cannot attend appointments. In such cases the agoraphobia obviously has to be treated first. Much more problematic, but unusual, are cases of obsessive–compulsive disorder in which the compulsions affect the patient's eating in such a way as to maintain the eating disorder. For example, we had one patient whose concerns about contamination centered on food and contributed to her eating very little. Such patients either need to have the anxiety disorder addressed first or the two disorders treated in tandem (by the same therapist). The latter option is difficult and requires an especially skilled and experienced therapist capable of adapting CBT-E to accommodate the obsessive–compulsive disorder and its treatment.

3. *Are the features of the co-existing disorder likely to dissipate if the eating disorder is successfully treated?*

   - Secondary anxiety features will dissipate if the eating disorder is successfully treated, and sometimes this is true of co-existing anxiety disorders such as generalized anxiety disorder.

Some patients have an anxiety disorder that is quite separate from the eating disorder in the sense that it does not interact with it nor will it affect treatment. In our experience, patients with posttraumatic stress disorder (PTSD) often fall into this group. In such cases we discuss with patients which problem they would like to address first, as in general it is unwise to engage in two psychological treatments at one time. Usually, but not invariably, they choose to address the eating problem first. In this case we agree that we will reassess the co-existing problem at the end of treatment and, if appropriate, arrange for it to be treated then. (We adopt the same strategy with patients who have a history of sexual or physical abuse and would like help for this.)

Substance Misuse

Substance misuse is not uncommon among patients with eating disorders, although in our experience it is largely confined to those who binge eat. It mainly involves excessive alcohol intake, although some patients use recreational drugs (e.g., marijuana, ecstasy) to an extent, and a small proportion take cocaine or amphetamines. In the latter case, the drug may be used partly as a means of weight control.

Again, applying the three questions listed at the outset:

1. *Are the features of the co-existing disorder directly attributable to the eating disorder or its consequences?*

   - This does not often apply other than in cases in which the substance is being used to control weight. Mood intolerance may be present in some cases and maintain both the eating disorder and the substance misuse (see Chapter 10). These patients generally engage in intermittent bouts of substance misuse (e.g., non-social binge drinking) rather than having a steady high intake. They may also have a history of other forms of dysfunctional mood modulatory behavior, particularly self-injury.

2. *Are the features of the co-existing disorder likely to interfere with the successful treatment of the eating disorder?*

   - Frequent intoxication during the day almost invariably interferes with treatment. It is our practice to explain this to patients and ask them to think it over. Somewhat to our surprise, quite a few patients not only decide that they must give up or markedly reduce their intake of the substance (usually alcohol) in question but readily succeed in doing so. They state that overcoming their eating disorder is so important that they just have to control their substance use. Other patients are unable or unwilling to do this. We recommend that such patients get specialist help for their substance misuse prior to beginning CBT-E. If the substance misuse is intermittent, we generally address it in the context of treating the eating disorder. This usually works well.

3. *Are the features of the co-existing disorder likely to dissipate if the eating disorder is successfully treated?*

   - This is often the case if the substance misuse is mild or intermittent.

As regards cigarette smoking, it is not generally addressed in treatment because it is rarely an obstacle to change. However, smoking used to resist eating should be discouraged and healthier alternatives found. (See the "Regular eating" intervention, page 79.) Trying to stop smoking while tackling the eating disorder is inadvisable as it is too ambitious a goal. This is best done afterward.

Other Axis I Psychiatric Disorders

Patients with eating disorders are not immune from having co-existing psychiatric disorders other than those already discussed. For example, we have encountered patients with schizophrenia, conversion disorder, hypochondriasis and body dysmorphic disorder. Again, answers to the three critical questions need to be sought when deciding how best to understand and manage such comorbidity.

Personality Disorders

As was stressed in Chapter 2 (page 16), it is difficult to assess the personality of patients with eating disorders because many of the features of interest are directly affected by the presence of an eating disorder. In our view making personality disorder diagnoses is particularly problematic as most patients will have had no period of adulthood free from the influence of the eating disorder. For this and other reasons, it is not our practice to do so.

We do, of course, see the types of patients who are given personality disorder diagnoses. Patients who engage in self-injury or substance misuse often attract the diagnosis of borderline personality disorder, whereas we view many of them as having mood intolerance and interpersonal difficulties. We manage them along the lines described in Chapters 10 and 13. Patients with clinical perfectionism are sometimes viewed as having obsessive–compulsive personality disorder. Their management was discussed in Chapter 13. Patients with core low self-esteem may receive a diagnosis of avoidant personality disorder or dependent personality disorder. Their management was also discussed in Chapter 13.

Co-Existing General Medical Disorders

Obesity

Obesity is the general medical disorder most commonly seen among patients with an eating disorder, although the combination is not as common as might be thought because it is largely confined to patients with binge eating disorder. Occasionally one meets a patient with bulimia nervosa who has a BMI over 30.0, but this is unusual.

Faced with a patient with both an eating disorder and obesity, it is crucial that the therapist and patient are clear about the goals of treatment. There are two basic options. Treatment can focus on weight loss and this might, or might not, simultaneously result in cessation of the binge eating. For example, it has been found that behavioral weight loss treatments have a substantial effect on the binge eating of patients with binge eating disorder, and we have developed a cognitive behavioral variant of these approaches that explicitly addresses binge eating while also focusing on achieving weight loss (Cooper, Fairburn, & Hawker, 2003). Weight loss treatments are inadvisable with patients with bulimia nervosa, however, as they intensify dietary restraint, one of the major causes of their binge eating (see page 18).

The other option is to treat the eating disorder first, the goal being to give patients control over their eating, and then they can consider tackling their weight. This is our preferred strategy, both with patients who have bulimia nervosa and with those with binge eating disorder. If this is the strategy being used, patients must understand that treatment is unlikely to have much impact on their weight. In the case of binge eating disorder this is because their excess energy intake comes largely from the way that they eat outside their binges, rather than from the binges themselves. With patients who have bulimia nervosa there may be some weight loss, but this is not a goal of the treatment.

If the second strategy is being adopted, then CBT-E is a good treatment option, although as mentioned in Chapter 4 (page 43), guided cognitive behavioral self-help is emerging as a good cost-effective alternative for many cases of binge eating disorder. Full-scale CBT-E is perhaps best suited for those patients with obesity who have prominent eating disorder psychopathology, such as mood-triggered eating or extreme concerns about appearance.

In the main the treatment of these patients proceeds in much the same way as with patients who do not have obesity. However, certain points are worth noting (and are discussed in detail in Cooper et al., 2003):

- *Some of these patients are prone to under-report their food intake and binge eating.* There are patients whose records seem implausible, given their weight and propensity to binge eat. This apparent under-reporting is difficult to address. Confrontation is not appropriate. Rather, it seems better to adopt a perplexed non-judgmental stance, perhaps adding that it would be helpful to treatment if there were more day-to-day problems to discuss and tackle.

- *Central to addressing binge eating is the "Regular eating" intervention and the strategies and procedures directed at event- and mood-triggered eating.* These are likely to be the main focus of the treatment of these patients and are described in Chapters 6 and 10 respectively. "Binge analysis" is especially important when tackling residual binges (see page 139).

- *Addressing dietary restraint, and food avoidance in particular, is not incompatible with healthy eating.* This is true in general but needs to be stressed with these patients. Some patients will not have any dietary rules, but those who do need to address them because they are likely to contribute to their binge eating. There is a risk, however, that encouraging these patients to break their dietary rules will be taken as endorsement of overeating and the consumption of a high-fat diet. This is to misunderstand the principles underpinning the procedure (see page 127), which are completely compatible with healthy eating.

- *Concerns about shape must be addressed.* Therapists sometimes think that it is understandable for overweight patients to dislike their appearance and therefore their concerns do not need to be addressed. This is quite wrong. Not everyone who is overweight is distressed about their appearance. If patients are highly concerned about the way that they look, this should be a focus of treatment whatever the patient's actual size. The strategies and procedures described in Chapter 8 should be followed as assiduously with overweight patients as with any others. Body checking, body avoidance and feeling fat may all need to be addressed, and focusing on marginalized domains of life is important too. Many of these patients put their life "on hold" thinking that they will address difficulties in their personal or interpersonal life once they have lost weight. This is a mistake as it is detrimental to their self-esteem and serves to perpetuate their concerns about their appearance. (See Cooper et al. [2003] for further information on addressing the shape concerns of people with obesity.)

- *Body acceptance should be a goal of treatment.* As noted by Wilson (2004), a balance has to be struck between acceptance and change. While we should strive to change things that are changeable and are doing ourselves or others harm, we should accept those things that cannot be changed without undue cost. This is especially true of body weight which is under strong physiological control. Doing so is made difficult by the impression given in the media and by weight loss organizations that one can control one's weight. This is true in the short term but certainly not true in the long run (Cooper et al., 2010). Patients with obesity need help to appreciate this.

- *Patients should be educated about healthy ways to lose weight.* Having addressed their eating disorder, patients are often eager to move directly on to losing weight. This is inadvisable. We recommend that for the first 20 weeks after treatment (i.e., until the post-treatment review) they focus on maintaining their progress. Then at the review appointment they can decide with their therapist whether or not they want to attempt to lose weight. The therapist's aim in this review should be to ensure that the patient has realistic weight goals and a weight loss plan that is unlikely to result in a deterioration in the eating disorder. In this context the notion of "binge-proof dieting" should be mentioned; that is, a style of moderate dietary restriction that has no inherent rules but is instead characterized by flexible dietary guidelines.

Diabetes Mellitus and Other General Medical Disorders

Eating disorders may co-exist with other general medical disorders and the two may interact in a detrimental way. This is best exemplified by type 1 diabetes (insulin-dependent diabetes) which, when it co-exists with an eating disorder, greatly complicates treatment. Diabetes will therefore be used to illustrate the principles that should be adopted when using CBT-E to treat patients who have a general medical disorder.

When evaluating patients with an eating disorder and a general medical condition therapists should keep the following six questions in mind:

1. *Am I sufficiently knowledgeable about the medical disorder to conduct a proper assessment and treatment?*

    - Non-medical therapists may need to educate themselves about the disorder using standard medical textbooks or reliable websites, and may also want to consult with medical colleagues. Some knowledge of the literature on the combination of the two disorders is also highly desirable.

2. *Are the two disorders interacting in any way and, if so, is there a two-way interaction?*

    - In the case of diabetes there is often a two-way interaction. First, many patients with eating disorders manipulate their insulin intake as a means of weight control. More specifically, they purposefully take too little insulin thereby losing sugar in their urine. Second, the hunger produced by injected insulin can make it particularly difficult for them to resist eating.

3. *Is the combination of the two disorders particularly harmful or dangerous?*

    - This is quite definitely so in the case of diabetes where glycemic control is often compromised by the presence of the eating disorder. Furthermore, by under-using insulin these patients put themselves at immediate risk of diabetic coma and, in the long term, of all the serious complications of diabetes.

4. *Are the physicians who are managing the general medical disorder aware of the eating disorder and its likely impact on the patient's condition?*

    - If not, it should be explained to the patient that the physicians should be informed. It is almost invariably inappropriate to accede to patients' requests to keep the eating disorder secret. This is unquestionably so in the case of diabetes.

5. *Are there properties of the general medical disorder or its treatment that are likely to complicate the treatment of the eating disorder, and vice versa?*

- Again, this is definitely so in the case of diabetes. The hunger that may follow injecting insulin may make it difficult for patients to follow the "Regular eating" intervention (see page 75), and the diabetic dietary regime may clash with what needs to be done to overcome the eating disorder (e.g., the addressing of food avoidance; see page 128). Conversely, the treatment of the eating disorder may result in a temporary decline in glycemic control. When such interactions are possible, it is essential that the therapist maintains close contact with the team that is managing the general medical disorder.

6. *Does CBT-E need to be adapted to accommodate the general medical disorder?*

- In the case of diabetes this is definitely the case. For example, the recording should include details of insulin usage and blood sugar levels. Also, it is best not to work within the usual fixed time frame as these patients' progress is often erratic and unpredictable.

In practice, diabetes is an extreme example of the complications that arise from the co-existence of an eating disorder and a general medical condition. With other disorders such interactions are either less marked and noxious (e.g., in the case of co-existing celiac disease, irritable bowel syndrome, food intolerance, food allergy) or there are none at all. In these cases CBT-E may not need to be modified at all, although liaison with the relevant physician is always important.

Life Events and Crises

Life Events and Crises Prior to Treatment

One obstacle to starting CBT-E is the presence of an ongoing life event or crisis. Some events will just pass (e.g., a major work commitment) and it is simply a matter of delaying treatment until they are over, whereas others may need to be addressed. Certain life difficulties are more pressing than the eating problem and have to take precedence over its treatment; for example, we were recently referred a patient who had just been made homeless. Other difficulties that we have encountered include the unexpected breakup of a long-term relationship, the death of a close relative, and suddenly becoming unemployed. In each case we helped the patient deal with the crisis before starting CBT-E. We find that this often does not take long, and it certainly serves to engage the patient.

Life Events and Crises during Treatment

CBT-E remains focused on the eating disorder more or less whatever happens in the patient's life. However, major crises during treatment cannot be ignored; for example, the parents of one our younger patients disappeared unexpectedly, leaving the patient at a loss as to what to do. Under such circumstances we arrange one or more "crisis sessions" devoted exclusively to the crisis and its resolution, in addition to the ongoing CBT-E sessions. Very occasionally the crisis is so serious that we suspend CBT-E for some weeks because continuing seems inappropriate or impossible. We do the same if the patient develops a psychiatric problem that is interfering with treatment, usually a clinical depression. Once the problem has been addressed, we resume treatment with an initial "catch-up" session to re-orient the patient.

A particular type of life event that commonly occurs during treatment is a vacation, "festivity" or celebration (e.g., Thanksgiving, Christmas, birthdays, weddings). These pose particular problems because they may involve close contact with people with whom the patient may have a difficult relationship; there is the expectation that everyone will enjoy themselves; and large meals may be a component. At the same time treatment may be disrupted. These events need to be thought through carefully in advance. Sometimes the patient's aim should be merely to "survive" without letting his or her progress be jeopardized. Rarely is it appropriate to introduce new procedures at these times, although patients may be able to capitalize on the change in circumstances to try new ways of eating and new forms of clothing. We try to maintain therapeutic contact over these periods, if necessary via planned telephone calls or e-mail-based sessions.

Recommended Reading

Co-Existing Psychiatric Disorders

Fluoxetine Bulimia Nervosa Collaborative Study Group. (1992). Fluoxetine in the treatment of bulimia nervosa: A multicenter, placebo-controlled, double blind trial. *Archives of General Psychiatry, 49,* 139–147.

Franko, D. L., & Keel, P. K. (2006). Suicidality in eating disorders: Occurrence, correlates, and clinical implications. *Clinical Psychology Review, 26,* 769–782.

Godart, N. T., Perdereau, F., Rein, Z., Berthoz, S., Wallier, J., Jeammet, P., et al. (2007). Comorbidity studies of eating disorders and mood disorders: Critical review of the literature. *Journal of Affective Disorders, 97,* 37–49.

Lilenfeld, L. R. R., Wonderlich, S., Riso, L. P., Crosby, R., & Mitchell, J. (2006). Eating disorders and personality: A methodological and empirical review. *Clinical Psychology Review, 26,* 299–320.

Touyz, S., Swinbourne, J., Hunt, C., Abbott, M., Clare, T., & Russell, J. (2007). The prevalence of co-morbid eating disorders and anxiety disorders: Do individuals with co-morbid diagnoses display more severe symptoms? *Australian and New Zealand Journal of Psychiatry, 41,* A92.

Co-Existing General Medical Disorders

Allison, K. C., & Stunkard, A. J. (2005). Obesity and eating disorders. *Psychiatric Clinics of North America, 28,* 55–67.

Cooper, Z., Doll, H. A., Hawker, D. M., Byrne, S., Bonner, G., Eeley, E., O'Connor, M. E., & Fairburn, C. G. (2010). Testing a new cognitive behavioural treatment for obesity: A randomized controlled trial with three-year follow-up. *Behaviour Research and Therapy, 48,* 706–713.

Cooper, Z., Fairburn, C. G., & Hawker, D. M. (2004). *Cognitive-behavioral treatment of obesity: A clinician's guide.* New York: Guilford Press.

Hill, A. J. (2007). Obesity and eating disorders. *Obesity Reviews, 8,* 151–155.

Powers, P. S. (1997). Management of patients with comorbid medical conditions. In D. M. Garner & P. E. Garfinkel (Eds.), *Handbook of treatment for eating disorders* (2nd ed., pp. 424–436). New York: Guilford Press.

Other Articles of Relevance to Chapter 16

Wilson, G. T. (2004). Acceptance and change in the treatment of eating disorders: The evolution of manual-based cognitive-behavioral therapy. In S. C. Hayes, V. M. Follette, & M. Linehan (Eds.), *Mindfulness and acceptance: Expanding the cognitive-behavioral tradition* (pp. 243–266). New York: Guilford Press.

POSTSCRIPT

Looking Forward

Christopher G. Fairburn

Over the 30 years since this treatment was originally developed (as a treatment for bulimia nervosa) much has changed. It has been extensively evaluated, made more effective, and modified so that it is now suitable for all forms of eating disorder. This is progress indeed. But much remains to be done. Three priorities stand out in my view.

First, the treatment needs to be made still more effective. Not everyone gets better. We need to understand why this is the case and modify the treatment accordingly. One's "treatment failures" (and here I am referring to the *treatment failing*, not the patient) are always more informative than one's successes. I am not someone who thinks that the answer necessarily lies within the realm of CBT. It is important to keep an open mind.

The second priority is to see if it is possible to simplify the treatment, either overall or for use with certain subgroups of patients. To do this requires an understanding of how it works and what are its active ingredients. On the basis of such knowledge key ingredients could be enhanced and redundant ones dropped. To date, few researchers have addressed fundamental questions of this sort.

Third, there is a need to disseminate the treatment. There are many therapists who would like to be trained in CBT-E, and this number is likely to grow, yet there are no empirically tested means of providing the necessary training or supervision. Conferences and workshops whet the appetite, but can do little more. Detailed written guidance (such as provided in this book) has the potential to be more helpful, but it is clearly not sufficient on its own. Herein lies another major challenge.

Recommended Reading

Kraemer, H. C., Wilson, G. T., Fairburn, C. G., & Agras, W. S. (2002). Mediators and moderators of treatment effects in randomized clinical trials. *Archives of General Psychiatry, 59,* 877–883.

APPENDICES

Eating Disorder Examination (Edition 16.0D)

Christopher G. Fairburn, Zafra Cooper
and Marianne E. O'Connor

Overview of EDE 16.0D

The 16th edition of the EDE is the latest version of this widely used instrument. It differs from the version that is generally used (EDE 12.0D; Fairburn & Cooper, 1993) in the following major ways:

1. There is an additional way of rating the Dietary Restraint subscale items such that restraint for the purpose of gaining a sense of control in general may be rated in addition to restraint intended to influence shape or weight. This is in order to detect a type of restraint seen mainly in younger patients and in the earlier stages of an eating disorder (see page 12). It is also seen in non-Western cases. Thus two Dietary Restraint subscale scores may be computed as well as a combined one.
2. There is a "binge eating disorder" module based on the research criteria in DSM-IV (American Psychiatric Association, 1994).
3. A distinction is drawn between compensatory and non-compensatory forms of purging (see page 11).
4. There is a new "Importance" item designed to detect the over-evaluation of control over eating per se (see page 12).

In all other significant respects the instrument is the same as EDE 12.0D and it generates EDE 12.0D-compatible data.

For further information about the EDE, see Fairburn and Cooper (1993). For full details about the differences between EDE 12.0D and EDE 16.0D, see the list at the end of the EDE schedule (page 307). Note that there is a version of the EDE designed specifically for use with children and adolescents (Bryant-Waugh, Cooper, Taylor, & Lask, 1996). If either version of the EDE is going to be used for research purposes, training is essential.

Recommended Reading

American Psychiatric Association. (1994). *Diagnostic and statistical manual of mental disorders* (4th ed.). Washington, DC: Author.

Bryant-Waugh, R. J., Cooper, P. J., Taylor, C. L., & Lask, B. D. (1996). The use of the Eating Disorder Examination with Children: A pilot study. *International Journal of Eating Disorders, 19*, 391–397.

Cooper, Z., & Fairburn, C. G. (1987). The Eating Disorder Examination: A semi-structured interview for the assessment of the specific psychopathology of eating disorders. *International Journal of Eating Disorders, 6*, 1–8.

Fairburn, C. G., & Beglin, S. J. (1994). Assessment of eating disorder psychopathology: Interview or self-request questionnaire? *International Journal of Eating Disorders, 16*, 363–370.

Fairburn, C. G., & Cooper, Z. (1993). The Eating Disorder Examination (12th ed.). In C. G. Fairburn & G. T. Wilson (Eds.), *Binge eating: Nature, assessment and treatment* (pp. 317–360). New York: Guilford Press.

Grilo, C. M. (2005). Structured instruments. In J. E. Mitchell & C. B. Peterson (Eds.), *Assessment of eating disorders* (pp. 120–128). New York: Guilford Press.

General Guidelines for Interviewers

The EDE is an *investigator-based interview.* This may be contrasted with respondent-based interviews in which the participant's answers to specified questions are rated without additional questioning. Respondent-based interviews are, in essence, verbally administered self-report questionnaires. They work well where the concepts being assessed are simple and there is general agreement as to their meaning, but they are unsatisfactory when the concepts are complex or key terms do not have a generally accepted specific meaning. With investigator-based interviews, interviewers need training to ensure that they fully understand the concepts being assessed. The structure in such interviews lies in the detailed specifications provided for the interviewer of the concepts to be rated and the rating scheme, rather than in the precise wording of individual questions. In summary, investigator-based interviews such as the EDE require that interviewers be trained both in the technique of interviewing and in the concepts and rules governing the ratings.

When using the EDE, it is essential that the participant understands the purpose of the interview. The interviewer should explain why the interview is being conducted and, before starting formal questioning, should aim to establish good rapport. The interviewer and participant together should be trying to obtain an accurate picture of the participant's current eating behavior and attitudes. It is important to explain that a standard set of questions is being asked and that some may not apply. Participants also need to know in advance how long the interview will take. At a minimum this will be 45 minutes, but it can take as long as an hour and a quarter. (EDE interviews should rarely be allowed to take longer than this since otherwise interviewer and participant fatigue will affect the quality of the ratings.)

The interviewer should explain that the interview mainly focuses on the preceding 4 weeks (28 days), although if the interview is also being used for diagnostic purposes certain questions extend out to cover the previous 3 months.[1] To help the participant accurately recall the primary period of interest, time should be devoted at the beginning of the interview to the identification of events that have taken place during these 28 days. For example, the interviewer should estab-

---

[1] The DSM-IV research diagnostic criteria for the provisional new diagnosis of binge eating disorder encompass a 6-month time frame. Interviewers wanting to elicit these diagnostic criteria should refer to the "Binge Eating Disorder Module" (see page 285), which opens with an orientation to this extended period of time.

lish whether the participant has been at home or away and what has happened on each of the four weekends. It can be helpful referring to a prepared calendar to locate the 4 weeks in question (see below). If the interview is also being used for diagnostic purposes (see sections demarcated by horizontal lines in the interview schedule) events of note in (28-day) months 2 and 3 (counting back from the present 28 days) should also be noted together with their boundaries. Rarely should the orientation to the time frame be allowed to take more than 10 minutes.

Each of the items in the EDE has one or more (asterisked) obligatory questions in bold type that must be asked. Special emphasis should be placed upon the words and phrases that are italicized. The obligatory questions should be supplemented with additional questions of the interviewer's choice. The phrase "over the past 4 weeks" that precedes most obligatory questions may be varied as seems appropriate (e.g., "over the past month" or "over the past 28 days") and inserted at any point within the question, but otherwise the obligatory questions should be asked as specified in the schedule. The items in the interview may be covered in any order, although for most purposes the sequence presented in the schedule will be found to be satisfactory. It is perfectly appropriate to return to earlier items if further information emerges during the interview that is of relevance to prior ratings. The interview should never be undertaken in the absence of the full schedule, as even the most experienced interviewers need to refer to the questions, definitions, and rating schemes.

The interviewer should pay careful attention to everything that the participant says. The interview should never be hurried. It should proceed at a steady, relaxed pace with the interviewer not moving on to the next item until he or she is satisfied that all the necessary information has been obtained. The interviewer should not be rushed along by rapid, and possibly impatient, replies. Apparently glib answers that do not seem to have been given thought should be sensitively explored. Conversely, participants who are loquacious and overly detailed in their replies need to be kept to the point. Care must always be taken to ensure that the participant understands what information the interviewer is trying to elicit. It is good practice to check back with the participant before making each rating.

The physical circumstances under which the interview is conducted are also important. The interviewer and participant need to be comfortably seated, and the interviewer needs to have the schedule in front of him or her together with the rating sheet. There should be as few distractions as possible, and except under unusual circumstances no one else should be present since otherwise participants tend not be to be frank and forthcoming.

Guidelines for making ratings are provided for most items. Ratings should be made as the interview proceeds (although certain calculations may be delayed until afterward). The instructions for making the ratings are given in square brackets and they are followed by the rating scheme itself. Frequency ratings should be based on a 28-day month: if a feature is not present, rate 0; if a feature is present on up to and including 5 days, rate 1; if it is present half the time, rate 3; if it is present almost every day (with up to and including 5 exceptions), rate 5; if it is present every day, rate 6. Some items are rated on a 7-point severity scale ranging from 0 to 6. In these cases 0 represents the absence of the feature in question and 6 represents its presence to an extreme degree; a rating of 1 should be made only if the feature is barely present, and a rating of 5 should be made only if the feature is present to a degree not quite severe enough to justify a rating of 6. A rating of 3 should be used for degrees of severity midway between 0 and 6. *If it is difficult to decide between two ratings, the lower rating (i.e., the less symptomatic) should be chosen.* (The exception is the first item "Pattern of eating" in which higher scores are [with the exception of nocturnal eating] less symptomatic.) This general rating scheme is summarized in Table A.1.

TABLE A.1. The EDE Rating Scheme

Severity ratings	Frequency ratings
0 — Absence of the feature	0 — Absence of the feature
1 — Feature almost, but not quite, absent	1 — Feature present on 1–5 days
2 —	2 — Feature present on 6–12 days
3 — Severity midway between 0 and 6	3 — Feature present on 13–15 days
4 —	4 — Feature present on 16–22 days
5 — Severity almost meriting a rating of 6	5 — Feature present on 23–27 days
6 — Feature present to an extreme degree	6 — Feature present every day

Rate *8* if, despite adequate questioning, it is impossible to decide upon a rating. Experienced interviewers will find that they rarely need to use this rating. If it is difficult to choose between two ratings, the lower (i.e., less symptomatic) rating should be made.

Rate *9* for missing values (or "not applicable").

Scoring

The EDE, and its self-report version, the EDE-Q, generate two types of data. First, they provide frequency data on key behavioral features of eating disorders in terms of number of episodes of the behavior and in some instances number of days on which the behavior has occurred. Second, they provide subscale scores reflecting the severity of aspects of the psychopathology of eating disorders. The subscales are Restraint, Eating Concern, Shape Concern and Weight Concern. To obtain a particular subscale score, the ratings for the relevant items (listed below) are added together and the sum divided by the total number of items forming the subscale. If ratings are available only on some items, a score may nevertheless be obtained by dividing the resulting total by the number of rated items so long as more than half the items have been rated. To obtain an overall or "global" score, the four subscales scores are summed and the resulting total divided by the number of subscales (i.e., four). Subscale scores are reported as means and standard deviations.

Subscale Items (the numbers are the item number on the EDE-Q 6.0):
Restraint
1 Restraint over eating
2 Avoidance of eating
3 Food avoidance
4 Dietary rules
5 Empty stomach

Eating Concern
7 Preoccupation with food, eating or calories
9 Fear of losing control over eating
19 Eating in secret
21 Social eating
20 Guilt about eating

Shape Concern

6 Flat stomach

8 Preoccupation with shape or weight

23 Importance of shape

10 Fear of weight gain

26 Dissatisfaction with shape

27 Discomfort seeing body

28 Avoidance of exposure

11 Feelings of fatness

Weight Concern

22 Importance of weight

24 Reaction to prescribed weighing

8 Preoccupation with shape or weight

25 Dissatisfaction with weight

12 Desire to lose weight

Community Norms

The data in Table A.2 are from a community-based sample of 243 young women assessed using the EDE and EDE-Q (see Fairburn & Beglin, 1994).

TABLE A.2. EDE and EDE-Q Community Norms

Measure	Mean	*SD*	*N*
EDE Interview			
Global EDE (four subscales)	0.932	0.805	243
Restraint subscale	0.942	1.093	243
Eating Concern subscale	0.266	0.593	243
Shape Concern subscale	1.339	1.093	243
Weight Concern subscale	1.181	0.929	243
EDE-Q			
Global EDE-Q (four subscales)	1.554	1.213	241
Restraint subscale	1.251	1.323	241
Eating Concern subscale	0.624	0.859	241
Shape Concern subscale	2.149	1.602	241
Weight Concern subscale	1.587	1.369	241

Eating Disorder Examination (Edition 16.0D)

The Interview Schedule

ORIENTATION TO THE TIME PERIOD

What we are going to do is a partially structured interview in which I will ask you about your eating habits and your feelings about your shape and weight. Because a standard set of questions is going to be asked, please note that some may not apply to you.

Most of the questions focus on the past 4 weeks (that is, the last 28 days), but there will be some that extend out to cover the previous 3 months. I know this will test your memory because the weeks tend to blend together.

What I have done to help you is to make this calendar for the last 28 days [show the blank calendar — see below]; it ends on yesterday because today is not over yet. So it goes from yesterday (day and date) to (day and date). I know it seems strange to have the weekends in the middle, but that is just the way it has worked out.

And here are the dates for the 2 months before that, (date) to (date). And to help you remember these periods, I have noted down the holidays (e.g., Labor Day, Thanksgiving).

What I would like you to do now is tell me about any events that have happened in the past 28 days because this will help us discuss these 4 weeks. Have there been any events out of the ordinary .... such as celebrations of any type, trips away or days off work? Then we can note these down on the calendar.

[These should be noted on the calendar (see Table A.3), thereby allowing the interviewer and participant to use it as an *aide memoire*.]

TABLE A.3. EDE Calendar

Calendar

Month 2 from .... to ....

    Events ....

Month 3 from .... to ....

    Events ....

Months 4–6★ from .... to ....

    Events ....

★This period is only of relevance if the DSM-IV research diagnostic criteria for binge eating disorder are being elicited. It is best to postpone focusing on months 4–6 until the beginning of the binge eating disorder module (see page 285).

Introductory Questions

[Having oriented the participant to the specific time period being assessed, it is best to open the interview by asking a number of introductory questions designed to obtain a general picture of the participant's eating habits. Suitable questions are suggested below.]

To begin with I should like to get a general picture of your eating habits over the last 4 weeks. What has been your usual eating pattern?

Have your eating habits varied much from day to day?

Have weekdays differed from weekends?

[The definition (and number) of weekdays and weekend days that best fits the patient's lifestyle needs to be established at this point (e.g., check if the participant's days off work regularly fall on weekdays).]

Have there been any days when you haven't eaten anything?

[Ask about months 2 and 3]

What about the previous 2 months (specify months) .... Were your eating habits much the same or were they different?

PATTERN OF EATING

*I would like to ask about your pattern of eating. Over the past 4 weeks which of these meals or snacks have you eaten on a regular basis?

— Breakfast   [   ]
— Mid-morning snack   [   ]
— Lunch (mid-day meal)   [   ]
— Mid-afternoon snack   [   ]
— Evening meal   [   ]
— Evening snack   [   ]
— Nocturnal eating (i.e., an episode of eating after the participant has been to sleep)   [   ]

[Rate each meal and snack separately, usually accepting the participant's classification (within the guidelines above). Ask about weekdays and weekends separately. Meals or snacks should be rated even if they lead to a "binge." "Brunch" should generally be classed as lunch. With the exception of nocturnal eating, rate up (i.e., give a higher rating) if it is difficult to choose between two ratings. Rate 8 if meals or snacks are difficult to classify (e.g., due to shift work).]

0 — Meal or snack not eaten
1 — Meal or snack eaten on 1–5 days
2 — Meal or snack eaten on less than half the days (6–12 days)
3 — Meal or snack eaten on half the days (13–15 days)
4 — Meal or snack eaten on more than half the days (16–22 days)
5 — Meal or snack eaten almost every day (23–27 days)
6 — Meal or snack eaten every day

[If participants report having had episodes of nocturnal eating, ask about their level of awareness (alertness) at the time and their recall of the episodes afterward.]

When you ate ......, how awake were you and how well could you recall the episode the next day?

0 — no nocturnal eating
1 — nocturnal eating with no impairment of awareness (alertness) or recall
2 — nocturnal eating with impairment of awareness (alertness) or recall

                                                                                                              [   ]

PICKING (NIBBLING)

*Over the past 4 weeks have you picked at (nibbled) food between meals and snacks? By "picking" (nibbling) I mean eating in an unplanned and repetitious way.

What about when cooking?

What have you typically eaten at these times?

Why would you not call these episodes snacks?

Have you known in advance how much you were going to eat?

[Rate the number of days on which picking (nibbling) has occurred. To count as picking (or nibbling) the episode of eating should have been unplanned, the amount eaten should have been uncertain at the time that the episode started, and the eating should have had a repetitious element to it. Typically what is eaten is incomplete (i.e., it constitutes part of something or a less-than-usual amount), but the total amount consumed should not have been minute (e.g., not simply one edge of a piece of toast). In general, participants themselves should view the episodes as examples of "picking" ("nibbling").

Picking (nibbling) may be contrasted with eating a "snack." A snack is an episode of eating in which the amount eaten was modest (smaller than a meal), known at the outset with some certainty, and did not have the repetitious element associated with picking. Episodes of picking which merge into snacks, meals or "binges" should not be rated. The rating of picking may require the re-rating of snacks.]

0 — No picking (nibbling)
1 — Picking (nibbling) on 1–5 days
2 — Picking (nibbling) on less than half the days (6–12 days)
3 — Picking (nibbling) on half the days (13–15 days)
4 — Picking (nibbling) on more than half the days (16–22 days)
5 — Picking (nibbling) almost every day (23–27 days)
6 — Picking (nibbling) every day

[　]

RESTRAINT OVER EATING (Restraint subscales)

★Over the past 4 weeks have you been *consciously trying* to restrict (cut back) the over-all amount that you eat, whether or not you have succeeded?

What have you been trying to do?

Has this been to influence your shape or weight, or to avoid triggering an episode of overeating?

[Rate the number of days on which the participant has *consciously attempted* to restrict his or her *overall* food intake (i.e., energy intake), whether or not he or she has succeeded. The restriction should have affected a *range of food items* and not just certain specific foods (cf., "Food avoidance"). This restriction should have been intended either to influence shape, weight or body composition, or to avoid triggering an episode of overeating, although this may not have been the sole or main reason. It should have consisted of planned attempts at restriction, rather than spur-of-the-moment attempts such as the decision to resist a second helping.]

0 — No attempt at restraint
1 — Attempted to exercise restraint on 1–5 days
2 — Attempted to exercise restraint on less than half the days (6–12 days)
3 — Attempted to exercise restraint on half the days (13–15 days)
4 — Attempted to exercise restraint on more than half the days (16–22 days)
5 — Attempted to exercise restraint almost every day (23–27 days)
6 — Attempted to exercise restraint every day

[ ]

Some people *consciously* try to restrict their eating for another reason — to give them a sense of being in control — of being in control in general.

Over the past 4 weeks has this applied to you?

[Rate again *only* taking this reason into account.] [ ]

[Also rate number of days on which one or other, or both, of these reasons has applied.] [ ]

AVOIDANCE OF EATING   (Restraint subscales)

*Over the past 4 weeks have you gone for periods of 8 or more *waking* hours without eating anything?

Has this been to influence your shape or weight, or to avoid triggering an episode of overeating?

[Rate the number of days on which there has been at least 8 hours abstinence from eating food (soup and milkshakes count as food, whereas drinks in general do not) during waking hours. It may be helpful to illustrate the length of time (e.g., 9 A.M.–5 P.M.). The abstinence must have been at least partly *self-imposed* rather than being due to force of circumstances. It should have been intended to influence shape, weight or body composition, or to avoid triggering an episode of overeating, although this may not have been the sole or main reason (i.e., fasting for religious or political reasons would not count). Note that the rating should be consistent with those made earlier for "Pattern of eating."]

0 — No such days
1 — Avoidance on 1–5 days
2 — Avoidance on less than half the days (6–12 days)
3 — Avoidance on half the days (13–15 days)
4 — Avoidance on more than half the days (16–22 days)
5 — Avoidance almost every day (23–27 days)
6 — Avoidance every day

[ ]

Some people avoid eating in this way ..... for 8 or more waking hours ..... for another reason — to give them a sense of being in control — of being in control in general.

Over the past 4 weeks has this applied to you?

[Rate again *only* taking this reason into account.]   [ ]

[Also rate number of days on which one or other, or both, of these reasons has applied.]   [ ]

EMPTY STOMACH   (Restraint subscales)

★Over the past 4 weeks have you wanted your stomach to *be empty*?

Has this been to influence your shape or weight, or to avoid triggering an episode of overeating?

[Rate the number of days on which the participant has had a *definite desire* to have a completely empty stomach for reasons to do with dieting, shape or weight. This desire should not simply be a response to episodes of perceived overeating; rather, it should exist between any such episodes. The rating of "Empty stomach" should not be confused with a desire for the stomach to *feel empty* or *be flat* (cf., "Flat stomach."]

0 — No definite desire to have an empty stomach
1 — Definite desire on 1–5 days
2 — Definite desire on less than half the days (6–12 days)
3 — Definite desire on half the days (13–15 days)
4 — Definite desire on more than half the days (16–22 days)
5 — Definite desire almost every day (23–27 days)
6 — Definite desire every day

[   ]

Some people want to have an empty stomach for another reason — to give them a sense of being in control — of being in control in general.

Over the past 4 weeks has this applied to you?

[Rate again *only* taking this reason into account.]   [   ]

[Also rate number of days on which one or other, or both, of these reasons has applied.]   [   ]

FOOD AVOIDANCE   (Restraint subscales)

*Over the past 4 weeks have you *tried* to avoid eating any foods that you like, whether or not you have succeeded?

What foods? Have you been attempting to exclude them altogether?

Has this been to influence your shape or weight, or to avoid triggering an episode of overeating?

[Rate the number of days on which the participant has *actively attempted to avoid eating specific foods* (which he or she likes, or has liked in the past) whether or not he or she succeeded. The goal should have been to *exclude the foods altogether* and not merely to restrict their consumption. Drinks do not count as food. The avoidance should have been planned and intended either to influence shape, weight or body composition, or to avoid triggering an episode of overeating, although this may not have been the sole or main reason.]

0 — No attempts to avoid foods
1 — Attempted to avoid foods on 1–5 days
2 — Attempted to avoid foods on less than half the days (6–12 days)
3 — Attempted to avoid foods on half the days (13–15 days)
4 — Attempted to avoid foods on more than half the days (16–22 days)
5 — Attempted to avoid foods almost every day (23–27 days)
6 — Attempted to avoid foods every day

[ ]

Some people avoid eating certain foods for another reason — to give them a sense of being in control — of being in control in general.

Over the past 4 weeks has this applied to you?

[Rate again *only* taking this reason into account.]   [ ]

[Also rate number of days on which one or other, or both, of these reasons has applied.]   [ ]

DIETARY RULES   (Restraint subscales)

★Over the past 4 weeks have you tried to follow certain *definite* rules regarding your eating; for example, a calorie limit, pre-set quantities of food, or rules about what you should — or should not — eat, or when you should eat? What have you been trying to do?

If answered negatively:

Have there been occasions when you have been aware that you may have broken a dietary rule that you have set for yourself?

Have these rules been designed to influence your shape or weight, or to avoid triggering an episode of overeating?

Have they been definite rules or general guidelines? Examples of definite rules would be "I must not eat eggs" or "I must not eat cake," whereas you could have the general guideline "I should try to eat healthy food."

[Dietary rules should be rated as present if the participant has been attempting to follow "definite" (i.e., specific) dietary rules regarding his or her food intake. The rules should be self-imposed, although originally they may have been prescribed (i.e., prescribed rules can be rated if they have been adopted by the participant). They should have concerned what the participant should have eaten or when eating should have taken place. They might consist of a calorie limit (e.g., below 1,200 kcals), not eating before a certain time of day, not eating specific foods (cf., "Food avoidance"), or not eating at all. They should have been specific rules and not general guidelines. If the participant is aware that he or she has occasionally broken a personal dietary rule, this indicates that one or more specific rules have been present. In such cases the interviewer should ask in detail about the transgression in an attempt to identify the underlying rule. The rules should have been intended to influence shape, weight or body composition, although this may not have been the sole or main reason.

Rate 0 if no dietary rule can be identified. If there has been more than one rule straddling different time periods within the 4 weeks, these periods should be combined to make the rating.]

0 — Has not attempted to obey such rules
1 — Attempted to obey such rules on 1–5 days
2 — Attempted to obey such rules on less than half the days (6–12 days)
3 — Attempted to obey such rules on half the days (13–15 days)
4 — Attempted to obey such rules on more than half the days (16–22 days)
5 — Attempted to obey such rules almost every day (23–27 days)
6 — Attempted to obey such rules every day

[   ]

Some people attempt to follow dietary rules for another reason — to give them a sense of being in control — of being in control in general. Over the past 4 weeks has this applied to you?

[Rate again *only* taking this reason into account.]   [   ]

[Also rate number of days on which one or other, or both, of these reasons has applied.]   [   ]

PREOCCUPATION WITH FOOD, EATING OR CALORIES

(Eating Concern subscale)

*Over the past 4 weeks have you spent much time between meals thinking about food, eating, or calories? ....

*..... Has thinking about food, eating, or calories *interfered* with your ability to concentrate on things that you are actively engaged in, for example, working, following a conversation or reading? What has it affected?

[This definition of preoccupation requires the presence of concentration impairment. Concentration is regarded as impaired if there have been *intrusive thoughts about food, eating or calories that have interfered with activities one is actively engaged in* rather than one's mind simply drifting off the matter at hand. Rate the number of days on which this has happened, whether or not bulimic episodes occurred.]

0 — No concentration impairment
1 — Concentration impairment on 1–5 days
2 — Concentration impairment on less than half the days (6–12 days)
3 — Concentration impairment on half the days (13–15 days)
4 — Concentration impairment on more than half the days (16–22 days)
5 — Concentration impairment almost every day (23–27 days)
6 — Concentration impairment every day

[ ]

FEAR OF LOSING CONTROL OVER EATING

(Eating Concern subscale)

*Over the past 4 weeks have you been *afraid* of losing control over eating?

[Rate the number of days on which a *definite fear* (common usage) of losing control over eating has been present, irrespective of whether the participant has felt that he or she has been in control. "*Loss of control*" *involves a sense that one will not be able to resist or stop eating*. If the participant feels unable to answer this question because he or she has already totally lost control, rate 9.]

0 — No fear of losing control over eating
1 — Fear of losing control over eating present on 1–5 days
2 — Fear of losing control over eating present on less than half the days (6–12 days)
3 — Fear of losing control over eating present on half the days (13–15 days)
4 — Fear of losing control over eating present on more than half the days (16–22 days)
5 — Fear of losing control over eating present almost every day (23–27 days)
6 — Fear of losing control over eating present every day

[ ]

BULIMIC EPISODES AND OTHER EPISODES OF OVEREATING

(Diagnostic item)

Classificatory Scheme

[Four forms of episodic "overeating" are distinguished. The distinction is based upon the presence or absence of two characteristics:

1. **Loss of control** (required for both types of "bulimic episode")
2. **The consumption of what would generally be regarded as a "large" amount of food** (required for "objective bulimic episodes" and "objective overeating").

The classificatory scheme is summarized below.

	"Large" amount eaten (EDE definition)	*Amount eaten not "large" but viewed by participant as excessive*
"Loss of control" present	Objective bulimic episodes	Subjective bulimic episodes
No "loss of control"	Objective overeating	Subjective overeating

Guidelines for Proceeding through the Overeating Section

The interviewer should ask about each form of overeating. It is important to note that *the four forms of overeating are not mutually exclusive*: It is possible for participants to have had several different forms within the time period being considered. With some participants it is helpful to explain the classificatory scheme.

There are five steps in making this series of ratings:
1. In general it is best to start by asking the asterisked questions to identify the various types of perceived or true overeating that have occurred over the previous 28 days.
2. Each form should be noted down on the blank section of the coding sheet.
3. Then detailed information should be obtained about a *representative example* of each form of overeating to decide whether or not it involved eating a "large" amount of food and whether or not there was "loss of control" (as defined below).
4. The next task is to establish for each form of overeating the number of days on which it occurred and the total number of occasions. Where there is possibility of overlap (i.e., two types of episode may have occurred on the same day), this should be clarified since this will affect the "days" ratings.
5. Finally, check with the participant to ensure that no misunderstandings have arisen (e.g., that no types of episode have been omitted).

It is advisable to make comprehensive notes.

Definition of Key Terms

"Loss of control." The interviewer should ask the participant whether he or she experienced a sense of loss of control over eating at any point in the episode. If this is clearly described, "Loss of control" should be rated as present. Similarly, if the participant describes having felt "driven" or "compelled" to eat, "Loss of control" should be rated as present.

If the participant reports having had no sense of loss of control yet describes having felt unable to stop eating once eating had started or having felt unable to prevent the episode from occurring, "Loss of control" should be rated as present. If participants report that they are no longer trying to control their eating because overeating is inevitable, "Loss of control" should once again be rated as present. Thus "Loss of control" may be rated positively even if the episode had been planned (i.e., the participant knew that he or she was going to overeat and had made provision for this).

The decision whether or not "Loss of control" was present should be made by the interviewer; it does not require the agreement of the participant. If the interviewer remains in doubt, "Loss of control" should be rated as absent.

"Large amount of food." The decision whether or not the amount eaten was "large" should also be made by the interviewer; it does not require the agreement of the participant. The notion of "large" may refer to the amount of any particular type of food consumed or the overall quantity of food eaten. The amount should have been unequivocally large but it does not have to have been enormous. In deciding whether the amount was "large," *the interviewer must take into account what would be the usual amount eaten under the circumstances.* This requires some knowledge of the eating habits of the participant's general, but not necessarily immediate, social group (e.g., those of female students, women in their 50s) as well as circumstances that tend to influence eating (e.g., Thanksgiving Day, Christmas Day). What else was eaten during the day is not taken into account when making this rating, nor is the speed of eating or whether or not the participant subsequently spat out or vomited the food.

If the interviewer remains in doubt, the amount should not be classified as "large."

Interviewers should not share with the patient their view on the amount eaten and they should avoid using potentially emotive terms such as such as "binge" and "large."

The number of episodes of overeating. When calculating the number of episodes of overeating, the participant's definition of separate episodes should be accepted unless, within a period of eating, there was an hour or more when the participant was not eating. In this case the initial episode should be regarded as having been completed. An exception is if the episode was temporarily interrupted by an outside event and then restarted afterward, and it was experienced as one single episode (somewhat like operating the pause button on a recorder). When estimating the length of any gap, do not count the time spent vomiting. *Note that "purging" (self-induced vomiting or laxative misuse) is not used to define the end of individual episodes of overeating.*

Questions for Identifying Bulimic Episodes
and Other Episodes of Overeating

[See preceding section "Guidelines for Proceeding Through the Overeating Section." The asterisked questions should be asked in every case.]

MAIN PROBE QUESTIONS (to get the overall picture)

*I would like to ask you about any episodes of overeating, or loss of control over eating, that you might have had over the past 4 weeks.

*Different people mean different things by overeating. I would like you to describe any times when you have *felt* that you have eaten, or might have eaten, too much at one time.

*And any times you have felt you have lost control over eating?

ADDITIONAL PROBE QUESTIONS

*Have there been any times when you have felt that you have eaten too much, but others might not agree?

*Have there been any times when you have felt that you have eaten an ordinary amount of food but others might have regarded you as having overeaten?

[N.B.: For subjective bulimic episodes to be eligible, they must have been viewed by the participant as having involved eating an excessive amount of food (i.e., they involved "overeating").]

SUBSIDIARY PROBE QUESTIONS (to classify any episodes of overeating)

To assess the amount of food eaten:
Typically what have you eaten at these times?

For subjective bulimic episodes (i.e., where the amount is not viewed by the interviewer as "large")
Did you view this amount as excessive?

To assess the social context:
What were the circumstances?
What were others eating at the time?

To assess "loss of control":
Did you have a sense of loss of control at the time?
Did you feel you could have stopped eating once you had started?
Did you feel you could you have prevented the episode from starting?

[For objective bulimic episodes, subjective bulimic episodes and episodes of objective overeating the following two ratings should be made:

1. Number of days (rate 00 if none)
2. Number of episodes (rate 000 if none)

In general, it is best to calculate the number of days first and then the number of episodes.

Rate 777 if the number of episodes is so great that their frequency cannot be calculated. Episodes of subjective overeating are not rated.]

Objective bulimic episodes

days [　][　]

episodes [　][　][　]

Subjective bulimic episodes

days [　][　]

episodes [　][　][　]

Episodes of objective overeating

days [　][　]

episodes [　][　][　]

[Ask about each of the preceding 2 months referring back to the relevant dates and any events of note. For objective and subjective bulimic episodes, rate the number of episodes over the preceding 2 months and the number of days on which they occurred. Rate 0s if none and 9s if not asked.]

Objective bulimic episodes

days — month 2 [　][　]

month 3 [　][　]

episodes — month 2 [　][　][　]

month 3 [　][　][　]

Subjective bulimic episodes

days — month 2 [　][　]

month 3 [　][　]

episodes — month 2 [　][　][　]

month 3 [　][　][　]

[Also rate the longest continuous period in weeks free (not due to force of circumstances) from objective bulimic episodes over the past 3 months. Rate 99 if not applicable.]

[　][　]

DSM-IV "BINGE EATING DISORDER" MODULE

[Only enter this DSM-IV module if objective bulimic episodes have been present over the preceding 12 weeks. Use a respondent-based interviewing style, rather than the investigator-based style of the EDE.

In line with the DSM-IV research criteria for "binge eating disorder," a 6-month assessment needs to be made of the number of *days* (N.B.: not episodes) on which objective bulimic episodes have occurred. Therefore, having focused initially on the preceding two 28-day months (months 2 and 3), the interviewer needs to move back to the three earlier 28-day months (months 4–6). To help patients recall this far back, they need to be told the specific dates in question. They also need help to recall the specific time period (along the lines specified earlier).]

★**What about the 3 months prior to the 3 months that we have been talking about** (specify the beginning and end dates)? ....

.... **Did you have episodes like** .... (describe a representative objective bulimic episode)?

Did you have any other equivalent episodes .... (refer, if applicable, to other types of objective bulimic episode that the participant reported)?

Did they occur more or less often than in the past 28 days?

Let's estimate together, on average over the past 6 months (specify months), **how many days per week have you had episodes like** .... (refer to the representative objective bulimic episode)?

[Estimate the average number of days per week on which objective bulimic episodes have occurred over the past 6 months (i.e., rate between 0 and 7). Rate 9 if not asked.]

[ ]

Features Associated with Binge Eating

[Only rate these items if, on average over the past 6 months, there have been at least two days per week on which episodes of binge eating have occurred. Otherwise rate 9.]

During these episodes (refer to objective bulimic episodes that are *representative* of those over the past 6 months), have you *typically* ....

... **Eaten much more rapidly than normal?**   [ ]
... **Eaten until you have felt uncomfortably full?**   [ ]
... **Eaten large amounts of food when you haven't felt physically hungry?**   [ ]
... **Eaten alone because you have felt embarrassed about how much you were eating?**   [ ]
... **Felt disgusted with yourself, depressed or very guilty?**   [ ]

[Rate each feature individually using the binary scheme below.]
  0 — Feature not present
  1 — Feature present

Distress about Binge Eating

In general, over the past 6 months how distressed or upset have you felt about these episodes (refer to objective bulimic episodes that are *representative* of those over the past 6 months)?

[Rate the presence of marked distress about the binge eating. This may stem from the actual behavior itself or its potential effect on body shape and weight.]
  0 — No marked distress
  1 — Marked

[ ]

DIETARY RESTRICTION OUTSIDE BULIMIC EPISODES   (Diagnostic item)

[RETURN TO THE 3-MONTH TIME FRAME and EDE STYLE OF QUESTIONING. Only rate this item if there have been at least 24 objective bulimic episodes over the past 3 months.]

Outside the times when you have lost control over eating ..... (refer to objective and subjective bulimic episodes), ... **how much have you been actually restricting (limiting) the amount that you eat? What have you eaten on a typical day?**

Has this been to influence your shape or weight?

[Ask about actual food intake outside the objective and subjective bulimic episodes. *Rate a typical day (whether or not it involves an episode of overeating).* The dietary restriction should have been intended to influence shape, weight or body composition, although this may not have been the sole or main reason. Rate each of the past 3 months separately. Rate 9 if not asked.]

0 — No extreme restriction outside objective and subjective bulimic episodes
1 — Extreme restriction outside objective and subjective bulimic episodes (i.e., purposeful low
    energy intake [e.g., < 1,200 kcals])
2 — No eating outside objective and subjective bulimic episodes (i.e., purposeful "fasting")

month 1 [ ]
month 2 [ ]
month 3 [ ]

SOCIAL EATING   (Eating Concern subscale)

*Outside the times when ..... (refer to any objective bulimic episodes and episodes of objective overeating), **over the past 4 weeks have you been concerned about other people seeing you eat?**

How concerned have you been? Has this concern led you to avoid such occasions? Could it have been worse?

[N.B.: This is the first severity item. Rate the degree of concern about eating normal or less than normal amounts of food in front of others. *Do not consider objective bulimic episodes or episodes of objective overeating.* Also, do not consider concern restricted to family members who are aware that the participant has an eating problem. On the other hand the concern can stem from idiosyncratic eating habits (e.g., very slow eating; eating fewer courses than others; eating different types of food) or allied behavior such as indecision when ordering in a restaurant. One index of the severity of such concern is whether it has led to avoidance. In common with all severity items, the rating should generally represent the *mode for the entire month.* If the possibility of eating with others has not arisen, rate 9.]

0 — No concern about being seen eating by others and no avoidance of such occasions.
1 —
2 — Has felt slight concern at being seen eating by others
3 —
4 — Has felt definite concern at being seen eating by others
5 —
6 — Has felt extreme concern at being seen eating by others

[   ]

EATING IN SECRET   **(Eating Concern subscale)**

*Outside the times when ..... (refer to any objective bulimic episodes and episodes of objective overeating), **over the past 4 weeks have you eaten in secret?**

[Rate the number of days on which there has been at least one episode of secret eating. *Do not consider objective bulimic episodes or episodes of objective overeating.* Secret eating refers to eating that is furtive and that the participant wishes to conceal because he or she does not want to be seen eating (i.e., it is not simply eating alone). Do not rate secrecy that stems from a desire not to be interrupted or a wish not to share food. Sensitivity about eating in front of others will have been rated under "Social eating" but it can result in eating in secret. If the possibility of eating with others has not arisen, rate 9.]

0 — Has not eaten in secret
1 — Has eaten in secret on 1–5 days
2 — Has eaten in secret on less than half the days (6–12 days)
3 — Has eaten in secret on half the days (13–15 days)
4 — Has eaten in secret on more than half the days (16–22 days)
5 — Has eaten in secret almost every day (23–27 days)
6 — Has eaten in secret every day

[   ]

GUILT ABOUT EATING   **(Eating Concern subscale)**

*Outside the times when ..... (refer to any objective and subjective bulimic episodes), **over the past 4 weeks have you felt guilty after eating?**

Have you felt that you have done something wrong? Why?

On what *proportion* of the times that you have eaten have you felt guilty?

[N.B.: This rating is based on occasions. Rate the *proportion of times* that feelings of guilt have followed eating. *Do not consider objective or subjective bulimic episodes,* but do consider other episodes of overeating. These feelings of guilt should relate to the effects of eating on shape, weight or body composition. *Distinguish guilt from regret*: Guilt refers to a feeling that one has done wrong.]

0 — No guilt after eating
1 —
2 — Has felt guilty after eating on less than half the *occasions*
3 —
4 — Has felt guilty after eating on more than half the *occasions*
5 —
6 — Has felt guilty after eating on every *occasion*

[   ]

SELF-INDUCED VOMITING   (Diagnostic item)

⋆Over the past 4 weeks have you made yourself sick as a means of controlling your shape or weight?

[Rate the number of discrete episodes of self-induced vomiting. If the participant denies that the vomiting is under his or her control, determine whether it has the characteristics that would be expected were it not self-induced (e.g., unpredictability, occurrence in public). If the available evidence suggests that the vomiting is under the participant's control (i.e., it is self-induced), then rate it as such. Accept the participant's definition of an episode. Rate 777 if the number of episodes is so great that it cannot be calculated. Rate 000 if no vomiting.]

[ ][ ][ ]

Outside the times when ..... (refer to objective and subjective bulimic episodes), **over the past 4 weeks how many times have you made yourself sick as a means of controlling your shape or weight?**

[Rate the number of episodes of "non-compensatory" self-induced vomiting. Accept the participant's definition of an episode. Rate 000 if no vomiting.]

[ ][ ][ ]

[Ask about the preceding 2 months. Estimate the number of discrete episodes of self-induced vomiting over each of the 2 preceding months.]

month 2 [ ][ ][ ]
month 3 [ ][ ][ ]

[Ask about the 3 months prior to that (to make a diagnosis of binge eating disorder). Estimate the number of discrete episodes of self-induced vomiting over these 3 months.]

months 4–6 [ ][ ][ ]

LAXATIVE MISUSE   **(Diagnostic item)**

*Over the past 4 weeks have you taken laxatives as a means of controlling your shape or weight?

[Rate the number of episodes of laxative-taking as a means of controlling shape, weight or body composition. This should have been the *main* reason for the laxative-taking, although it may not have been the sole reason. Only rate the taking of substances with a true laxative effect. Rate 00 if there was no laxative use or there is doubt whether the laxative-taking was primarily to influence shape, weight or body composition.]

[ ][ ][ ]

[Rate the average number of laxatives taken on each occasion. Rate 999 if not applicable. Rate 777 if not quantifiable, e.g., use of bran.]

[ ][ ][ ]

[Note the type of laxative taken.]

Outside the times when ..... (refer to objective and subjective bulimic episodes), **over the past 4 weeks how many times have you taken laxatives as a means of controlling your shape or weight?**

[Rate the number of episodes of "non-compensatory" laxative misuse. Accept the participant's definition of an episode. Rate 000 if no laxative misuse.]

[ ][ ][ ]

[Ask about the preceding 2 months. Estimate the number of episodes of laxative misuse over each of the 2 preceding months.]

month 2 [ ][ ][ ]
month 3 [ ][ ][ ]

[Ask about the 3 months prior to that. Estimate the number of episodes of laxative misuse over these 3 months.]

months 4–6 [ ][ ][ ]

DIURETIC MISUSE   (Diagnostic item)

★Over the past 4 weeks have you taken diuretics as a means of controlling your shape or weight?

[Rate the number of episodes of diuretic-taking as a means of controlling shape, weight or body composition. This should have been the *main* reason for the diuretic-taking, although it may not have been the sole reason. Only rate the taking of substances with a true diuretic effect. Rate 000 if there was no diuretic use or there is doubt whether the diuretic-taking was primarily to influence shape, weight or body composition.]

[ ][ ][ ]

[Rate the average number of diuretic taken on each occasion. Rate 999 if not applicable.]

[ ][ ][ ]

[Note the type of diuretic taken.]

Outside the times when ..... (refer to objective and subjective bulimic episodes), **over the past 4 weeks how many times have you taken diuretics as a means of controlling your shape or weight? ?**

[Rate the number of episodes of "non-compensatory" diuretic misuse. Accept the participant's definition of an episode. Rate 000 if no diuretic misuse.]

[ ][ ][ ]

[Ask about the preceding 2 months. Estimate the number of episodes of diuretic misuse over each of the 2 preceding months.]

month 2 [ ][ ][ ]
month 3 [ ][ ][ ]

[Ask about the 3 months prior to that. Estimate the number of episodes of diuretic misuse over these 3 months.]

months 4–6 [ ][ ][ ]

291

DRIVEN EXERCISING (Diagnostic item)

*Over the past 4 weeks have you exercised as a means of controlling your weight, altering your shape or amount of fat, or burning off calories?

*Have you felt driven or compelled to exercise?

Typically, what form of exercise have you taken? How hard have you exercised? Have you pushed yourself?

Have you exercised even when it might interfere with other commitments or do you harm?

Have there been times when you have been unable to exercise for any reason? How has this made you feel?

[Rate the number of days on which the participant has engaged in "driven" exercising. Such exercising should have been intense in character and have had a "compulsive" quality to it. The participant may describe having felt compelled to exercise. Other indices of this compulsive quality are exercising to the extent that it significantly interferes with day-to-day functioning (e.g., such that it prevents attendance at social commitments or it intrudes on work or exercising when it might do one harm, e.g., when possibly injured). Another suggestive feature is having a strong negative reaction to being unable to exercise. Only rate driven exercising that was *predominantly* intended to use calories or change shape, weight or body composition. Exercising that was exclusively intended to enhance health or fitness should not be rated. Rate 00 if no such driven exercising.]

[ ][ ]

[Rate the *average* amount of time (in minutes) per day spent exercising in this way. Only consider days on which the participant has exercised. Rate 999 if no such exercising.]

[ ][ ][ ]

[Ask about the preceding 2 months. Rate the number of days on which the participant has exercised in this manner over each of the 2 preceding months. If not asked, rate 99.]

month 2 [ ][ ]
month 3 [ ][ ]

OTHER EXTREME WEIGHT-CONTROL BEHAVIOR

*Over the past 4 weeks have you done anything else to control your shape or weight?

[Rate other noteworthy (i.e., potentially effective) dysfunctional forms of weight-control behavior (e.g., spitting, insulin under-use, thyroid medication misuse). Rate number of days and nature of the behavior. Rate 00 if no such behavior.]

month 1 [   ] [   ]

month 2 [   ] [   ]
month 3 [   ] [   ]

PERIODS OF ABSENCE OF EXTREME WEIGHT-CONTROL BEHAVIOR

[Only ask this question if at least one of the five main methods of weight-control behavior has been rated positively at the specified severity level over the past 3 months. The five forms of behavior are as follows:

— Fasting (a rating of 1 or 2 on "Dietary restriction outside bulimic episodes")
— Self-induced vomiting (on average at least twice a week)
— Laxative misuse (on average at least twice a week)
— Diuretic misuse (on average at least twice a week)
— Driven exercise — Ignore in this context]

Over the past 3 months has there been a period of 2 or more weeks when you have not. ....

[Ask as for individual items. Ascertain the number of consecutive weeks over the past 3 months "free" (i.e., not at or above threshold levels) from all five forms of extreme weight-control behavior. Do not rate abstinence due to force of circumstance. Rate 99 if not applicable.]

[   ] [   ]

I am now going to ask you some questions about your shape and weight. ....

DISSATISFACTION WITH WEIGHT   (Weight Concern subscale)

★**Over the past 4 weeks have you been dissatisfied with your weight (..... the number on the scale)? What has this been like?**

Why have you been dissatisfied with your weight? Have you been so dissatisfied that it has made you unhappy? Could you have felt worse? How long has this feeling lasted?

[Only rate dissatisfaction due to weight being regarded as too high. Assess the participant's attitude to his or her weight and rate accordingly. In common with all severity items, the rating should generally represent the *mode for the entire month*. Only rate 4, 5 or 6 if there has been distress. Do not prompt with the terms "slight," "moderate" or "marked." This rating can be made with participants who do not know their exact weight. Only rate 9 with participants who are totally unaware of their weight.]

0 — No dissatisfaction
1 —
2 — Slight dissatisfaction (no associated distress)
3 —
4 — Moderate dissatisfaction (some associated distress)
5 —
6 — Marked dissatisfaction (extreme concern and distress; weight totally unacceptable)

[ ]

DESIRE TO LOSE WEIGHT   (Weight Concern subscale)

★**Over the past 4 weeks have you wanted to weigh less (again I am referring to the number on the scale)?**

Have you had a *strong desire* to lose weight?

[Rate the number of days on which there has been a *strong desire* to lose weight. This rating can be made with participants who do not know their exact weight. Only rate 9 with participants who are totally unaware of their weight.]

0 — No strong desire to lose weight
1 — Strong desire on 1–5 days
2 — Strong desire on less than half the days (6–12 days)
3 — Strong desire on half the days (13–15 days)
4 — Strong desire on more than half the days (16–22 days)
5 — Strong desire almost every day (23–27 days)
6 — Strong desire every day

[ ]

DESIRED WEIGHT

*On average, over the past month what weight have you wanted to be?

[Rate weight in kilograms. Rate 888 if the participant is not interested in his or her weight. Rate 777 if no specific weight would be low enough. Rate 666 if the participant is primarily interested in his or her shape but has some concern about weight (but not a specific weight). Rate 555 if cannot be rated.]

[ ][ ][ ]

WEIGHING

*Over the past 4 weeks how often have you weighed yourself?

[Calculate the approximate frequency that the participant has weighed him- or herself. If the participant has not weighed him- or herself determine whether this is the result of avoidance. Rate 777 if it is due to avoidance.]

[ ][ ][ ]

REACTION TO PRESCRIBED WEIGHING   (Weight Concern subscale)

*Over the past 4 weeks how would you have felt if you had been asked to weigh yourself once each week for the subsequent 4 weeks ..... just once a week; no more often and no less often?

[Rate the strength of negative reaction to the prospect of having to weigh once weekly (no more often, no less often) over the subsequent 4 weeks. This assumes that the participant would thereby be made aware of his or her weight. Positive reactions should be rated 9. In common with all severity items, the rating should generally represent the *mode for the entire month*. Ask the participant to describe in detail how he or she would have reacted and rate accordingly. Check whether other aspects of the participant's life would have been influenced. Do not prompt with the terms "slight," "moderate" or "marked." If the participant would not have complied with such weighing because it would have been extremely disturbing, rate 6.]

0 — No reaction
1 —
2 — Slight reaction
3 —
4 — Moderate reaction (definite reaction, but manageable)
5 —
6 — Marked reaction (pronounced reaction that would affect other aspects of the participant's life)

[ ]

SENSITIVITY TO WEIGHT GAIN

*Over the past 4 weeks what amount of weight gain, over a period of 1 week, would have *definitely* upset you?

[Ascertain what weight gain (from the participant's average weight over the past 4 weeks) would have led to a *marked negative reaction*. Check several numbers. Be particularly careful to code the number correctly. This should represent the average degree of sensitivity for the entire month.]

0 — 7 lb or 3.5 kg (or more) would have generated a marked negative reaction, or no amount of weight gain would generate this type of reaction

1 — 6 lb or 3 kg would have generated a marked negative reaction

2 — 5 lb or 2.5 kg would have generated a marked negative reaction

3 — 4 lb or 2 kg would have generated a marked negative reaction

4 — 3 lb or 1.5 kg would have generated a marked negative reaction

5 — 2 lb or 1 kg would have generated a marked negative reaction

6 — 1 lb or 0.5 kg (i.e., any weight gain) would have generated a marked negative reaction

[   ]

DISSATISFACTION WITH SHAPE   (Shape Concern subscale)

*Over the past 4 weeks have you been dissatisfied with your overall shape (your figure)? What has this been like?

Why have you been dissatisfied with your shape? Have you been so dissatisfied that it has made you unhappy? Could you have felt worse? How long has this feeling lasted?

[Only rate dissatisfaction with overall shape or figure because it is viewed as too large. This dissatisfaction may include concerns about relative proportions of the body but not dissatisfaction restricted to specific body parts. Do not rate concerns about body tone. Assess the participant's attitude to his or her shape and rate accordingly. In common with all severity items, the rating should generally represent the *mode for the entire month*. Only rate 4, 5 or 6 if there has been associated distress. Do not prompt with the terms "slight," "moderate" or "marked." Reports of disgust or revulsion should be rated 6.]

0 — No dissatisfaction with shape

1 —

2 — Slight dissatisfaction with shape (no associated distress)

3 —

4 — Moderate dissatisfaction with shape (some associated distress)

5 —

6 — Marked dissatisfaction with shape (extreme concern and distress; shape totally unacceptable)

[   ]

PREOCCUPATION WITH SHAPE OR WEIGHT

(Shape and Weight Concern subscales)

*Over the past 4 weeks have you spent much time thinking about your shape or weight? ....

*..... Has thinking about your shape or weight *interfered* with your ability to concentrate on things that you are actively engaged in, for example, working, following a conversation or reading? What has it affected?

[This definition of preoccupation requires concentration impairment. Concentration is regarded as impaired if there have been *intrusive thoughts about shape or weight that have interfered with activities one is actively engaged in* rather than one's mind simply drifting off the matter at hand. Rate the number of days on which this has happened, whether or not bulimic episodes occurred.]

0 — No concentration impairment
1 — Concentration impairment on 1–5 days
2 — Concentration impairment on less than half the days (6–12 days)
3 — Concentration impairment on half the days (13–15 days)
4 — Concentration impairment on more than half the days (16–22 days)
5 — Concentration impairment almost every day (23–27 days)
6 — Concentration impairment every day

[   ]

IMPORTANCE OF WEIGHT, SHAPE AND STRICT CONTROL OVER EATING
(Diagnostic items, Weight and Shape Concern subscales)

Weight

★I am now going to ask you a rather complex question — you may not have thought about this before. Over the past 4 weeks has your *weight* (the number on the scale) been important in influencing how you feel about (judge, think, evaluate) yourself as a person?

★..... If you imagine the things that influence how you feel about (judge, think, evaluate) yourself — such as (your performance at work, being a parent, your marriage, how you get on with other people) — and put these things in order of importance, where does your weight fit in?

(If, over the past 4 weeks, your weight had changed in any way, would this have affected how you felt about yourself?)

(Over the past 4 weeks has it been important to you that your weight does *not* change? Have you been making sure that it does not change?)

Shape

★What about your shape? How has it compared in importance with your weight in influencing how you feel about yourself?

[N.B.: Make all the unadjusted "shape" and "weight" ratings at this point.]

Strict Control over Eating

★What about *maintaining strict control* over your eating? How has it compared in importance with your weight and shape in influencing how you feel about yourself?

[First gauge the degree of importance the participant has placed on body weight and its position in his or her scheme for self-evaluation. The rating can be made with participants who do not know their exact weight — the importance of their presumed weight can be rated. To make the rating, comparisons need to be made with other aspects of the participant's life that are of importance in his or her scheme for self-evaluation (e.g., quality of relationships, being a parent, performance at work or in leisure activities) including body shape and maintaining strict control over eating. In common with all severity items, the rating should generally represent the *mode for the entire month*.

The three "Importance" items can be difficult to rate. It is best to start by discussing weight and then address shape. At this point ratings of the importance of weight and shape should be made. Then, maintaining strict control over eating should be added to the equation and the importance of all three domains rated (i.e., importance of weight and shape are rated twice).

When starting with weight, it is recommended that the two mandatory probe questions be asked in tandem. Then the interviewer should help the participant formulate his or her answer. After that it is good practice to repeat the two probe questions to ensure that the participant has fully grasped the concept that is being assessed. The questions in parentheses should only be asked if the participant is denying that weight is important yet his or her behavior suggests otherwise. Do not prompt with the terms "some," "moderate" or "supreme."]

0 — No importance

1 —

2 — Some importance (definitely an aspect of self-evaluation)

3 —

4 — Moderate importance (definitely one of the main aspects of self-evaluation)

5 —

6 — Supreme importance (nothing is more important in the participant's scheme for self-evaluation)

Weight (unadjusted rating) [   ]

Shape (unadjusted rating) [   ]

[Ask about each of the preceding 2 months. Rate 9 if not asked.]

Weight (unadjusted) month 2 [   ]

Weight (unadjusted) month 3 [   ]

Shape (unadjusted) month 2 [   ]

Shape (unadjusted) month 3 [   ]

Maintaining strict control over eating [   ]

Weight (adjusted for strict control over eating) [   ]

Shape (adjusted for strict control over eating) [   ]

FEAR OF WEIGHT GAIN (**Diagnostic item, Shape Concern subscale**)

*Over the past 4 weeks have you been *afraid* that you might gain weight?

[With participants who have recently gained weight the question may rephrased as "**..... have you been afraid that you might gain *more* weight?**"]

How afraid have you been?

[Rate the number of days on which a *definite fear* (common usage) has been present. Exclude reactions to actual weight gain.]

0 — No definite fear of weight gain
1 — Definite fear of weight gain on 1–5 days
2 — Definite fear of weight gain on less than half the days (6–12 days)
3 — Definite fear of weight gain on half the days (13–15 days)
4 — Definite fear of weight gain on more than half the days (16–22 days)
5 — Definite fear of weight gain almost every day (23–27 days)
6 — Definite fear of weight gain every day

[ ]

[With participants whose weight might make them eligible for the diagnosis of anorexia nervosa, ask about each of the preceding 2 months. Rate 9 if not asked.]

month 2 [   ]
month 3 [   ]

DISCOMFORT SEEING BODY   (Shape Concern subscale)

*Over the past 4 weeks have you felt uncomfortable seeing your body, for example, in the mirror, in shop window reflections, while undressing, or while taking a bath or shower?

What have you felt like at these times? Could you have felt worse? Have you avoided seeing your body?

[Only rate discomfort about overall shape or figure because it is viewed as too large. The discomfort should not stem from sensitivity about specific aspects of appearance (e.g., acne) or from modesty. One index of the severity of such discomfort is whether it has led to avoidance (ask for examples, e.g., when washing). In common with all severity items, the rating should generally represent the *mode for the entire month*.]

0 — No discomfort about seeing body
1 —
2 — Some discomfort about seeing body
3 —
4 — Definite discomfort about seeing body
5 —
6 — Extreme discomfort about seeing body (e.g., viewed as loathsome)

[   ]

DISCOMFORT ABOUT EXPOSURE   (Shape Concern subscale)

*Over the past 4 weeks have you felt uncomfortable about *others seeing your body*, for example, in communal changing rooms, when swimming, or when wearing clothes that show your shape? What about your partner or friends seeing your body?

What have you felt like at these times? Could you have felt worse?

Have you avoided others seeing your body? Have you chosen to wear clothes that disguise your shape?

[Only rate discomfort arising from concerns about overall shape or figure (because it is viewed as too large). Do not consider discomfort restricted to family members who are aware that the participant has an eating problem. The discomfort should not stem from sensitivity about specific aspects of appearance (e.g., acne) or from modesty. One index of the severity of such discomfort is whether it has led to avoidance (ask for examples, e.g., when dressing). If the possibility of exposure has not arisen, rate 9. In common with all severity items, the rating should generally represent the *mode for the entire month*.]

0 — No discomfort about others seeing body
1 —
2 — Some discomfort about others seeing body
3 —
4 — Definite discomfort about others seeing body
5 —
6 — Extreme discomfort about others seeing body   [   ]

FEELING FAT   (Diagnostic item, Shape Concern subscale)

*Over the past 4 weeks have you "felt fat"? [With participants who have already acknowledged such feelings, this question may need to be prefaced by an apology.]

[Rate the number of days on which the participant has "felt fat" in general (not with respect to a particular body part) accepting his or her use of this expression. Distinguish "feeling fat" from feeling bloated premenstrually, unless this is experienced as feeling fat.]

0 — Has not felt fat
1 — Has felt fat on 1–5 days
2 — Has felt fat on less than half the days (6–12 days)
3 — Has felt fat on half the days (13–15 days)
4 — Has felt fat on more than half the days (16–22 days)
5 — Has felt fat almost every day (23–27 days)
6 — Has felt fat every day

                                                                    [ ]

[With participants whose weight might make them eligible for the diagnosis of anorexia nervosa, ask about each of the preceding 2 months. Rate 9 if not asked.]

                                                    month 2 [   ]
                                                    month 3 [   ]

REGIONAL FATNESS

*Over the past month have you felt that any *particular part* of your body is too fat?

[Rate the number of days on which the participant has thought that one or more specific parts of his or her body are definitely too "fat." This does not preclude also thinking that his or her entire body is too "fat."]

0 — No regional fatness
1 — Regional fatness on 1–5 days
2 — Regional fatness on less than half the days (6–12 days)
3 — Regional fatness on half the days (13–15 days)
4 — Regional fatness on more than half the days (16–22 days)
5 — Regional fatness almost every day (23–27 days)
6 — Regional fatness every day

                                                                    [ ]

VIGILANCE ABOUT SHAPE

*Over the past 4 weeks have you been actively monitoring your shape ..... for example, by scrutinizing yourself in the mirror, by measuring or pinching yourself, or by repeatedly checking that certain clothes fit?

[Rate the number of days on which the participant has *actively monitored* his or her shape with the intention of detecting any changes. The participant should believe that the method used is capable of detecting change.]

0 — No vigilance
1 — Vigilance on 1–5 days
2 — Vigilance on less than half the days (6–12 days)
3 — Vigilance on half the days (13–15 days)
4 — Vigilance on more than half the days (16–22 days)
5 — Vigilance almost every day (23–27 days)
6 — Vigilance every day

[   ]

FLAT STOMACH   (Shape Concern subscale)

*Over the past 4 weeks have you had a definite desire to have a completely flat stomach?

[Rate the number of days on which the participant has had a *definite desire to have a flat or concave stomach*. Demonstrate by holding a pen vertically. Participants who already have a flat stomach can be rated, whereas the desire to have a "flatter" (i.e., less protruding) stomach should not be rated.]

0 — No definite desire to have a flat stomach
1 — Definite desire to have a flat stomach on 1–5 days
2 — Definite desire to have a flat stomach on less than half the days (6–12 days)
3 — Definite desire to have a flat stomach on half the days (13–15 days)
4 — Definite desire to have a flat stomach on more than half the days (16–22 days)
5 — Definite desire to have a flat stomach almost every day (23–27 days)
6 — Definite desire to have a flat stomach every day

[   ]

BODY COMPOSITION

*Over the past 4 weeks have you thought about the actual composition of your body ..... the percentage of fat as compared with muscle ..... the way you are under the skin?

How concerned have you been about the composition of your body?

[Rate the strength of the participant's concern about the proportion of fat in his or her body. *Do not rate concern about "being fat" or concerns about particular parts of the body.* Do not prompt with the terms "slight," "moderate" or "marked." In common with all severity items, the rating should generally represent the *mode for the entire month.*]

0 — No concern about body composition
1 —
2 — Slight concern about body composition (aware of the notion, but it is not of personal importance to the participant)
3 —
4 — Moderate concern about body composition (clearly interested in composition of body and regularly thinks about it)
5 —
6 — Marked concern about body composition (extreme interest in actual make-up of body and frequently thinks about it)   [   ]

WEIGHT AND HEIGHT   **(Diagnostic item)**

[The participant's weight and height should be measured.]   Weight in kg [   ][   ][   ]
Height in cm [   ][   ][   ]

MAINTAINED LOW WEIGHT   (Diagnostic item)

[Rate for participants whose weight might make them eligible for the diagnosis of anorexia nervosa. If in doubt, make this rating.]

Over the past three months have you been trying to lose weight?

If no: **Have you been trying to make sure that you do not gain weight?**

[Rate presence of attempts either to lose weight or to avoid weight gain. Rate 9 if not asked.]

0 — No attempts either to lose weight or to avoid weight gain over the past 3 months
1 — Attempts either to lose weight or to avoid weight gain over the past 3 months for reasons concerning shape or weight
2 — Attempts either to lose weight or to avoid weight gain over the past 3 months for other reasons

[   ]

MENSTRUATION   (Diagnostic item)

*Have you missed any menstrual periods over the past few months?

How many periods have you had?

*Are you taking an oral contraceptive (the "pill")?

[With post-menarchal females, rate number of menstrual periods over the past 3 and 6 months. Rate 33 if the participant has never menstruated; rate 44 if she has been taking an oral contraceptive during the months in question; rate 55 if she has been pregnant or breast feeding; rate 66 if she is not menstruating because of a gynecological procedure (e.g., a hysterectomy); rate 77 if she is clearly post-menopausal; and rate 88 if participant is male.]

months 0–3 [   ][   ]
months 0–6 [   ][   ]

END OF EDE SCHEDULE

Differences between EDE 16.0D and EDE 12.0D

New Items in EDE-16.0D
Picking (nibbling)
Binge eating disorder module:
    Average frequency (days per week) over past 6 months
    Associated features
        — eating more rapidly
        — eating until full
        — eating when not hungry
        — eating alone
        — feeling disgust
    Distress about binge eating
Other extreme methods for controlling shape or weight
Weighing
Sensitivity to weight gain
Maintaining strict control over eating
Regional fatness
Vigilance about shape
Body composition

Modification to EDE-12.0D Items
Nocturnal eating
    — level of alertness
Restraint over eating
    — to give sense of control
    — shape and weight/sense of control
Avoidance of eating
    — to give sense of control
    — shape and weight/sense of control
Empty stomach
    — to give sense of control
    — shape and weight/sense of control
Food avoidance
    — to give sense of control
    — shape and weight/sense of control
Dietary rules
    — to give sense of control
    — shape and weight/sense of control
Importance of weight
    — adjusted for control
Importance of shape
    — adjusted for control
Subjective bulimic episodes
    — number of days in month 2
    — number of days in month 3

— number of episodes in month 2

— number of episodes in month 3

Self-induced vomiting

— episodes independent of objective and subjective bulimic episodes

— number of episodes in months 4–6

Laxative misuse

— episodes independent of objective and subjective bulimic episodes

— number of episodes in months 4–6

Diuretic misuse

— episodes independent of objective and subjective bulimic episodes

— number of episodes in months 4–6

Items Dropped from EDE-12.0D

Self-induced vomiting, Laxative misuse and Diuretic misuse

— 4 weeks (number of days)

Items Re-Named in EDE-16.0D

"Intense exercising to control shape and weight" changed to "Driven exercising"

"Avoidance of exposure" changed to "Discomfort about exposure"

"Feelings of fatness" changed to "Feeling fat"

Change in Scoring

For severity items, ratings now based on mode over the previous 28 days rather than mean

APPENDIX B

Eating Disorder Examination Questionnaire (EDE-Q 6.0)

Christopher G. Fairburn and Sarah Beglin

Introduction

The EDE-Q 6.0 (Fairburn & Beglin, 1994) is a self-report version of the Eating Disorder Examination (EDE), the well-established investigator-based interview (Fairburn & Cooper, 1993). It is scored in the same way as the EDE (see page 268). Its performance has been compared with that of the EDE and other instruments in numerous studies (see Peterson & Mitchell, 2005): In some respects it performs well, but in others it does not. Community norms are available for adults (see page 269 and Mond et al., 2006) and adolescents (Carter, Stewart, & Fairburn, 2001).

Recommended Reading

Carter, J. C., Stewart, D. A., & Fairburn, C. G. (2001). Eating Disorder Examination Questionnaire: Norms for adolescent girls. *Behaviour Research and Therapy, 39,* 625–632.

Fairburn, C. G., & Beglin, S. J. (1994). Assessment of eating disorder psychopathology: Interview or self-report questionnaire? *International Journal of Eating Disorders, 16,* 363–370.

Fairburn, C. G., & Cooper, Z. (1993). The Eating Disorder Examination (12th ed.). In C. G. Fairburn & G. T. Wilson (Eds.), *Binge eating: Nature, assessment, and treatment.* (pp. 317–360). New York: Guilford Press.

Mond, J. M., Hay, P. J., Rodgers, B., & Owen, C. (2006). Eating Disorder Examination Questionnaire (EDE-Q): Norms for young adult women. *Behaviour Research and Therapy, 44,* 53–62.

Peterson, C. B., & Mitchell, J. E. (2005). Self-report measures. In J. E. Mitchell & C. B. Peterson (Eds.), *Assessment of eating disorders* (pp. 120–128). New York: Guilford Press.

Studies of the EDE-Q

Binford, R. B., Le Grande, D., & Jellar, C. (2005). Eating Disorder Examination versus Eating Disorder Examination Questionnaire in adolescents with full and partial-syndrome bulimia nervosa and anorexia nervosa. *International Journal of Eating Disorders, 37,* 44–49.

Carter, J. C., Aime, A. A., & Mills, J. S. (2001). Assessment of bulimia nervosa: A comparison of interview and self-report questionnaire methods. *International Journal of Eating Disorders, 30,* 187–192.

Carter, J. C., Stewart, D. A., & Fairburn, C. G. (2001). Eating Disorder Examination Questionnaire: Norms for young adolescent girls. *Behaviour Research and Therapy, 39,* 625–632.

Decaluwe, V., & Braet, C. (2004). Assessment of eating disorder psychopathology in obese children and adolescents: Interview versus self-report questionnaire. *Behaviour Research and Therapy, 42,* 799–811.

Engelsen, B. K., & Laberg, J. C. (2001). A comparison of three questionnaires (EAT-12, EDI, and EDE-Q) for assessment of eating problems in healthy female adolescents. *Nordic Journal of Psychiatry, 55,* 129–135.

Goldfein, J. A., Devlin, M. J., & Kamenetz, C. (2005). Eating Disorder Examination Questionnaire with and without instruction to access binge eating in patients with binge eating disorder. *International Journal of Eating Disorders, 37,* 107–111.

Grilo, C. M., Masheb, R. M., & Wilson, G. T. (2001). A comparison of different methods for assessing the features of eating disorders in patients with binge eating disorder. *Journal of Consulting and Clinical Psychology, 69,* 317–322.

Kalarchian, M. A., Wilson, G. T., Brolin, R. E., & Bradley, L. (2000). Assessment of eating disorders in bariatric surgery candidates: Self-report questionnaire versus interview. *International Journal of Eating Disorders, 28,* 465–469.

Luce, K. H., & Crowther, J. H. (1999). The reliability of the Eating Disorder Examination—Self-report questionnaire version (EDE-Q). *International Journal of Eating Disorders, 25,* 349–351.

Mond, J. M., Hay, P. J., Rodgers, B., & Owen, C. (2006). Eating Disorder Examination Questionnaire (EDE-Q): Norms for young adult women. *Behaviour Research and Therapy, 44,* 53–62.

Mond, J. M., Hay, P. J., Rodgers, B., Owen, C., & Beumont, R. J. V. (2004). Validity of the Eating Disorder Examination Questionnaire (EDE-Q) in screening for eating disorders in community samples. *Behaviour Research and Therapy, 42,* 551–567.

Passi, V. A., Bryson, S. W., & Lock, J. (2003). Assessment of eating disorders in adolescents with anorexia nervosa: Self-report questionnaire versus interview. *International Journal of Eating Disorders, 33,* 45–54.

Peterson, C. B., Crosby, R. D., Wonderlich, S. A., Joiner, T., Crow, S. J., Mitchell, J. E., Bardone-Cone, A. M., Klein, M., & Le Grande, D. (2007). Psychometric properties of the Eating Disorder Examination Questionnaire: Factor structure and internal consistency. *International Journal of Eating Disorders, 40,* 386–389.

Reas, D. L., Grilo, C. M., & Masheb, M. (2006). Reliability of the Eating Disorder Examination—Questionnaire in patients with binge eating disorder. *Behaviour Research and Therapy, 44,* 43–51.

Sysko, R., Walsh, B. T., Fairburn, C. G. (2005). Eating Disorder Examination Questionnaire as a measure of change in patients with bulimia nervosa. *International Journal of Eating Disorders, 37,* 100–106.

Wilfley, D. E., Schwartz, M. B., Spurrell, E. B., & Fairburn, C. G. (1997). Assessing the specific psychopathology of binge eating disorder patients: Interview or self-report? *Behaviour Research and Therapy, 35,* 1151–1159.

Wolk, S. L., Loeb, K. L., & Walsh, B. T. (2005). Assessment of patients with anorexia nervosa: Interview versus self-report. *International Journal of Eating Disorders, 29,* 401–408.

Eating Questionnaire

Instructions: The following questions are concerned with the past 4 weeks (28 days) only. Please read each question carefully. Please answer all the questions. Thank you.

Questions 1–12: Please circle the appropriate number on the right. Remember that the questions only refer to the past 4 weeks (28 days) only.

On how many of the past 28 days . . .	No days	1–5 days	6–12 days	13–15 days	16–22 days	23–27 days	Every day
1. Have you been deliberately *trying* to limit the amount of food you eat to influence your shape or weight (whether or not you have succeeded)?	0	1	2	3	4	5	6
2. Have you gone for long periods of time (8 waking hours or more) without eating anything at all in order to influence your shape or weight?	0	1	2	3	4	5	6
3. Have you *tried* to exclude from your diet any foods that you like in order to influence your shape or weight (whether or not you have succeeded)?	0	1	2	3	4	5	6
4. Have you *tried* to follow definite rules regarding your eating (for example, a calorie limit) in order to influence your shape or weight (whether or not you have succeeded)?	0	1	2	3	4	5	6
5. Have you had a definite desire to have an *empty* stomach with the aim of influencing your shape or weight?	0	1	2	3	4	5	6
6. Have you had a definite desire to have a *totally flat* stomach?	0	1	2	3	4	5	6
7. Has thinking about *food, eating or calories* made it very difficult to concentrate on things you are interested in (for example, working, following a conversation, or reading)?	0	1	2	3	4	5	6
8. Has thinking about *shape or weight* made it very difficult to concentrate on things you are interested in (for example, working, following a conversation, or reading)?	0	1	2	3	4	5	6
9. Have you had a definite fear of losing control over eating?	0	1	2	3	4	5	6
10. Have you had a definite fear that you might gain weight?	0	1	2	3	4	5	6
11. Have you felt fat?	0	1	2	3	4	5	6
12. Have you had a strong desire to lose weight?	0	1	2	3	4	5	6

Questions 13–18: Please fill in the appropriate number on the right. Remember that the questions only refer to the past 4 weeks (28 days).

Over the past 4 weeks (28 days) . . .

13. Over the past 28 days, how many *times* have you eaten what other people would regard as an *unusually large amount of food* (given the circumstances)?	....
14. On how many of these times did you have a sense of having lost control over your eating (at the time that you were eating)?	....
15. Over the past 28 days, on how many *days* have such episodes of overeating occurred (i.e., you have eaten an unusually large amount of food *and* have had a sense of loss of control at the time)?	....
16. Over the past 28 days, how many *times* have you made yourself sick (vomit) as a means of controlling your shape or weight?	....
17. Over the past 28 days, how many *times* have you taken laxatives as a means of controlling your shape or weight?	....
18. Over the past 28 days, how many *times* have you exercised in a "driven" or "compulsive" way as a means of controlling your weight, shape or amount of fat, or to burn off calories?	....

Questions 19–21: Please circle the appropriate number. *Please note that for these questions the term "binge eating" means* **eating what others of your age and gender would regard as an unusually large amount of food for the circumstances, accompanied by a sense of having lost control over eating.**

	No days	1–5 days	6–12 days	13–15 days	16–22 days	23–27 days	Every day
19. Over the past 28 days, on how many days have you eaten in secret (i.e., furtively)? ..... Ignore episodes of binge eating	0	1	2	3	4	5	6

	None of the time	A few of the times	Less than half	Half of the times	More than half	Most of the time	Every time
20. On what proportion of the times that you have eaten have you felt guilty (felt that you've done wrong) because of its effect on your shape or weight? ..... Ignore episodes of binge eating	0	1	2	3	4	5	6

	Not at all		Slightly		Moderately		Markedly
21. Over the past 28 days, how concerned have you been about other people seeing you eat? ..... Ignore episodes of binge eating	0	1	2	3	4	5	6

Questions 22–28: Please circle the appropriate number on the right. Remember that the questions only refer to the past 4 weeks (28 days).

Over the past 28 days . . .	Not at all	Slightly		Moderately		Markedly
22. Has your *weight* (number on the scale) influenced how you think about (judge) yourself as a person?	0	1	2	3	4	5	6
23. Has your *shape* influenced how you think about (judge) yourself as a person?	0	1	2	3	4	5	6
24. How much would it have upset you if you had been asked to weigh yourself once a week (no more, or less, often) for the next 4 weeks?	0	1	2	3	4	5	6
25. How dissatisfied have you been with your *weight* (number on the scale)?	0	1	2	3	4	5	6
26. How dissatisfied have you been with your *shape*?	0	1	2	3	4	5	6
27. How uncomfortable have *you* felt seeing your body (for example, seeing your shape in the mirror, in a shop window reflection, while undressing or taking a bath or shower)?	0	1	2	3	4	5	6
28. How uncomfortable have you felt about *others* seeing your body (for example, in communal changing rooms, when swimming, or wearing tight clothes)?	0	1	2	3	4	5	6

What is your weight at present? (Please give your best estimate.) ....

What is your height? (Please give your best estimate.) ....

If female: Over the past 3–4 months have you missed any menstrual periods? ....

    If so, how many? ....

    Have you been taking the "pill"? ....

THANK YOU

Clinical Impairment Assessment Questionnaire (CIA 3.0)

Kristin Bohn and Christopher G. Fairburn

Nature and Use of the CIA

The Clinical Impairment Assessment questionnaire (CIA) is a 16-item self-report measure of the severity of psychosocial impairment due to eating disorder features. It focuses on the past 28 days. The 16 items cover impairment in domains of life that are typically affected by eating disorder psychopathology: mood and self-perception, cognitive functioning, interpersonal functioning and work performance. The purpose of the CIA is to provide a simple single index of the severity of psychosocial impairment secondary to eating disorder features.

The CIA is designed to be completed immediately after filling in a measure of current eating disorder features that covers the same time frame (e.g., the Eating Disorder Examination questionnaire, EDE-Q; see page 309). This ensures that patients have their eating disorder features "at the front of their mind" when filling in the CIA.

The CIA is intended to assist in the clinical assessment of patients both before and after treatment. It is also suitable for use in epidemiological studies.

Status of the CIA

Tests of reliability, validity, sensitivity to change and the instrument's ability to predict case status have been conducted, all of which support its use (Bohn et al., 2008; see below).

Scoring of the CIA

Each item is rated on a Likert scale with the response options being "Not at all," "A little," "Quite a bit" and "A lot." These responses are scored 0, 1, 2 and 3 respectively with a higher rating indicating a higher level of impairment. Since it is the purpose of the CIA to measure the *overall severity* of secondary psychosocial impairment, a global CIA impairment score is calculated. To obtain the global CIA impairment index the ratings on all the items are added together with prorating of missing ratings so long as at least 12 of the 16 items have been rated. The resulting score ranges from 0 to 48 with a higher score being indicative of a higher level of secondary psychosocial impairment.

References

Bohn, K., Doll, H. A., Cooper, Z., O'Connor, M. E., Palmer, R. L., & Fairburn, C. G. (2008). The measurement of impairment due to eating disorder psychopathology. *Behaviour Research and Therapy, 46,* 1105–1110.

Fairburn, C. G., & Beglin, S. J. (2008). Eating Disorder Examination Questionnaire (EDE-Q 6.0). In C. G. Fairburn, *Cognitive behavior therapy and eating disorders* (pp. 309–313). New York: Guilford Press.

INSTRUCTIONS

Please place an "X" in the column which best describes how your eating habits, exercising or feelings about your eating, shape or weight have affected your life over the past 4 weeks (28 days). Thank you.

	Over the past 28 days, to what extent have your . . . eating habits . . . exercising or feelings about your eating, shape or weight . . .	Not at all	A little	Quite a bit	A lot
1	. . . made it difficult to concentrate?				
2	. . . made you feel critical of yourself?				
3	. . . stopped you going out with others?				
4	. . . affected your work performance (if applicable)?				
5	. . . made you forgetful?				
6	. . . affected your ability to make everyday decisions?				
7	. . . interfered with meals with family or friends?				
8	. . . made you upset?				
9	. . . made you feel ashamed of yourself?				
10	. . . made it difficult to eat out with others?				
11	. . . made you feel guilty?				
12	. . . interfered with your doing things you used to enjoy?				
13	. . . made you absent-minded?				
14	. . . made you feel a failure?				
15	. . . interfered with your relationships with others?				
16	. . . made you worry?				

Index